CASE REVIEW
Spine Imaging
THIRD EDITION

Efrat Saraf-Lavi, MD
Associate Professor of Clinical Radiology
Neuroradiology Section,
Medical Director of Applebaum MRI Center
University of Miami, Miller School of Medicine
Miami, Florida

CASE REVIEW

Spine Imaging

THIRD EDITION

CASE REVIEW SERIES

ELSEVIER
SAUNDERS

1600 John F. Kennedy Blvd.
Ste 1800
Philadelphia, PA 19103-2899

SPINE IMAGING: CASE REVIEW, Third Edition   ISBN: 978-1-4557-5116-7
Copyright © 2014, 2008, 2001 by Saunders, an imprint of Elsevier Inc.

Notices

Library of Congress Cataloging-in-Publication Data
Saraf-Lavi, Efrat, author.
  Spine imaging : case review / Efrat Saraf-Lavi. -- Third edition.
      p. ; cm. -- (Case review series)
  Preceded by: Spine imaging : case review / Brian C. Bowen, Alfonso Rivera, Efrat Saraf-Lavi. 2nd ed. c2008.
  Includes bibliographical references and indexes.
  ISBN 978-1-4557-5116-7 (paperback : alk. paper)
  I. Bowen, Brian C. Spine imaging. Preceded by (work): II. Title. III. Series: Case review series.
  [DNLM: 1. Spinal Diseases--radiography--Case Reports. 2. Diagnostic Imaging--methods--Case Reports. WE 725]
  RD768
  616.7'30754--dc23   2013035842

Senior Content Strategist: Don Scholz
Content Development Specialist: Katy Meert
Publishing Services Manager: Jeff Patterson
Senior Project Manager: Mary G. Stueck
Design Direction: Steven Stave

Printed in the United States of America

Last digit is the print number: 9 8 7 6 5 4 3 2 1

To my dear parents,
my companion Randy,
and my amazing boys
Koren and Ariel

I have been very gratified by the popularity and positive feedback that the authors of the *Case Review* series have received for their volumes. Reviews in journals and on-line sites, as well as word-of-mouth comments, have been uniformly favorable. The authors have done an outstanding job in filling the niche of an affordable, easy-to-access, case-based learning tool that supplements the material in *The REQUISITES* series. I have been told by residents, fellows, and practicing radiologists that the *Case Review* series books are ideal for studying for oral Board examinations and subspecialty certification tests.

Although some students learn best in a noninteractive study book mode, others need the stimulation of being quizzed. The format of the *Case Review* series (which consists of showing a few images needed to construct a differential diagnosis and then asking a few clinical and imaging questions) was designed to simulate the Board examination experience. The only difference is that the *Case Review* books provide the correct answer and immediate feedback. The limit and range of the reader's knowledge are tested through scaled cases ranging from relatively easy to very difficult. The *Case Review* series also offers a brief discussion of each case, a link back to the pertinent volume of *The REQUISITES,* and up-to-date references from the literature.

Because of the popularity of on-line learning, we have published new editions on the Web. We also have adjusted to the new Boards examination format, which will be electronic and largely case-based. We are ready for the new Boards! The *Case Review* questions have been reframed into multiple-choice format, the links are dynamic to on-line references, and feedback is interactive with correct and incorrect answers. Personally, I am very excited about the future. Join us.

David M. Yousem, MD, MBA

I am happy to present for your reading pleasure the third edition of *Spine Imaging: Case Review,* by Dr. Efrat Saraf-Lavi. Dr. Saraf-Lavi has updated the cases, reformatted the material for on-line education, introduced new techniques and new entities, and made this an outstanding resource for residents and fellows in neuroradiology preparing for the new end-of-residency Board examinations, as well as neuroradiology subspecialty Boards. The University of Miami's neuroradiology team is world renowned in spine imaging, and Dr. Saraf-Lavi provides a level of expertise unmatched by many programs elsewhere in the world. I congratulate her for leading the efforts to make *Spine Imaging* an anchor of the *Case Review* series. I am especially pleased that her material will be in support of *Neuroradiology: The REQUISITES,* which I have co-authored. It's an honor to have that affiliation. Enjoy!

David M. Yousem, MD, MBA

The third edition of *Spine Imaging* has been updated from the previous editions and is tailored to fit the latest computer-based certifying examination format. The cases included in the third edition were selected to comply with the American Board of Radiology study guide for the spine. Each case contains a set of spine images and four related multiple-choice questions. The first question is the differential diagnosis for the case, and more than one answer may be correct. For the remaining three questions, only one answer is correct. On the following page are the answers to the questions as well as teaching points and comments on the case, including background, histopathology, imaging findings, and management. Literature references and a cross-reference to the parent textbook (*Neuroradiology: The REQUISITES*, Third Edition) are provided. Nearly all the cases in the third edition are either a new diagnostic entity with new images and text or a similar diagnostic entity as in the second edition with new images and text. A few cases use the same images as in the second edition but with revised text. Many of the entities discussed in the third edition are covered in more depth than in the previous edition. The literature references have been updated, and the text addresses patient management, which is often asked during the Board examination.

My goal has been to increase the diversity of cases and the information content of each case, providing additional insights for all readers but especially those who are preparing for examinations such as the Diagnostic Radiology Core and Certifying Examinations, Neuroradiology Subspecialty Examination (CAQ), and Maintenance of Certification (MOC). This edition also provides images of higher quality and resolution, and the cases were selected on the basis of criticisms, comments, and recommendations that the author has received from residents and fellows over the past 3 years.

Efrat Saraf-Lavi, MD

ACKNOWLEDGMENTS

I am both honored and especially grateful to David Yousem, who offered me the opportunity to write the third edition of *Spine Imaging* and to continue the work of individuals who labored so diligently on the first two editions. I would to thank managing editor, Gina Donato, who guided me through the final stages of the manuscript, seamlessly bringing together the case material. I extend a special and deep appreciation to Brian Bowen, my teacher, my mentor, my colleague, and my friend who authored the first edition and co-authored the second edition of the *Case Review Series*. His wisdom and achievements inspired me to continue his work with the *Case Review Series* and to make it as professional and useful as possible to residents, fellows, and colleagues. I would like to single out Armando Ruiz for contributing and writing five of the cases in the book. I also want to thank my colleague, Charif Sidani, and our program residents, Maria Juliana Borja and Harry G. Greditzer, for contributing two cases each to the book.

I want to thank my colleagues in the Neuroradiology section at the University of Miami, Miller School of Medicine who pointed out interesting cases to include and continue to provide an environment that encourages dialogue and critical assessment of spine imaging methods and results during our biweekly division conferences. As a professional group of colleagues at the medical school, we continue to benefit from our close working relationship with faculty members in the Departments of Neurological Surgery, Neuroradiology, and Orthopedic Surgery, as well as researchers at the interdisciplinary Miami Project to Cure Paralysis. These and other individuals have contributed directly or indirectly to the materials in the third edition.

Finally, I want to thank Robert Quencer, chairman of the Department of Radiology at the University of Miami, Miller School of Medicine, former editor-in-chief of the *American Journal of Neuroradiology,* and a former president of the American Society of Neuroradiology, who gave his valuable time to review the cases. His comments and suggestions were incisive and added an additional level of editorial scrutiny, and his contributions have resulted in a more readable and informative third edition, which is more contemporary in educational scope.

Efrat Saraf-Lavi, MD

Opening Round

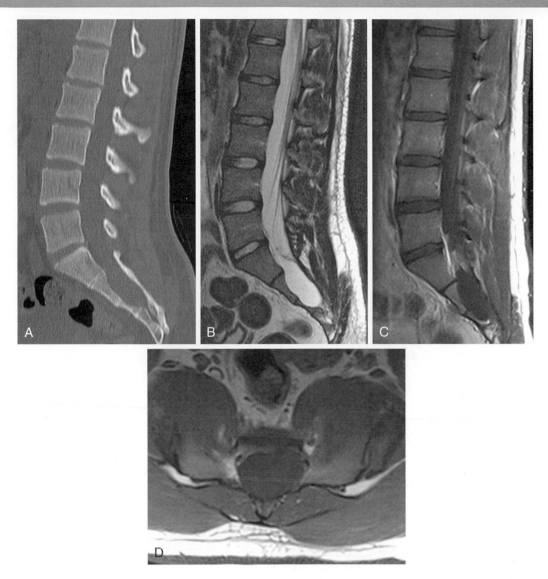

History: A patient presents with left lower extremity pain and numbness.

1. What should be included in the differential diagnosis? (Choose all that apply.)
   a. Tarlov cyst
   b. Epidural abscess
   c. Chordoma
   d. Ependymoma
   e. Cystic schwannoma

2. What are the typical signal characteristics of a Tarlov cyst on MRI?
   a. Hyperintense on T1-weighted images and hyperintense on T2-weighted images
   b. Hypointense on T1-weighted images and hypointense on T2-weighted images
   c. Hyperintense on T1-weighted images and hypointense on T2-weighted images
   d. Hypointense on T1-weighted images and hyperintense on T2-weighted images

3. Which of the following sequences would be used to differentiate a Tarlov cyst from a cystic schwannoma?
   a. T1-weighted
   b. T1-weighted with contrast agent administration
   c. T2-weighted
   d. Short tau inversion recovery (STIR)

4. Tarlov cyst is classified as which type of meningeal cyst?
   a. Type IA
   b. Type IB
   c. Type II
   d. Type III

Tarlov Cyst

1. a and e

2. d

3. b

4. c

References

Nabors MW, Pait TG, Byrd EB, et al: Updated assessment and current classification of spinal meningeal cysts, *J Neurosurg* 68(3):366-377, 1988.

Paulsen RD, Call GA, Murtagh FR: Prevalence and percutaneous drainage of cysts of the sacral nerve root sheath (Tarlov cysts), *AJNR Am J Neuroradiol* 15(2):293-297, 1994.

Cross-Reference

Neuroradiology: The REQUISITES, 3rd ed, p 551.

Comment

Background

Tarlov cysts, or perineural cysts, occur in approximately 4.6% to 9% of adults. They are most often located at S2 and S3 and are usually incidental findings on CT and MRI.

Pathophysiology

Nabors and colleagues divided spinal meningeal cysts into three categories: type I is an intraspinal extradural meningeal cyst without spinal nerve root fibers, type II is an intraspinal extradural meningeal cyst with spinal nerve root fibers, and type III is a spinal intradural meningeal cyst (arachnoid cyst). Type I comprises two subgroups: type IA is an intraspinal extradural arachnoid cyst, and type IB is a sacral meningocele. There are two kinds of type II cysts: Tarlov cysts, which are located distal to the nerve root ganglion and occur almost exclusively in the sacrum, and meningeal diverticula, which occur proximal to the nerve root ganglion and largely communicate with the subarachnoid space. The latter most commonly occur in the thoracic spine, followed by the lumbar and cervical spine.

Although most Tarlov cysts are asymptomatic, symptomatic cysts may grow over time secondary to CSF hydrostatic and pulsatile forces, leading to increasing symptoms. As the mass enlarges, sensory nerve root fibers are compressed, causing pain or other sensory disturbances. Because of the anatomic location of the cysts near other pathology in the lumbar spine, such as degenerative disk disease, it may be difficult to determine whether the cyst is responsible for symptoms.

Imaging

Plain radiographs may reveal erosion of the sacrum, bone scalloping, or a rounded paravertebral shadow. On CT, Tarlov cysts are isodense with CSF and often demonstrate osseous erosion and sacral bone scalloping (Fig. A). CT myelography is effective in demonstrating the presence of communication between the cyst and the spinal subarachnoid space. MRI is the preferred initial imaging modality, owing to its capacity to delineate bone and pedicle erosion, sacral canal widening, and neural foraminal enlargement, as well as the relationship of the cyst to the thecal sac (Figs. B-D). The final diagnosis is based on histopathologic evidence of spinal nerve root fibers within the cyst wall or cavity.

Management

Consensus is lacking on the optimal management of symptomatic Tarlov cysts. Nonsurgical management includes medical treatment with anti-inflammatory drugs and physical therapy or percutaneous cyst drainage. Surgery should be reserved for the subset of patients in whom conservative measures elicit no response. Surgical management includes cyst resection at the neck, cyst wall resection, and cyst fenestration.

Notes

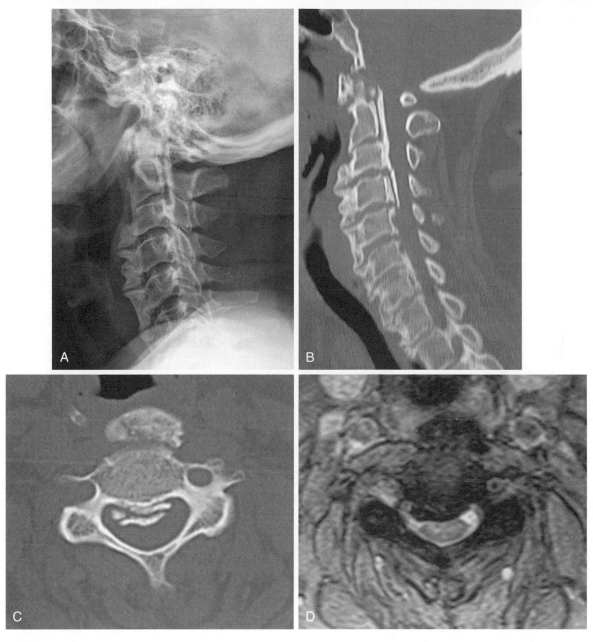

History: A 55-year-old man presents with myelopathy.

1. What should be included in the differential diagnosis? (Choose all that apply.)
   a. Bridging osteophytes
   b. Ossification of ligamentum flavum
   c. Ossification of the posterior longitudinal ligament (OPLL)
   d. Calcified meningioma

2. Which vertebral levels are most severely involved with OPLL?
   a. C2-C4
   b. C4-C6
   c. C7-T2
   d. T3-T5

3. Which one of the four types of OPLL, according to the classification based on CT appearance, may be difficult to differentiate from an osteophyte?
   a. Type I
   b. Type II
   c. Type III
   d. Type IV

4. Which imaging technique is preferred for diagnosing OPLL?
   a. Plain radiographs
   b. CT
   c. MRI
   d. Ultrasound

Ossification of the Posterior Longitudinal Ligament

1. a and c

2. b

3. d

4. b

References

Koyanagi I, Iwasaki Y, Hida K, et al: Magnetic resonance imaging findings in ossification of the posterior longitudinal ligament of the cervical spine, *J Neurosurg* 88(2):247-254, 1988.

Nagata K, Sato K: Diagnostic imaging of cervical ossification of the posterior longitudinal ligament. In Yonenobu K, Nakamura K, Toyama Y, editors: *OPLL: Ossification of the posterior longitudinal ligament*, Tokyo, 2006, Springer Japan.

Cross-Reference

Neuroradiology: The REQUISITES, 3rd ed, p 531.

Comment

Background and Clinical Findings

OPLL generally produces severe central canal stenosis and significant myelopathy. Patients typically present in the sixth decade with upper and lower extremity weakness, dysesthesias, and neck pain.

Pathophysiology

OPLL begins with calcification and progresses to frank ossification, first in the upper cervical spine and later in the lower cervical and upper thoracic spine. OPLL can be associated with ligamentum flavum calcification or ossification and, when combined, these processes may result in circumferential compression of the cord. Association of OPLL with diffuse idiopathic skeletal hyperostosis, as seen in this case (Figs. A and B), has also been reported.

Imaging

CT scans and plain films are probably preferable to MRI to identify subtle calcification or ossification. Four types of OPLL have been proposed on the basis of the CT appearance: (1) continuous, in which confluent lesions extend over several vertebral bodies (27% of cases); (2) segmental, which consists of one or several separate lesions behind the vertebral bodies (39%); (3) mixed continuous and segmental (29%) (see Fig. B); and (4) circumscribed, in which lesions are mainly located posterior to a disk space (5%). The shape of OPLL on axial images varies and may be mushroom-like, cubic, round, or tandem (Fig. C). MRI is valuable for identifying cord compression (Fig. D). The ossified ligament may have fatty marrow and increased signal on T1-weighted images and on T2-weighted fast-spin-echo images. An important finding on CT or MRI is that the calcification or ossification usually occurs along the length of the ligament and can be seen at the level of the pedicles; this helps differentiate OPLL from osteophytes and calcified herniated disks, which should be present at the level of the disk space only.

Management

Numerous studies have shown clinical benefits when multi-level disease is treated with a canal-expansive laminoplasty procedure. This procedure usually includes levels C3-C7.

Notes

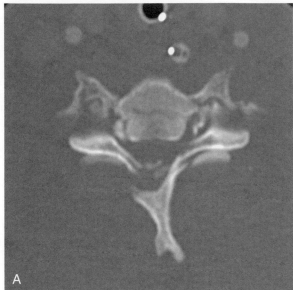

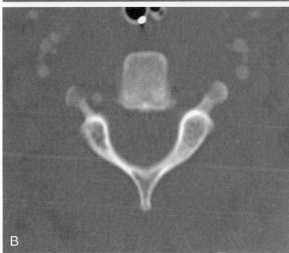

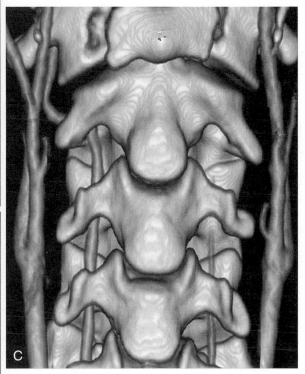

History: A 24-year-old man was found unconscious after diving from a boat.

1. What should be included in the differential diagnosis? (Choose all that apply.)
   a. Left vertebral artery pseudoaneurysm
   b. Left vertebral artery occlusion
   c. Left vertebral artery dissection
   d. Left vertebral artery aneurysm
   e. Left carotid artery occlusion

2. What is the most common mechanism associated with traumatic vertebral artery occlusion?
   a. Distractive flexion injury
   b. Unilateral facet dislocation
   c. Compression fracture
   d. Hyperextension injury

3. Fracture of which of the following vertebral structures would most likely explain injury to the vertebral artery?
   a. Spinous process
   b. Transverse foramen
   c. Transverse process
   d. Lamina

4. Which of the following statements regarding traumatic vascular injuries to the neck is true?
   a. In penetrating neck trauma, vertebral artery injury is more common than carotid injury.
   b. Vertebral artery injury is more common than carotid injury in cervical blunt trauma.
   c. Most injuries to the vertebral artery occur near its origin (V1 segment).
   d. Extremity weakness is the most common complaint in patients with symptomatic vertebral artery injury.

Traumatic Vertebral Artery Occlusion

1. b and c

2. a

3. b

4. b

References

Chokshi F, Munera F, Rivas L, et al: 64-MDCT angiography of blunt vascular injuries to the neck, *AJR Am J Roentgenol* 196(3):W309-W315, 2011.

Taneichi H, Suda K, Kajino T, et al: Traumatically induced vertebral artery occlusion associated with cervical spine injuries: Prospective study using magnetic resonance angiography, *Spine (Phila Pa 1976)* 30(17):1955-1962, 2005.

Torina P, Flanders A, Carrino J, et al: Incidence of vertebral artery thrombosis in cervical spine trauma: Correlation with severity of spinal cord injury, *AJNR Am J Neuroradiol* 26(10):2645-2651, 2005.

Cross-Reference

Neuroradiology: The REQUISITES, 3rd ed, pp 156-157.

Comment

Anatomy

The vertebral artery is anatomically divided into four segments: segment V1, from its origin at the subclavian artery to the level of the transverse foramen at C6 or C7; segment V2, the transforaminal course from C6 to C1 (see Fig. C); segment V3, from C1 to the dura; and segment V4, from the dura to its termination in the basilar artery. The transforaminal segment is the most commonly injured secondary to stretching of the artery or displaced fractures of the foramen (Fig. A).

Pathophysiology

Vascular injuries to the neck may be due to blunt or penetrating trauma. With the advent of helical CT and the increased use of magnetic resonance angiography (MRA), traumatic vertebral artery injury has proved to be more common than previously reported—seen in 25% of cases of acute major cervical trauma. Distraction flexion injury has been identified as the most common spinal mechanism of injury. Vascular lesions to the vertebral arteries include occlusion, pseudoaneurysm, dissection, transection, intimal flap, and arteriovenous fistula formation. The most common lesion in blunt neck trauma for both the carotid and the vertebral arteries is vascular occlusion (Figs. B and C), likely the result of intimal injury and subsequent thrombosis of the vessel.

Imaging

CT angiography plays a central role in the evaluation of acute trauma patients. The wide availability and fast acquisition of CT makes CT angiography the initial test of choice. The intravascular contrast agent allows the evaluation of vascular structures with an accuracy equivalent to that of catheter angiography in blunt neck trauma. MRI has also proved useful in evaluating vertebral artery injury, mainly in cases of vascular occlusion.

Management

Most vertebral artery injuries are clinically silent, and spontaneous recanalization of vascular occlusion has been documented. Infrequently, vertebrobasilar ischemia may occur, particularly in cases of inadequate collateral circulation. Given the poor prognosis of brainstem ischemia, early recognition and prompt management with anticoagulation, embolization, or surgical ligation are usually required to prevent secondary injury.

Notes

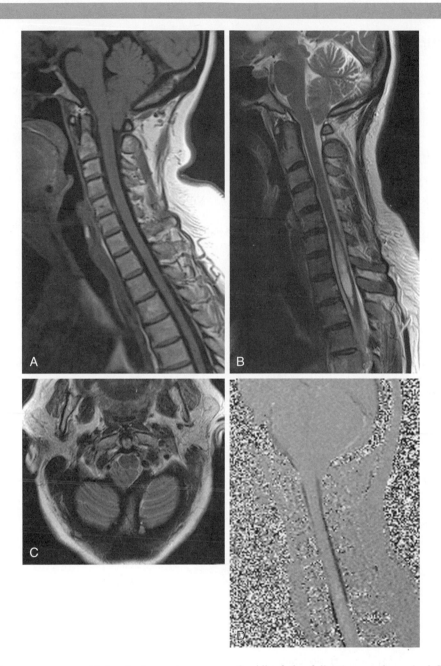

History: A 24-year-old man presents with headaches and dizziness.

1. What should be included in the differential diagnosis? (Choose all that apply.)
   a. Intracranial hypotension
   b. Dandy-Walker malformation
   c. Chiari I malformation
   d. Chiari II malformation
   e. Basilar invagination

2. All of the following congenital osseous abnormalities may be seen in association with Chiari I malformation *except:*
   a. Klippel-Feil anomalies
   b. Occipitalization of the atlas
   c. Os odontoideum
   d. Bifid C1 posterior arch

3. All of the following cerebrospinal fluid (CSF) flow abnormalities may be seen in Chiari I malformation *except:*
   a. Impaired CSF systolic (craniocaudal) pulsations
   b. Impaired CSF diastolic pulsations
   c. Pulsatile downward motion of the cerebellar tonsils
   d. Reduction of CSF flow in the retrocerebellar subarachnoid space

4. What measurement of tonsillar ectopia is considered abnormal in adults?
   a. When the tips of the tonsils extend less than 3 mm below a line drawn from the basion to the opisthion
   b. When the tips of the tonsils extend more than 5 mm below a line drawn from the basion to the opisthion
   c. When the tips of the tonsils extend more than 8 mm below a line drawn from the hard palate to the opisthion
   d. When the tips of the tonsils extend more than 5 mm below a line drawn from the hard palate to the opisthion

Chiari I Malformation

1. a and c

2. c

3. b

4. b

Reference

Sekula RF Jr, Arnone GD, Crocker C, et al: The pathogenesis of Chiari I malformation and syringomyelia, *Neurol Res* 33(3):232-239, 2011.

Cross-Reference

Neuroradiology: The REQUISITES, 3rd ed, pp 297-298.

Comment

Background

In Chiari I malformation, there is inferior displacement of the cerebellar tonsils, which is defined as tonsillar ectopia 5 mm or greater below the foramen magnum (Fig. A). The pathogeneses of Chiari I malformation and syringomyelia remain incompletely understood. A simple radiographic definition of Chiari I malformation is probably insufficient and does not predict treatment outcome. Syringomyelia has been reported to accompany symptomatic Chiari I malformation 40% to 80.5% of the time. Chiari I malformation–associated syringohydromyelia is usually cervical in location and has been attributed to abnormal CSF flow at the foramen magnum.

Clinical Findings

The most common symptom is suboccipital headache; this is exacerbated by increases in intracranial pressure, which typically occur when patients strain for any reason. Other symptoms include visual problems, hearing and equilibrium difficulty, swallowing dysfunction, and apnea. In cases of Chiari I malformation associated with a syrinx (Fig. B), patients may note weakness and paresthesias of the extremities and sensory changes elsewhere in the body. In contrast to the more severe Chiari II malformation, which typically manifests in infancy, syringohydromyelia 'associated with Chiari I malformation usually manifests later in life.

Imaging

MRI is the imaging modality of choice. To meet the criteria for congenital Chiari I malformation, tonsillar herniation should be primary. Asymmetric tonsillar herniation may be seen (Fig. C). Other features such as a pointed or peglike appearance of the tonsils, cervicomedullary kinking, and elongation of the fourth ventricle may be observed. CSF flow studies demonstrate a reduction of CSF flow in the foramen magnum (Fig. D) and posterior fossa, along with pulsatile downward motion of the cerebellar tonsils. These findings have been shown to resolve after cranial decompression.

Management

Current treatment is based on the presence of signs and symptoms of brainstem compression, syringohydromyelia, or both. Resection of the posterior margin of the foramen magnum from condyle to condyle, cervical laminectomy to expose the caudal limit of tonsillar herniation, and duroplasty produce a striking improvement in symptoms caused by brainstem compression. The procedure also leads to stabilization or improvement of symptoms caused by syringohydromyelia.

Notes

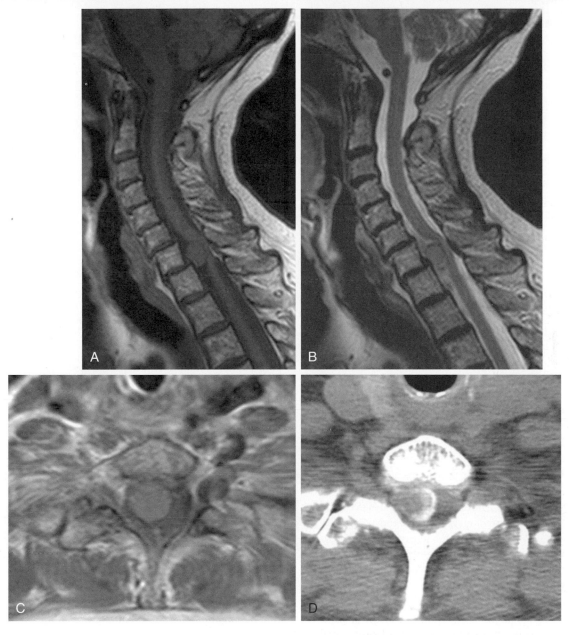

History: A 47-year-old woman presents with myelopathy.

1. What should be included in the differential diagnosis? (Choose all that apply.)
   a. Ependymoma
   b. Meningioma
   c. Schwannoma
   d. Lymphoma
   e. Chloroma

2. What is the location of this lesion?
   a. Intramedullary
   b. Intradural extramedullary
   c. Extradural
   d. Extraspinal

3. What is the most common intraspinal tumor?
   a. Ependymoma
   b. Meningioma
   c. Schwannoma
   d. Paraganglioma

4. Which of the following statements regarding spinal meningioma is *false?*
   a. Most meningiomas arise at the lumbar level.
   b. Spinal meningiomas occur most commonly in middle-aged women.
   c. Spinal meningiomas may have an epidural location.
   d. Calcifications are rarely visible on plain radiographs.

Calcified Intradural Meningioma

1. b

2. b

3. c

4. a

References

El Khamary SM, Alorainy IA: Case 100: Spinal epidural meningioma, *Radiology* 241(2):614-617, 2006.

Liu WC, Choi G, Lee SH, et al: Radiological findings of spinal schwannomas and meningiomas: Focus on discrimination of two disease entities, *Eur Radiol* 19(11):2707-2715, 2009.

Cross-Reference

Neuroradiology: The REQUISITES, 3rd ed, pp 560-561.

Comment

Background

Intraspinal meningiomas represent 25% to 46% of primary spinal neoplasms and are the second most common intraspinal tumor after schwannomas, which account for 30% of all primary spine neoplasms. They most often affect middle-aged women.

Histopathology

In genetic studies, investigators showed complete or partial loss of chromosome 22 in greater than 50% of patients with spinal meningiomas. The histologic types of spinal meningioma include fibroblastic, transitional, meningotheliomatous, and psammomatous; the last two histologic types are the most common. Because meningiomas have a dural base, approximately 85% project intradurally, whereas the remainder are either extradural or both intradural and extradural in location.

Imaging

MRI is the best imaging technique for diagnosing spinal meningiomas. MRI clearly delineates the location of the tumor and its relationship to the cord, which is useful in planning surgery. Meningiomas are usually isointense to gray matter on MRI but may be lower in signal intensity, depending on the extent of calcification. They are well circumscribed, tend to be located posterolaterally in the canal, and often show homogeneous enhancement (Figs. A-C). A "dural tail" may be present, although this finding is nonspecific. CT is useful in showing calcification (Fig. D), which helps differentiate meningiomas from schwannomas of the spine.

Management

The optimal treatment for primary spinal meningioma is total surgical resection. Tumor recurrence is rare; it occurs in cases of en plaque or infiltrating meningiomas and in partially resected lesions.

Notes

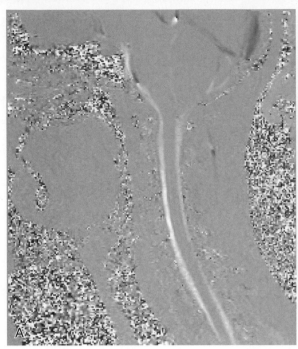 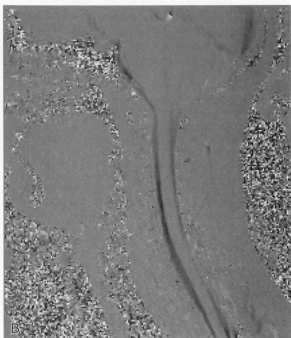

History: A healthy volunteer undergoes imaging.

1. What are these images called? (Choose the *best* answer.)
   a. Diffusion-weighted images
   b. Phase images
   c. Maximum-intensity projection images
   d. Susceptibility-weighted images
   e. Diffusion tensor images

2. What type of pulse sequence is used to obtain such images?
   a. Gradient echo
   b. Spin echo
   c. Time-of-flight
   d. Inversion recovery

3. What is the main use of this technique?
   a. To detect occult blood products
   b. To determine cerebrospinal fluid (CSF) velocities and volumetric flow rates
   c. To evaluate cord signal
   d. To evaluate for cord compression

4. All of the following lesions may be better characterized by this technique *except:*
   a. Syringohydromyelia
   b. Spinal meningeal cyst
   c. Subarachnoid cyst
   d. Spinal cord tumors

Cerebrospinal Fluid Flow Imaging

1. b

2. a

3. b

4. d

References

Hofkes SK, Iskandar BJ, Turski PA, et al: Differentiation between symptomatic Chiari I malformation and asymptomatic tonsillar ectopia by using cerebrospinal fluid flow imaging: Initial estimate of imaging accuracy, *Radiology* 245(2):532-540, 2007.

Levy LM: MR imaging of cerebrospinal fluid flow and spinal cord motion in neurologic disorders of the spine, *Magn Reson Imaging Clin N Am* 7(3): 573-587, 1999.

McGirt MJ, Nimjee SM, Fuchs HE, et al: Relationship of cine phase-contrast magnetic resonance imaging with outcome after decompression for Chiari I malformations, *Neurosurgery* 59(1):140-146, 2006.

Cross-Reference

Neuroradiology: The REQUISITES, 3rd ed, pp 297-298.

Comment

Background

Cine phase-contrast MRI has been used increasingly in the last decade to evaluate cranial and spinal CSF flow. The technique allows noninvasive flow quantification and has yielded considerable information on the physiology of the normal CSF circulation.

Imaging

The phase images shown here represent 2 of 32 cardiac-gated images reconstructed from data acquired during each cardiac cycle. With this "phase-contrast" technique, the images are obtained in cine mode by pixel-by-pixel computation of the phase difference between two interleaved acquisitions—one being flow compensated, and the other having a specific flow encoding. The flow encoding, or flow sensitivity, is usually adjusted by varying the gradient strength or duration. In this case, the flow-encoding gradient is in the superior-inferior (or cephalad-caudad) direction, which is also the read gradient direction. The size of the phase shift resulting from superior-inferior flow is proportional to primarily three factors: (1) the size of the flow-encoding gradient, (2) the magnitude of the CSF velocity in the superior-inferior direction, and (3) the square of echo time (TE). The flow-encoding gradient has been adjusted to give maximum phase shift to CSF moving with a velocity of 8 cm/sec in this case. Caudad flow induces a positive phase shift and is displayed as hyperintense, whereas cephalad flow induces a negative phase shift and appears hypointense relative to nonmoving background tissue (e.g., neck muscles).

The two images display a biphasic pattern of CSF flow in the cervical region—caudad flow in response to systole (Fig. A), and cephalad flow in response to diastole (Fig. B). The direction and amplitude of CSF flow vary along the spinal axis because of the effects of wave propagation and expansion and contraction of the epidural venous plexus; therefore, the flow pattern in the lumbar region differs from the pattern in the cervical region. The spinal cord also moves, albeit with a velocity at least 10 times less than that of CSF. Phase, or velocity, images (with appropriate setting of the motion-encoding gradient) can demonstrate both the magnitude and the direction of cord motion. Caudad motion of the cord occurs in early systole, at approximately the same time as the onset of caudad CSF flow. Spinal cord tethering is associated with decreased cord velocities relative to normal. In addition to the longitudinal (superior-inferior) component of cord and CSF motion, a smaller transverse component is present. In the case of postoperative scarring in the cervical canal, loss of transverse motion of the cord at the site of focal cord tethering has been demonstrated in addition to decreased longitudinal velocity.

Management

CSF flow analysis through the foramen magnum with phase-contrast cine MRI helps distinguish symptomatic Chiari I malformation from asymptomatic cerebellar ectopia and helps predict response to surgical decompression.

Notes

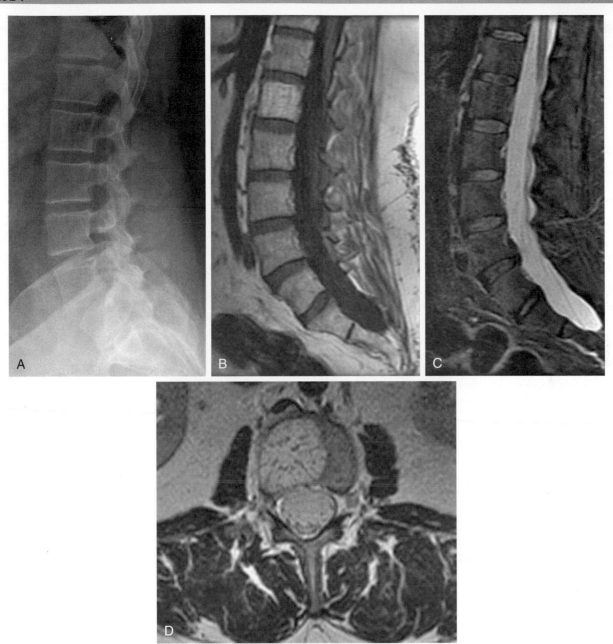

History: A 63-year-old man presents with a 2-year history of lower back pain.

1. What should be included in the differential diagnosis? (Choose all that apply.)
   a. Giant cell tumor
   b. Fat island
   c. Metastatic disease
   d. Plasmacytoma
   e. Hemangioma

2. The hyperintensity observed on the T1-weighted image is due to which of the following components of the lesion?
   a. Vessels
   b. Fat
   c. Cartilage
   d. Marrow edema

3. Which of the following statements regarding vertebral hemangioma management is *false?*
   a. Embolization is advocated before surgery for compressive lesions.
   b. Kyphoplasty is an effective treatment only in cases of pathologic fracture.
   c. No treatment is needed for asymptomatic vertebral hemangiomas.
   d. Painful lesions with minimal or no compression can be treated with embolization alone.

4. Which of the following imaging features is *not* associated with the development of symptoms?
   a. Complete vertebral body involvement
   b. Epidural mass
   c. Expanded osseous cortex with indistinct margins
   d. Location between L1 and L3

Benign Vertebral Hemangioma

1. b and e

2. b

3. b

4. d

References

Baudrez V, Galant C, Vande Berg BC: Benign vertebral hemangioma: MR-histological correlation, *Skeletal Radiol* 30(8):442-446, 2001.

Ropper AE, Cahill KS, Hanna JW, et al: Primary vertebral tumors: A review of epidemiologic, histological, and imaging findings. Part I: Benign tumors, *Neurosurgery* 69(6):1171-1180, 2011.

Cross-Reference

Neuroradiology: The REQUISITES, 3rd ed, p 567.

Comment

Background and Clinical Findings

Vertebral hemangiomas are benign vascular lesions of the vertebral column that occur in 10% of the general population, based on autopsy studies in adults. Incidence increases with age, and there is a slight female predominance. They are usually incidental, asymptomatic, and solitary; they become symptomatic in 1% of affected individuals. Symptoms include back pain and radicular pain. Symptoms are thought to develop by the following mechanisms: (1) vascular expansion of the vertebra, leading to direct compression of nerve roots, the thecal sac, or both; (2) subperiosteal extension, resulting in an extradural mass causing sac or cord compression; and (3) compression fractures secondary to replacement of bone by the hemangioma. Rarely, a vertebral hemangioma may cause bleeding with epidural hematoma or vascular steal with spinal cord ischemia. Pregnancy may contribute to the development of aggressive and symptomatic hemangiomas, possibly due to an increase in blood volume and cardiac output.

Histopathology

Histologically, hemangiomas result from the proliferation of normal capillary and venous structures. Approximately 20% to 30% of hemangiomas are multiple. The lesions are usually rounded, with discrete margins. They vary in size from less than a centimeter to replacing the entire vertebral body. Lesions are most commonly limited to the vertebral body; 10% to 15% extend into the posterior elements. Hemangiomas rarely arise primarily from the posterior elements.

Imaging

Vertebral hemangiomas exhibit a classic radiographic appearance of coarse vertical striations owing to the thickening of bony trabeculae. This appearance has been described as a characteristic "honeycomb" or "corduroy cloth" pattern; the overall density of the vertebral body is decreased because of the presence of fatty marrow (Fig. A). CT scan shows low attenuation interspersed with thickened bony trabeculae appearing as multiple dots, representing a cross section of reinforced trabeculae with a characteristic "salt-and-pepper" or "polka dot" appearance on axial images. Conventional MRI is less definitive. MRI-histologic correlation from autopsy specimens has shown that the signal intensity patterns observed on MRI are related to the relative proportion of fat, vessels, and interstitial edema. Areas with high signal intensity on T1-weighted images contain a larger proportion of marrow occupied by fat (Figs. B and C), whereas areas with high signal intensity on T2-weighted images contain a larger proportion of vessels and edema. These signal characteristics also differ from those of metastatic lesions, which have decreased signal intensity on T1-weighted images and increased signal intensity on T2-weighted images. As with CT scans, the thickened bony trabeculae on MRI axial images result in a "salt-and-pepper" or "polka dot" pattern (Fig. D). For more difficult indeterminate cases, CT can be used to problem-solve because it is more sensitive than MRI to the characteristic osseous remodeling of hemangiomas. If necessary, follow-up examinations can be performed to ensure stability. Angiography confirms the vascular nature of these tumors, and preoperative embolization is useful in many cases.

Management

Most patients with asymptomatic vertebral hemangiomas can be observed. Treatment options include surgery with decompression or resection and stabilization, transarterial embolization, vertebroplasty, kyphoplasty, and radiation therapy.

Notes

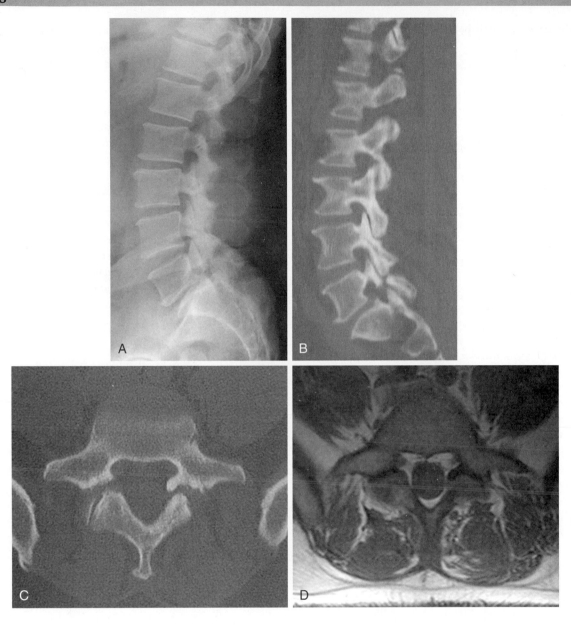

History: A 46-year-old patient presents with a history of low back pain and numbness.

1. What should be included in the differential diagnosis? (Choose all that apply.)
   a. Bilateral fracture and dislocation of the facet complex at L5-S1
   b. L5-S1 spondylolysis with spondylolisthesis
   c. Degenerative changes of the facet joints with resulting spondylolisthesis at L5-S1
   d. Congenital spinal canal stenosis
   e. Pathologic fracture of L5

2. What vertebral anomaly is more frequent in individuals with spondylolisthesis?
   a. Spina bifida
   b. Hemivertebra
   c. Butterfly vertebra
   d. Short anteroposterior dimensions of the vertebral body

3. Which of the following statements regarding spondylolysis is true?
   a. It occurs most commonly at L4.
   b. Involvement of the thoracic spine is common.
   c. Involvement of multiple levels is common.
   d. The process may be unilateral.

4. What is "pseudoherniation"?
   a. Disk herniation at the level above the spondylolisthesis
   b. Disk herniation above the level of spondylolisthesis
   c. Disk herniation into the vertebral body end-plate.
   d. Appearance of the posterior disk margin on axial images at the level of spondylolisthesis, giving the spurious impression that the disk is herniated

Spondylolytic Spondylolisthesis

1. b

2. a

3. d

4. d

References

Logroscino G, Mazza O, Aulisa G, et al: Spondylolysis and spondylolisthesis in the pediatric and adolescent population, *Childs Nerv Syst* 17(11):644-655, 2001.

Sairyo K, Katoh S, Takata Y, et al: MRI signal changes of the pedicle as an indicator for early diagnosis of spondylolysis in children and adolescents: A clinical and biomechanical study, *Spine (Phila Pa 1976)* 31(2):206-211, 2006.

Wiltse LL, Rothman SLG, Milanowska K, et al: Lumbar and lumbosacral spondylolisthesis. In Weinstein JN, Wiesel SW, editors: *The lumbar spine*, Philadelphia, 1990, Saunders, pp 471-499.

Cross-Reference

Neuroradiology: The REQUISITES, 3rd ed, pp 533-534.

Comment

Background

Spondylolisthesis refers to the slippage of one vertebral body with respect to the one beneath it. This condition most commonly occurs at the level of L5-S1, with L5 slipping over S1. There are six types of spondylolisthesis in the widely accepted classification of Wiltse: (I) congenital (dysplastic), (II) isthmic (spondylolytic), (III) degenerative, (IV) traumatic, (V) pathologic, and (VI) postsurgical. The incidence of isthmic spondylolisthesis (type II) is approximately 5%, based on autopsy studies. It is subdivided into two subtypes: IIA, in which the pars has a break (owing to a fatigue fracture), and IIB, in which the pars is elongated and thinned, without a break (owing to repeated microfractures and healing). Type IIA is the more common type in patients younger than 50 years.

Pathophysiology

Patients with spondylolysis have a defect in the pars interarticularis (portion of the neural arch that connects the superior and inferior articular facets). Spondylolysis is believed to be caused by repeated microtrauma, resulting in stress fracture of the pars interarticularis. It is especially common in adolescents participating in certain kinds of sports. It is also more prevalent in some populations, suggesting a hereditary component. Patients with bilateral pars defects can develop spondylolisthesis of varying degrees, which can progress over time.

Imaging

The initial evaluation of patients with suspected spondylolysis consists of plain radiography, including anteroposterior, lateral, and oblique views of the lumbar spine (Fig. A). Lateral views (see Fig. A) are most sensitive for detecting pars fractures, and oblique views are most specific. On oblique radiographs, the posterior elements have the appearance of a Scottie dog. A break in the pars interarticularis may have the appearance of a collar around the neck. Spondylolisthesis can be graded in the sagittal plane based on vertebral subluxation as a percentage of vertebral diameter. Slippage of 25% or less of the vertebral body width is termed a grade 1 spondylolisthesis; 25% to 50% is grade 2; 50% to 75% is grade 3; 75% to 100% is grade 4; and greater than 100% is termed spondyloptosis. The limitation of plain films is their inability to detect stress reactions in the pars interarticularis that have not progressed to complete fracture. If plain radiographs are negative or inconclusive, further imaging may be warranted.

CT scan can demonstrate minimal anterior slippage and allows direct identification of the pars defects (Figs. B and C), although it is not sensitive for detecting early acute stress reactions in the pars interarticularis when there is only marrow edema and microtrabecular fracture. These findings are easily observed on MRI. Some investigators and practicing radiologists believe that once normal radiographs have been obtained, MRI (Fig. D) should be next; however, identification of pars defects may be more difficult with MRI than with CT.

Management

Some patients with spondylolysis and spondylolisthesis remain asymptomatic, but most complain of symptoms ranging from low back pain to radiculopathy and neurogenic claudication. Many patients can be managed conservatively; however, in patients with significant slip progression or symptoms that do not respond to conservative treatment, surgery is indicated. The goal of surgery is to stabilize the spinal segment and decompress the posterior elements when needed.

Notes

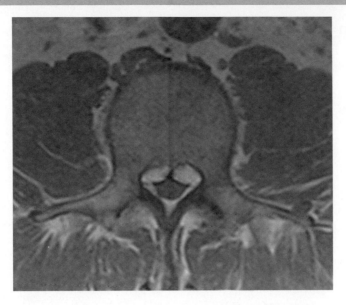

History: A 45-year-old man presents with back pain.

1. What should be included in the differential diagnosis? (Choose all that apply.)
   a. Normal epidural midline septum
   b. Epidural lipoma
   c. Epidural lipomatosis
   d. Prominent epidural veins
   e. Arachnoiditis or thecal scarring

2. Which part of the spine contains more fatty tissue in the epidural space?
   a. Cervical spine
   b. Thoracic spine
   c. Lumbar spine
   d. Sacral spine

3. What is the most likely migration path location for lumbar disks that are extruded or sequestered?
   a. Paramedian
   b. Midline
   c. Inferior
   d. Superior

4. Which of the following is *not* an attachment point of the posterior longitudinal ligament (PLL)?
   a. Annulus fibrosus
   b. Sagittal septum
   c. Lateral membranes
   d. Ligamentum flavum

Midline Epidural Septum

1. a and c

2. c

3. a

4. d

References

Scapinelli R: Anatomical and radiologic studies on the lumbosacral meningo-vertebral ligaments of humans, *J Spinal Disord* 3(1):6-15, 1990.

Schellinger D, Manz HJ, Vidic B, et al: Disk fragment migration, *Radiology* 175(3):831-836, 1990.

Cross-Reference

Neuroradiology: The REQUISITES, 3rd ed, pp 525, 527.

Comment

Anatomy

The sagittal midline septum consists of lamellae of compact collagen. At its anterior extent, the septum merges with the periosteum of the vertebral body (see the figure). The midline septum spans the anterior epidural space from the anterior surface of the thecal sac to the periosteum and divides the space into two compartments. The superior and inferior margins of these compartments are formed by the insertion of the PLL into the annulus fibrosus (i.e., no midline septum is opposite the disk space). The posterior margins of the anterior epidural space are formed by the PLL and the lateral membranes, which are fibrous bands that stretch laterally from the free edge of the PLL to the lateral wall of the canal. The midline septum and lateral membranes are also referred to as lumbosacral meningovertebral ligaments and, near the tip of the thecal sac, as the sacrodural ligaments of Trolard and Hofmann.

Imaging

The midline septum appears as a sagittally oriented hypointense band in the midline, perpendicular to the PLL (see the figure). The effect of the midline septum is to direct migrated disk extrusions and fragments into either the left-sided or the right-sided compartment.

Notes

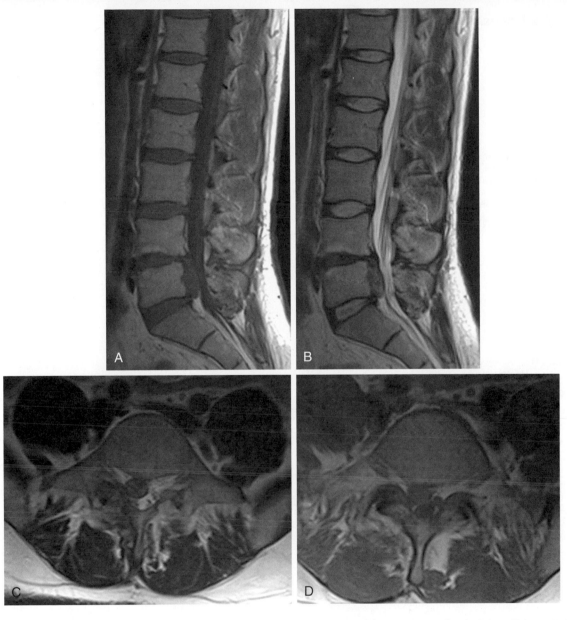

History: A 34-year-old man presents with back pain radiating to the right lower extremity that occurred after lifting his daughter.

1. What should be included in the differential diagnosis? (Choose all that apply.)
   a. Meningioma
   b. Disk protrusion
   c. Disk extrusion
   d. Diskitis osteomyelitis
   e. Epidural hematoma

2. All of the following are descriptive types of disk herniation characterized by a commonly used nomenclature on MRI *except:*
   a. Disk protrusion
   b. Disk extrusion
   c. Disk migration
   d. Sequestration

3. What is the frequency of a bulging disk on MRI among asymptomatic individuals?
   a. Less than 5%
   b. 25%
   c. 50%
   d. 90%

4. What is the most common location for disk herniation?
   a. Cervical spine
   b. Upper thoracic spine
   c. Lower thoracic spine
   d. Lumbar spine

Lumbar Disk Extrusion

1. c and e

2. c

3. c

4. d

References

Fardon DF, Milette PC, Combined Task Forces of the North American Spine Society, American Society of Spine Radiology, and American Society of Neuroradiology: Nomenclature and classification of lumbar disc pathology. Recommendations of the Combined Task Forces of the North American Spine Society, American Society of Spine Radiology, and American Society of Neuroradiology, *Spine (Phila Pa 1976)* 26(5):E93-E113, 2001.

Jensen MC, Brant-Zawadzki MN, Obuchowski N, et al: Magnetic resonance imaging of the lumbar spine in people without back pain, *N Engl J Med* 331(2):69-73, 1994.

Cross-Reference

Neuroradiology: The REQUISITES, 3rd ed, pp 525-526.

Comment

Background

Disk herniation is most common in the lumbar spine, followed by the cervical spine. Lumbar disk herniation is one of the most common causes of lower back pain and often causes leg pain as well.

Pathophysiology

In the nomenclature systems used to categorize degenerative disk pathology as displayed on MRI, disks extending beyond the interspace are categorized as bulging (symmetric, circumferential extension—50% to 100% of the circumference of the disk space), protruded (asymmetric or symmetric, focal extension, with a roughly conical shape pointing posteriorly, and residual low-signal-intensity annular fibers), or extruded (without or with caudad or cephalad extension, with complete rupture of annular fibers) (Figs. A-D). This nomenclature describes a sequestered disk as an extruded disk with a dissociated fragment ("free fragment").

Imaging

MRI is very sensitive in delineating lumbar disk herniation and its relationship to adjacent soft tissues. On MRI, disk extrusion appears as focal, asymmetric protrusions of disk material beyond the confines of the annulus. Extruded disks are usually hypointense on T2-weighted images; however, because disk herniations are often associated with a radial annular tear, high signal intensity in the posterior annulus is often seen.

Management

In most cases, spinal disk herniation does not require surgery. Nonsurgical methods of treatment are usually attempted first. Surgery is considered only as a last resort or if the patient has a significant neurologic deficit.

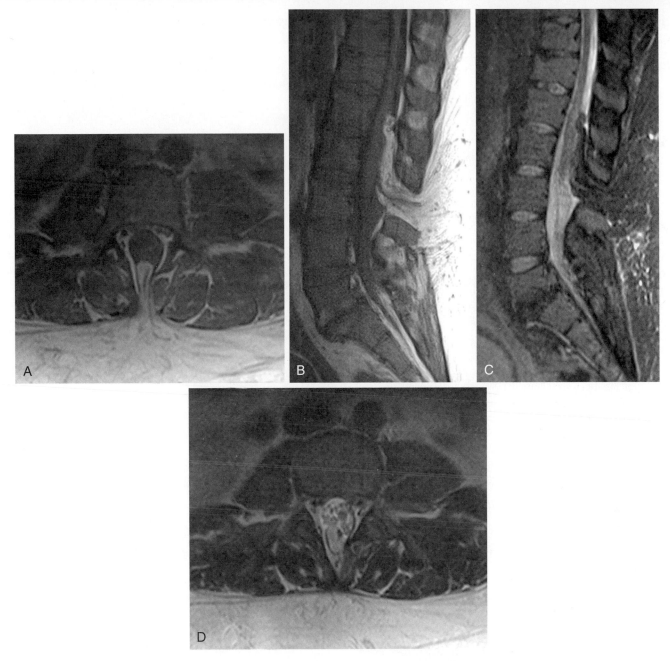

History: A 37-year-old pregnant woman is found to have a lipoma in the lower back on evaluation before epidural anesthesia.

1. What should be included in the differential diagnosis? (Choose all that apply.)
   a. Dermoid
   b. Lumbar teratoma
   c. Intradural lipoma
   d. Lipomyelomeningocele
   e. Epidural lipomatosis

2. Is lipomyelomeningocele classified as an open or closed spinal dysraphism?
   a. Open
   b. Closed
   c. Open in some cases and closed in others
   d. It is not classified as a dysraphism.

3. Which of the following statements regarding lipomyelo-meningocele is *false?*
   a. Lipomyelomeningoceles typically manifest early in life.
   b. Lipomyelomeningocele cannot be distinguished from intradural lipoma.
   c. MRI is the preferred imaging modality.
   d. Females are affected slightly more than males.

4. All of the following are closed spinal dysraphisms associated with a subcutaneous mass in the lower back *except:*
   a. Lipomyelocele
   b. Myelomeningocele
   c. Meningocele
   d. Myelocystocele

Lipomyelomeningocele

1. d

2. b

3. b

4. b

References

Rossi A, Biancheri R, Cama A, et al: Imaging in spine and spinal cord malformations, *Eur J Radiol* 50(2):177-200, 2004.

Sutton LN: Lipomyelomeningocele, *Neurosurg Clin N Am* 6(2):325-338, 1995.

Cross-Reference

Neuroradiology: The REQUISITES, 3rd ed, pp 313-314.

Comment

Background

Lipomyelomeningocele is a congenital lesion associated with spina bifida. These lesions usually become evident within the first few months to first years of life, but sometimes they are discovered in older children or adults.

Classification

A simple classification scheme for spinal dysraphisms by Rossi and colleagues categorizes them as either open, in which there is exposure of abnormal nervous tissues through a skin defect (myelomeningocele, myelocele), or closed, in which there is continuous skin coverage. Closed dysraphisms may be associated with a subcutaneous mass in the lower back (lipomyelocele, lipomyelomeningocele, meningocele, myelocystocele) or may occur without a mass (simple dysraphisms such as tight filum terminale, filar and intradural lipomas, persistent terminal ventricle, and dermal sinus; or complex dysraphisms such as diastematomyelia and caudal agenesis).

Imaging

MRI is the preferred imaging method for characterizing these complex malformations. Lipomyelomeningocele is distinguished from intradural lipoma by the presence of a widely bifid spinal canal and protrusion of the lipoma and dural sac through the defect (Fig. A). The term *lipomyeloschisis* encompasses both lesions and refers to a spectrum of conditions characterized by variable protrusion of the lipoma into the associated dorsal dysraphic defect.

For purposes of surgical management, lipomyelomeningoceles have been divided into lesions that insert caudally into the conus and lesions that attach to the dorsal surface of the conus. In the former, the lipoma may replace the filum terminale, or a separate filum may lie anteriorly. The nerve roots usually lie ventral to the lipoma. In this case, the lipoma attaches to the dorsal surface of the cord (Figs. A-C), with resulting cord tethering and a low position of the conus (Fig. D).

Management

Surgical treatment is indicated to prevent further neurologic decline. The goals of surgery are to release the attachment of the fat to the spinal cord (tethering) and reduce the bulk of the fatty tumor.

Notes

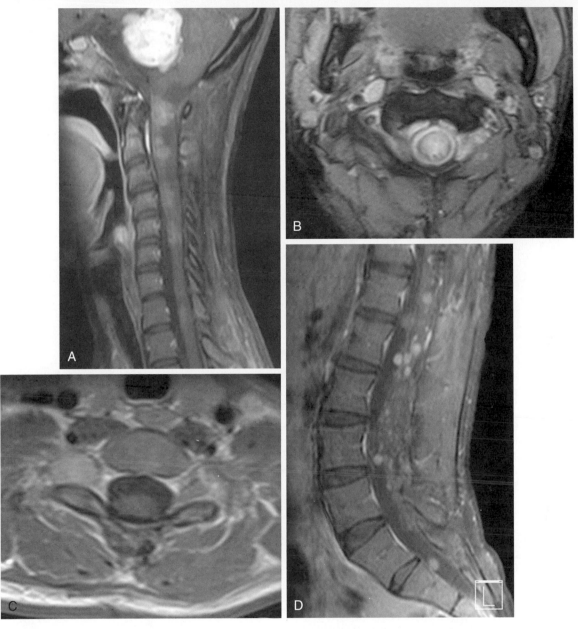

History: A 23-year-old woman presents with a history of deafness and multiple spinal tumors.

1. What should be included in the differential diagnosis? (Choose all that apply.)
   a. Neurofibromatosis type 1 (NF1)
   b. Neurofibromatosis type 2 (NF2)
   c. Multiple meningiomas
   d. Metastasis
   e. Sarcoidosis

2. What is the most common tumor associated with NF2?
   a. Ependymoma
   b. Meningioma
   c. Vestibular schwannoma
   d. Trigeminal nerve schwannoma

3. What is the most likely diagnosis for the intramedullary lesion in this patient with NF2?
   a. Astrocytoma
   b. Meningioma
   c. Hemangioblastoma
   d. Ependymoma

4. Which of the following imaging studies could be diagnostic?
   a. CT scan of the abdomen
   b. Ultrasound of the kidneys
   c. MRI of the internal auditory canals
   d. CT scan of the temporal bones

Neurofibromatosis Type 2

1. b

2. c

3. d

4. c

References

Mautner VF, Tatagiba M, Lindenau M, et al: Spinal tumors in patients with neurofibromatosis type 2: MR imaging study of frequency, multiplicity, and variety, *AJR Am J Roentgenol* 165(4):951-955, 1995.

Selch MT, Pedroso A, Lee SP, et al: Stereotactic radiotherapy for the treatment of acoustic neuromas, *J Neurosurg* 101(Suppl3):362-372, 2004.

Cross-Reference

Neuroradiology: The REQUISITES, 3rd ed, pp 64-65, 307-309.

Comment

Background

NF2 is an inherited autosomal dominant syndrome character-ized by the development of various tumors of the central and peripheral nervous systems. The mnemonic *MISME* (*m*ultiple *i*nherited *s*chwannomas, *m*eningiomas, and *e*pendymomas) is widely used to remember the components of the disease.

Histopathology

The genetic defect responsible for NF2 is a deletion of a por-tion of chromosome 22. The NF2 gene product serves as a tumor suppressor, and decreased function or decreased pro-duction of this protein results in a predisposition to tumor development.

Imaging

Imaging findings in NF2 include bilateral vestibular schwan-nomas, meningiomas, and schwannomas involving the cranial nerves. Spinal manifestations include meningiomas, ependy-momas (Figs. A and B), and nerve sheath tumors (Figs. C and D). Contrast-enhanced MRI of the brain and the entire spine is the modality of choice to screen for NF2. Contrast agent administration is important for detecting small schwannomas (see Fig. D) and intraparenchymal ependymomas (see Figs. A and B). High-resolution fast-spin-echo T2 cisternography can aid in evaluating the cranial nerves.

Management

Surgical resection of tumors is the mainstay of treatment; recent advances in surgery and stereotactic radiosurgery per-mit the preservation of hearing and facial nerve function. Resection of spinal cord tumors is often difficult, and com-plete resection is not always possible. The risks and benefits of surgery must be considered on an individual basis.

Notes

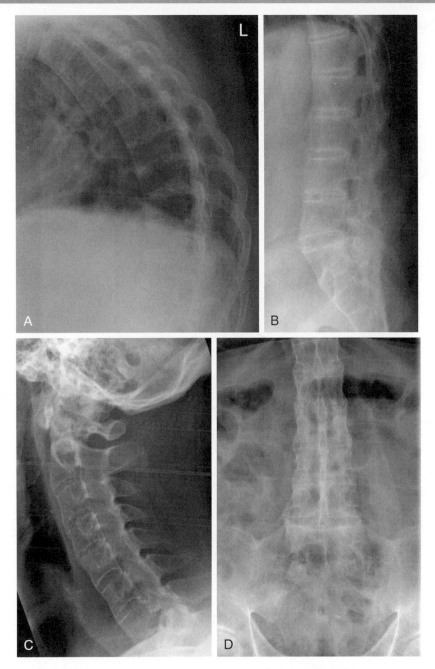

History: A 65-year-old man presents with long-standing stiffness and back pain.

1. What should be included in the differential diagnosis? (Choose all that apply.)
   a. Diffuse idiopathic skeletal hyperostosis
   b. Baastrup's disease
   c. Ankylosing spondylitis
   d. Rheumatoid arthritis
   e. Degenerative disk disease

2. What laboratory study may help narrow the differential diagnosis?
   a. HLA-A3
   b. HLA-B27
   c. HLA-DR2
   d. HLA-DR4

3. All of the following spine abnormalities are associated with ankylosing spondylitis *except:*
   a. Andersson lesion
   b. Dural ectasia or vertebral scalloping
   c. Increased incidence of spinal fractures
   d. Platybasia

4. All of the following signs may be seen in ankylosing spondylitis *except:*
   a. "Y" sign
   b. "Dagger" sign
   c. "Shiny corner" sign
   d. "Trolley-track" sign

Ankylosing Spondylitis

1. c

2. b

3. d

4. a

Reference
Jacobson JA, Girish G, Jiang Y, et al: Radiographic evaluation of arthritis: Inflammatory conditions, *Radiology* 248(2):378-389, 2008.

Cross-Reference
Neuroradiology: The REQUISITES, 3rd ed, p 534.

Comment

Background
Ankylosing spondylitis is the most common seronegative spondyloarthropathy and is more common in men than in women (male-to-female ratio 3:1). Disease onset occurs between the ages of 15 and 35 years, and more than 90% of patients are HLA-B27 positive.

Pathophysiology
Ankylosing spondylitis affects primarily the spine and sacroiliac joints, causing pain, stiffness, and a progressive thoracolumbar kyphotic deformity. In the late stage of the disease, the spine demonstrates progressive ossification of the annulus fibrosus (syndesmophyte formation), anterior longitudinal ligament, apophyseal joints, interspinous ligaments, and ligamentum flavum, resulting in a complete ankylosed spine, known as *bamboo spine*. The most serious complication of the disease is spinal fracture, which can occur with even minor trauma because of spinal rigidity and osteoporosis, especially in older patients or those with long-standing disease.

Imaging
Radiographic findings include osteopenia (Fig. A), fusion of the facet joints (Figs. B and C), and sacroiliac erosions and ankylosis, usually bilaterally symmetric (Fig. D). The radiographic signs of ankylosing spondylitis are due to enthesitis, particularly of the annulus fibrosus, resulting in syndesmophytes (Figs. A-D). Early radiographic signs include squaring of the vertebral bodies caused by erosion of the superior and inferior margins of these bodies, resulting in loss of the normal concave contour of their anterior surface (Figs. A-D).

Management
No definite disease-modifying treatment exists, although tumor necrosis factor-α antagonists appear to have potential as disease-modifying agents. Surgical treatment is reserved for complications related to ankylosing spondylitis.

Notes

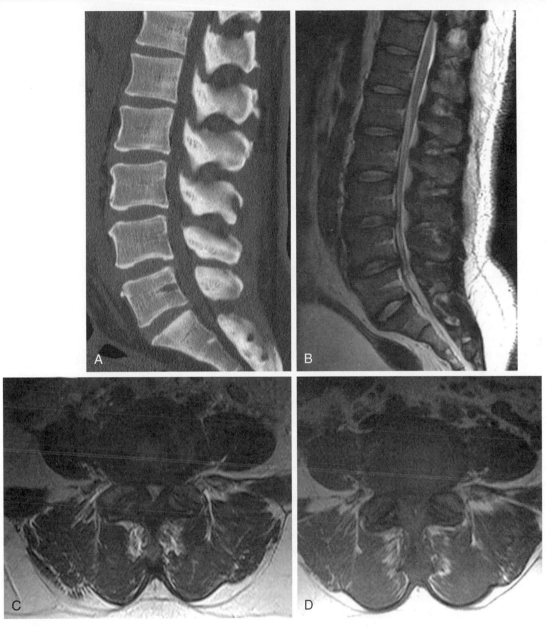

History: A 45-year-old man presents with low back pain and bilateral lower extremity pain.

1. What should be included in the differential diagnosis? (Choose all that apply.)
   a. Central stenosis
   b. Congenital stenosis
   c. Spondylolisthesis
   d. Lateral recess stenosis
   e. Baastrup's disease

2. Which vertebral structures typically appear shortened in patients with congenital narrowing of the lumbar canal?
   a. Laminae
   b. Pedicles
   c. Transverse processes
   d. Vertebral bodies

3. Which nerve root may be compromised as a result of lateral recess stenosis at the L4-5 level?
   a. L3 root
   b. L4 root
   c. L5 root
   d. S1 root

4. Which of the following degenerative changes does *not* cause spinal stenosis?
   a. Osteophyte
   b. Ligamentum flavum hypertrophy
   c. Synovial cyst
   d. Schmorl's node

Lumbar Spinal Stenosis

1. a, b, and d

2. b

3. c

4. d

References

Amundsen T, Weber H, Lilleas F, et al: Lumbar spinal stenosis: Clinical and radiologic features, *Spine (Phila Pa 1976)* 20(10):1178-1186, 1995.

Goh KJ, Khalifa W, Anslow P, et al: The clinical syndrome associated with lumbar spinal stenosis, *Eur Neurol* 52(4):242-249, 2004.

Comment

Background

Lumbar spinal stenosis often results from acquired degenerative changes; however, it may also be congenital in nature. In some patients, degenerative changes aggravate a congenitally narrow canal. Congenital canal stenosis may predispose a patient with mild degenerative changes to become symptomatic earlier. Lumbar spinal stenosis is classified by anatomy or etiology. Anatomic subclassifications include central canal and lateral recess stenosis.

Clinical Presentation

Common symptoms in patients with lumbar spinal stenosis include numbness, radicular pain, claudication, and motor weakness.

Imaging

Because MRI depicts the features directly, measurements of the dimensions of the bony canal on CT or radiography are no longer recommended. In the patient in this case, central stenosis is due to a combination of the degenerative bony (hypertrophic facet joints) and soft tissue (thickened ligamentum flavum, bulging annulus) changes and underlying congenital canal narrowing (Figs. A-C). Evidence of a congenital component is best shown on axial images that display developmentally shortened pedicles, but it can be inferred from the paucity of cerebrospinal fluid in the thecal sac over several vertebral levels, with minor spondylotic changes, on the sagittal T2-weighted image (Fig. B). Lumbar lateral stenosis (Fig. D) may be due to lateral recess stenosis (also present at L4-5), neural foraminal stenosis, or both. The causes of lateral recess stenosis are hypertrophy of the superior articular facet (most common), bulging or herniated disk, and vertebral body osteophyte.

Management

Treatment can be conservative or surgical. Conservative treatment includes physical therapy, bracing, and nonsteroidal anti-inflammatory drugs. Surgical decompression is indicated in patients with intractable pain, claudication, and neurologic deficit.

Notes

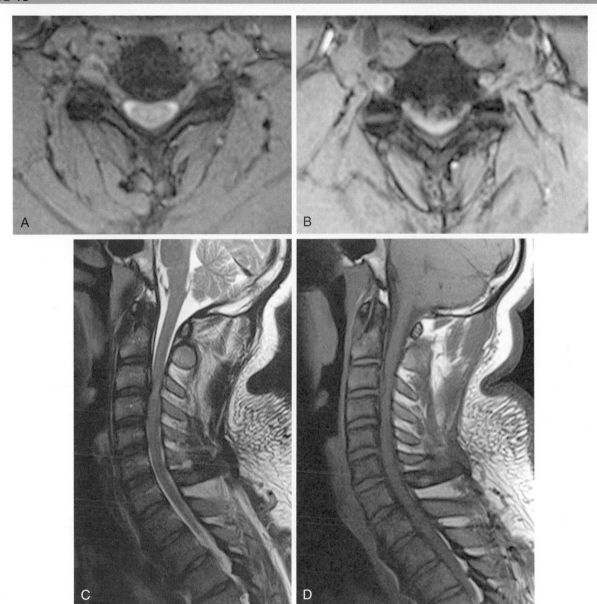

History: A 45-year-old man presents with a 6-month history of neck and upper extremity pain, right worse than left; numbness in the forearm and fingers; and difficulty performing fine motor tasks.

1. What should be included in the differential diagnosis? (Choose all that apply.)
   a. Diffuse idiopathic skeletal hyperostosis
   b. Central spinal stenosis
   c. Ankylosing spondylitis
   d. Congenital canal stenosis
   e. Rheumatoid arthritis

2. According to the classification of cervical canal stenosis by Muhle and colleagues, which grade defines complete obliteration of the subarachnoid space?
   a. Grade 0
   b. Grade 1
   c. Grade 2
   d. Grade 3

3. Which of the following statements regarding cervical spinal stenosis is true?
   a. Patients with spinal stenosis are less susceptible to traumatic cord injury.
   b. MRI can overestimate the degree of stenosis in the cervical region.
   c. Sagittal images in a patient with spinal stenosis typically show narrowing of the thecal sac involving one level.
   d. Stenosis usually involves the upper cervical region.

4. In which neck position is the degree of canal stenosis greater?
   a. Neutral position
   b. Flexion
   c. Extension
   d. The degree of canal stenosis does not change in different neck positions.

Cervical Spinal Stenosis

1. b and d

2. c

3. b

4. c

References

Muhle C, Metzner J, Weinert D, et al: Classification system based on kinematic MR imaging in cervical spondylitic myelopathy, *AJNR Am J Neuroradiol* 19(9):1763-1771, 1998.

Reul J, Gievers B, Weis J, et al: Assessment of the narrow cervical spinal canal: A prospective comparison of MRI, myelography, and CT-myelography, *Neuroradiology* 37(3):187-191, 1995.

Cross-Reference

Neuroradiology: The REQUISITES, 3rd ed, pp 535-537.

Comment

Background

Cervical myelopathy in older adults is most often secondary to cervical spinal stenosis. In patients with a congenitally narrow canal, mild degenerative changes are sufficient to cause spinal stenosis.

Pathophysiology

Hypertrophy of the ligamentum flavum, bony spondylitic hypertrophy, and bulging of the disk annulus contribute to the development of central spinal stenosis. Movement of the cervical spine exacerbates congenital or acquired spinal stenosis.

Imaging

MRI is the most commonly used imaging modality for the accurate evaluation of spinal canal stenosis, particularly axial T2-weighted images (Figs. A and B). Sagittal T2-weighted images typically show hourglass narrowing of the thecal sac involving multiple levels. Evidence of congenital stenosis can be inferred from the paucity of cerebrospinal fluid in the thecal sac over several levels with minor spondylotic changes (Figs. A and C). On T1-weighted images, canal stenosis results in scalloping of the ventral or dorsal cord contour (Fig. D).

Management

In patients with myelopathy secondary to cervical spinal stenosis, treatment is surgical decompression. Defining the extent of anterior, lateral, and posterior thecal sac compression is necessary to plan the surgical approach.

Notes

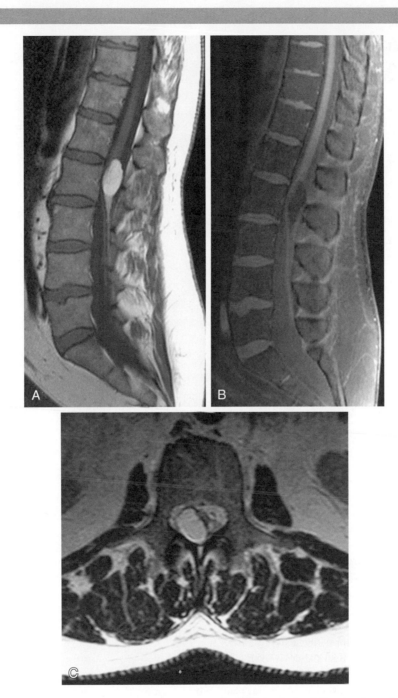

History: A 30-year-old man has a 2-year history of low back pain.

1. What should be included in the differential diagnosis? (Choose all that apply.)
   a. Dermoid
   b. Arachnoid cyst
   c. Lipoma
   d. Meningioma
   e. Subacute thrombus

2. What is the most common location of intradural lipomas?
   a. Cervical spine
   b. Thoracic spine
   c. Lumbar spine
   d. Sacral spine

3. Which of the following is *not* hyperintense on T1-weighted images?
   a. Subacute blood
   b. Melanin
   c. Proteinaceous fluid
   d. Coarse calcifications

4. Which of the following statements regarding spinal lipomas is *false*?
   a. The clinical presentation of spinal lipomas is mainly related to a tethered spinal cord.
   b. There is typically a dural defect related to the lipoma.
   c. Lipomas with intact dura mater involve predominantly the cervical and thoracic spinal cord.
   d. Spinal lipomas can grow when the patient's body weight increases.

Lipoma of the Conus Medullaris

1. a and c

2. b

3. d

4. a

References

Chapman P, Stieg PE, Magge S, et al: Spinal lipoma controversy, *Neurosurgery* 44(1):186-192, 1999.

Hsieh CT, Sun JM, Liu MY, et al: Lipoma of conus medullaris without spinal dysraphism in an adult, *Neurol India* 57(6):825-826, 2009.

Wykes V, Desai D, Thompson DN: Asymptomatic lumbosacral lipomas—a natural history study, *Childs Nerv Syst* 28(10):1731-1739, 2012.

Cross-Reference

Neuroradiology: The REQUISITES, 3rd ed, pp 564-565.

Comment

Background

Lipomas of the conus medullaris without spinal dysraphism are rare in adults. Most patients have symptoms for more than 2 years before the diagnosis. Although spinal lipomas are often discussed in the context of a tethered spinal cord, the clinical presentation of intradural spinal lipoma is related mainly to the mass effect, with resulting displacement of the conus or crowding of the nerve roots.

Pathophysiology

Although lipomas of the conus may appear intradural, it has been noted that these tumors usually have some connection with the dorsal thecal sac and are not completely intradural. Chapman and colleagues proposed an anatomic classification of lumbosacral lipomas based on the relationship of the lipoma to the conus medullaris. Dorsal lipomas are located entirely on the dorsal aspect of the lower spinal cord and always spare the conus. Caudal types are attached to the termination of the spinal cord and involve the tip of the conus. A transitional type represents a complex malformation that extends inferiorly from the dorsum of the terminal spinal cord to involve both the conus and elements of the cauda equina. This last type is frequently complicated by rotation of the neural placode to one side or the other, resulting in forward displacement and apparent shortening of the nerve roots. The dura mater is typically deficient dorsally and occasionally laterally, where the lipoma erupts through the spinal defect.

Imaging

MRI is the best diagnostic modality to evaluate spinal lipoma and delineate the adjacent neural structures (Figs. A-C). The fat component can be easily confirmed with fat-suppression images (see Fig. B).

Management

The goal of surgery is to release the tethered neural elements and remove the bulk of the lipoma, while preserving neurologic functions. Because the dorsal roots sometimes exit through the lateral aspect of the lipoma, a distinct plane between tumor and spinal cord may not be present, precluding complete resection of the tumor.

Notes

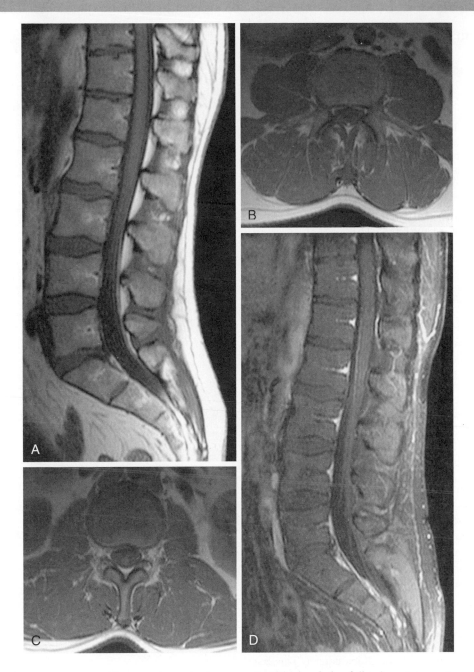

History: A 42-year-old man presents with severe lower back pain.

1. What should be included in the differential diagnosis? (Choose all that apply.)
   a. Subarachnoid hemorrhage
   b. Epidural lipomatosis
   c. Dural arteriovenous fistula
   d. Fatty filum terminale
   e. Dermoid

2. Which of the following conus tip positions is abnormal in an adult?
   a. T12
   b. L1
   c. L1-2
   d. L2-3

3. Which of the following statements regarding "tight filum terminale" syndrome is true?
   a. The conus tip is always in an abnormal position.
   b. Fatty tissue in the filum is always present.
   c. The filum is typically thickened.
   d. Surgery is not indicated.

4. Which congenital vertebral anomaly is strongly associated with tight filum terminale syndrome?
   a. Block vertebra
   b. Spina bifida
   c. Hemivertebra
   d. Butterfly vertebra

Fatty Filum Terminale

1. d

2. d

3. c

4. b

References

Brown E, Matthes JC, Bazan C 3rd, et al: Prevalence of incidental intraspinal lipoma of the lumbosacral spine as determined by MRI, *Spine (Phila Pa 1976)* 19(7):833-836, 1994.

McLone D, Thompson D: Lipomas of the spine. In McLone D, editor: *Pediatric neurosurgery*, Philadelphia, 2001, Saunders, pp 289-301.

Cross-Reference

Neuroradiology: The REQUISITES, 3rd ed, pp 317-318, 564-565.

Comment

Background

Lipoma (or fibrolipoma) of the filum has been found incidentally in 4% to 6% of normal adults on postmortem examination; however, the true incidence of fatty filum is unknown because the condition is frequently occult.

Embryology

In contrast to lipomas of the conus medullaris, lipomas of the filum develop as a result of a disorder of secondary neurulation. It is currently believed that progressive coalescence of vacuoles, which arise in the caudal cell mass during the fourth and fifth weeks of development, leads to the emergence of a central canal within the caudal cell mass. This canal coalesces with the neural tube formed by primary neurulation. The distal portion of the caudal cell mass regresses to become the terminal filum. The exact pathogenic mechanisms by which lipomas of the filum arise remain unknown, but impaired canalization of the caudal cell mass and persistence of cells capable of maturing into adipocytes are likely involved. This process occurs after disjunction of the cutaneous and neural ectoderm, and these lesions are skin covered and lacking cutaneous stigmata.

Imaging

If the lipoma is large enough, fat density can be seen on CT. MRI (Figs. A-D) shows linear soft tissue (Fig. A) following the fat signal on all pulse sequences and extending over a varying length.

Management

No treatment is indicated in asymptomatic patients. When patients have tethered cord syndrome and a low position of the conus, surgical intervention is considered.

Notes

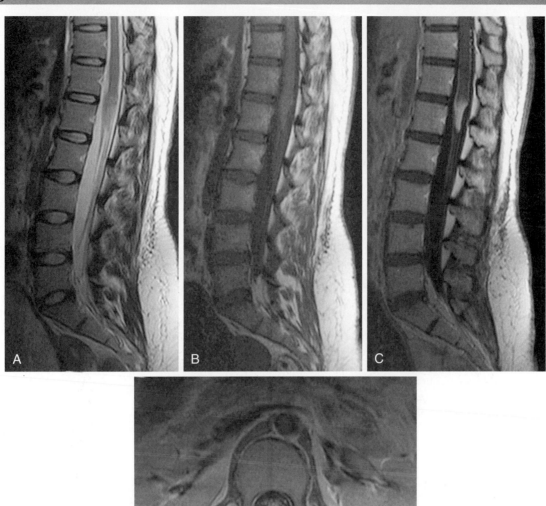

History: A 23-year-old woman presents with right buttock pain extending to the perineum.

1. What should be included in the differential diagnosis? (Choose all that apply.)
   a. Guillain-Barré syndrome
   b. Meningioma
   c. Cord infarct
   d. Tuberculosis
   e. Sarcoidosis

2. Which of the following infections is the least likely to produce a leptomeningitis and pachymeningitis enhancement pattern?
   a. Tuberculosis
   b. Fungal infection
   c. Toxoplasmosis
   d. Syphilis

3. Which of the following imaging studies would be least helpful as the next study in the evaluation of this patient?
   a. Chest x-ray
   b. Gallium scan
   c. MRI of the brain
   d. Ultrasound of the abdomen

4. Patients with sarcoidosis have an increased incidence of which of the following infections?
   a. Tuberculosis
   b. Group B streptococcus
   c. *Salmonella*
   d. Echinococcosis

Neurosarcoid Conus Medullaris

1. c, d, and e

2. c

3. d

4. a

Reference

Prelog K, Blome S, Dennis C: Neurosarcoidosis of the conus medullaris and cauda equina, *Australas Radiol* 47(3):295-297, 2003.

Cross-Reference

Neuroradiology: The REQUISITES, 3rd ed, pp 546, 547.

Comment

Background

Sarcoidosis is a multisystem noncaseating granulomatous disease of unknown etiology. It can affect patients of all ages and races but is most common in the third and fourth decades. African Americans and whites of northern European descent have the highest disease incidence, and women are more frequently affected than men. Neurosarcoidosis is uncommon and most frequently involves the brain basal leptomeninges. Spinal cord involvement is infrequent and is most commonly seen in the cervical and thoracic regions. Involvement of the conus is rare.

Histopathology

Definitive diagnosis of neurosarcoidosis requires the exclusion of other causes of neuropathy and the identification of noncaseating sarcoid granulomas by histologic analysis.

Imaging

Contrast-enhanced MRI is the most sensitive diagnostic tool for the assessment of neurosarcoidosis. Both intramedullary disease and extramedullary disease have been documented (Figs. A-D). Leptomeningeal disease is characteristic, but not specific, and the combination of cord parenchyma and surface or pial involvement is highly suggestive of sarcoidosis (see Figs. C and D).

Management

Diagnosis and early treatment of neurosarcoidosis with corticosteroids can minimize neurologic complications and decrease disease morbidity rates; however, with delayed diagnosis and treatment, the disease typically resolves only partially and may recur.

Notes

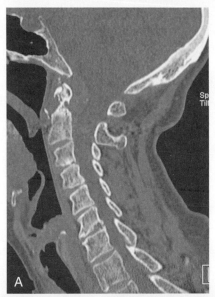

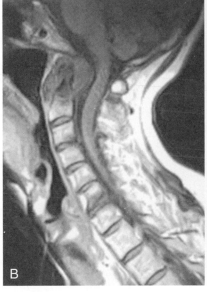

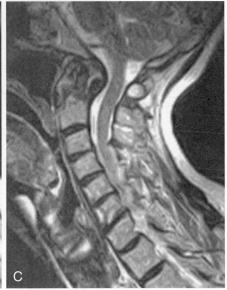

History: A 62-year-old woman with a 3-year history of progressive hand numbness and weakness presents with increased limitation of head rotation, stabbing neck pain, and occipital pain for the past 2 months.

1. What should be included in the differential diagnosis? (Choose all that apply.)
   a. Calcium pyrophosphate deposition disease
   b. Rheumatoid arthritis
   c. Chordoma
   d. Ankylosing spondylitis
   e. Plasmacytoma

2. Which MRI sequence is most helpful in distinguishing between joint effusion and pannus in patients with rheumatoid arthritis of the craniocervical region?
   a. Proton density
   b. T2-weighted
   c. T1-weighted
   d. T1-weighted with contrast enhancement

3. In which of the following synovium-lined articular capsules and bursae is pannus formation most common in patients with rheumatoid arthritis involving the cervical spine?
   a. Predental
   b. Supradental
   c. Retrodental
   d. Zygapophyseal

4. Which of the following statements regarding supradental fat is true?
   a. Supradental fat is preserved in patients undergoing hemodialysis.
   b. Supradental fat is often lost in patients with rheumatoid arthritis.
   c. Supradental fat disappears with age.
   d. Loss of supradental fat implies underlying atlantoaxial subluxation.

Adult Rheumatoid Arthritis

1. a, b, and e

2. d

3. c

4. b

Reference

Stiskal MA, Neuhold A, Szolar DH, et al: Rheumatoid arthritis of the cranio-cervical region by MR imaging: Detection and characterization, *AJR Am J Roentgenol* 165(3):585-592, 1995.

Cross-Reference

Neuroradiology: The REQUISITES, 3rd ed, pp 300, 301.

Comment

Background

Rheumatoid arthritis is a chronic systemic inflammatory disease; the cause is unknown. It is characterized by proliferative, hypervascularized synovitis resulting in bone erosion, cartilage damage, and joint destruction. The atlantoaxial joint is commonly involved because it contains multiple synovial joints, resulting in erosion of the stabilizing ligaments of the atlantoaxial articulation and instability that leads to cord compromise. Pannus may also erode the bone and compress the thecal sac and cord. Facet joints may be involved as well, leading to instability within the spinal axis.

Histopathology

Proliferative synovitis (rheumatoid pannus) is the earliest pathologic abnormality in rheumatoid arthritis. Pannus is an inflammatory exudate overlying the lining layer of synovial cells on the inside of a joint; however, histologic findings in rheumatoid arthritis patients with inflamed synovium may vary from a fibrinous fluid collection in the joint space to granulation tissue with abundant vessels to dense fibrous tissue without proliferating vessels or edema.

Imaging

CT is useful in diagnosing erosions of the odontoid process (Fig. A). MRI can visualize the extent of spinal cord compression, particularly when compression is due to pannus (Figs. B and C). Contrast-enhanced T1-weighted images of the craniocervical region may differentiate the various types of pannus, which have been divided into four groups on the basis of enhancement patterns: joint effusion, hypervascular pannus, hypovascular pannus, and fibrous pannus. These patterns have been detected even when plain radiographs are negative. Thickening of the ligaments and dura may also contribute to the masslike appearance of pannus.

Management

Treatment goals are to avoid irreversible neurologic deficit and prevent sudden death (reported in 10% of patients). In asymptomatic patients, early aggressive medical management is important because cervical spine involvement correlates with disease activity. Symptomatic patients often require surgery to relieve compression and establish stability.

Notes

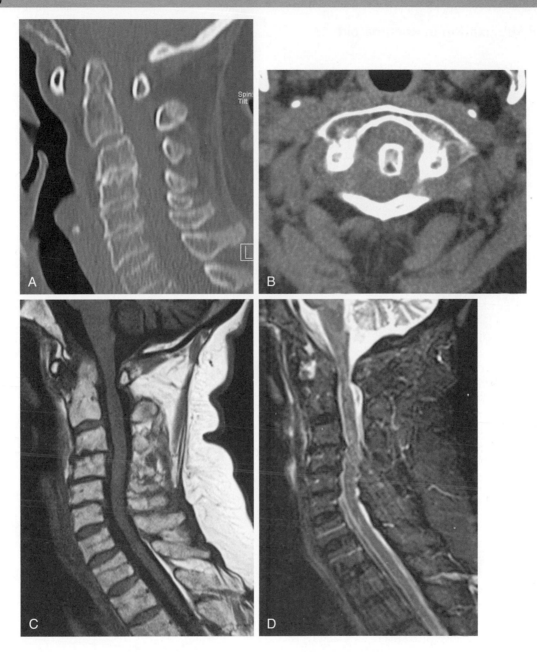

History: A 70-year-old woman presents with neck pain, Lhermitte's sign, and upper extremity numbness.

1. What should be included in the differential diagnosis? (Choose all that apply.)
   a. Hangman's fracture
   b. Rheumatoid arthritis
   c. Trauma
   d. Morquio syndrome
   e. Down syndrome

2. Which of the following types of subluxation or dislocation at the C1-2 level is most common in patients with rheumatoid arthritis?
   a. Anterior
   b. Posterior
   c. Lateral
   d. Vertical

3. Which of the following is an abnormal atlantodental interval in an adult?
   a. Greater than 1 mm
   b. Greater than 2 mm
   c. Greater than 3 mm
   d. Greater than 4 mm

4. What is the first imaging modality recommended in patients with rheumatoid arthritis suspected of having cervical involvement?
   a. Plain radiography
   b. CT scan
   c. MRI
   d. Diskography

Atlantoaxial Subluxation in Rheumatoid Arthritis

1. b, c, d, and e

2. a

3. c

4. a

References

Karhu JO, Parkkola RK, Koskinen SK: Evaluation of flexion/extension of the upper cervical spine in patients with rheumatoid arthritis: An MRI study with a dedicated positioning device compared to conventional radiographs, *Acta Radiol* 46(1):55-66, 2005.

Stiskal MA, Neuhold A, Szolar DH, et al: Rheumatoid arthritis of the cranio-cervical region by MR imaging: Detection and characterization, *AJR Am J Roentgenol* 165(3):585-592, 1995.

Cross-Reference

Neuroradiology: The REQUISITES, 3rd ed, pp 300, 301.

Comment

Background

Rheumatoid cervical spine involvement can be divided into three categories that may be seen in isolation or in combination. Atlantoaxial instability or atlantoaxial subluxation is the most common and can be fixed or reducible. Superior migration of the odontoid (also known as cranial settling) is the next most common abnormality. The third and least common deformity is subaxial subluxation, which may be seen at multiple levels and produces a stepladder appearance of the cervical spine.

Imaging

Lateral flexion and extension plain radiographs are initially obtained to evaluate the anterior atlantodental interval (posterior margins of the anterior C1 arch to the anterior aspect of the odontoid). An interval of more than 3 mm in adults and 4 mm in children is considered abnormal. CT scan (Figs. A and B) is performed to obtain a more accurate measurement in patients with abnormal radiographs. MRI (Figs. C and D) is performed to better visualize the pannus and to evaluate for cord compression or cord signal changes.

Management

Asymptomatic patients with atlantoaxial subluxation may be observed. In symptomatic patients, posterior atlantoaxial fusion can be performed if the subluxation is reducible. Patients with irreducible deformity can be treated with C1 laminectomy and transarticular stabilization.

Notes

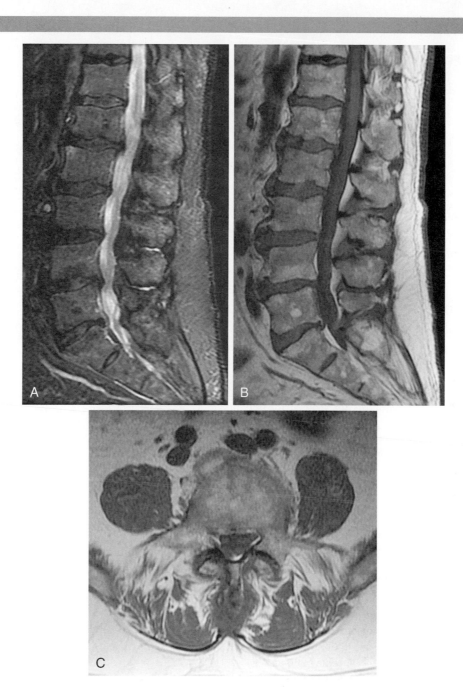

History: A 70-year-old man presents with back pain.

1. What should be included in the differential diagnosis? (Choose all that apply.)
   a. Infection
   b. Fibrosarcoma
   c. Baastrup's disease
   d. Compression fracture
   e. Leukemia

2. Which of the following imaging findings in this case is not associated with Baastrup's disease?
   a. Hyperintense signal on T2-weighted images in the interspinous bursa at L2-3
   b. Mild retrolisthesis of L3 on L4 and anterolisthesis of L4 on L5
   c. Hypertrophy of the spinous process
   d. Disk space narrowing at L2-3

3. Which of the following cysts is associated with Baastrup's disease?
   a. Posterior epidural cyst
   b. Synovial cyst
   c. Ligamentum flavum cyst
   d. Tarlov cyst

4. Which of the following statements regarding Baastrup's disease is true?
   a. Baastrup's disease occurs most commonly at L1-2.
   b. Patients with Baastrup's disease typically have localized lumbar pain that worsens on flexion and improves on extension.
   c. Fatty infiltration of the paraspinous muscles is often seen.
   d. Widening of the interspinous space is often seen.

Baastrup's Disease

1. a and c

2. d

3. a

4. c

References

Chen CKH, Yeh L, Resnick D, et al: Intraspinal posterior epidural cysts associated with Baastrup's disease: Report of 10 cases, *AJR Am J Roentgenol* 182(1):191-194, 2004.

Clifford PD: Baastrup disease, *Am J Orthop (Belle Mead NJ)* 36(10):560-561, 2007.

Rajasekaran S, Pithwa YK: Baastrup's disease as a cause of neurogenic claudication, *Spine (Phila Pa 1976)* 28(14):E273-E275, 2003.

Cross-Reference
Neuroradiology: The REQUISITES, 3rd ed, pp 533-534.

Comment

Background
Baastrup's disease is also known as "kissing spines." Patients typically have localized lumbar pain that worsens on extension and improves on flexion. The etiology of the pain is controversial. Some authors postulate that the pain is caused by direct contact between the spinous processes. Others hypothesize that the pain is caused by the associated findings (listhesis, facet hypertrophy, or disk herniation).

Pathophysiology
This process can result in degenerative hypertrophy, inflammatory changes, and pseudarthrosis with bursa formation between adjacent spinous processes.

Imaging
MRI usually demonstrates fluid in one or more interspinous bursae (Fig. A). Close approximation of the spinous processes with secondary flattening and hypertrophy (Figs. A-C) is frequently seen. Some patients develop an epidural cyst in the posterior spinal canal that communicates with the interspinous bursa. Baastrup's disease occurs most commonly at L3-4 and L4-5. Listhesis, or slippage of one vertebra on the subjacent vertebra, is frequently found.

Management
Treatment options include direct anesthetic injection or surgical excision of the spinous process.

Notes

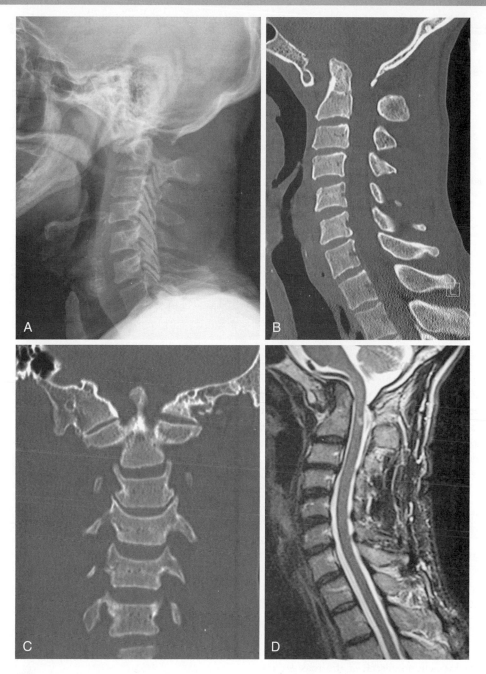

History: A 60-year-old man presents with neck pain.

1. What should be included in the differential diagnosis? (Choose all that apply.)
   a. Hangman's fracture
   b. Basilar invagination
   c. Platybasia
   d. Atlantoaxial subluxation
   e. Atlantooccipital assimilation

2. McGregor's line is drawn between which anatomic landmarks?
   a. Posterior edge of the hard palate and the opisthion
   b. Posterior edge of the hard palate and the undersurface of the occipital squamosal surface
   c. Basion and opisthion
   d. Tuberculum sella and basion

3. All of the following neural axis abnormalities are associated with basilar invagination *except:*
   a. Chiari I malformation
   b. Hydrocephalus
   c. Syringomyelia
   d. Dandy-Walker cyst

4. All of the following are causes of basilar impression *except:*
   a. Paget's disease
   b. Hypoparathyroidism
   c. Rickets
   d. Osteogenesis imperfecta

Atlantooccipital Assimilation with Basilar Invagination

1. b, d, and e

2. b

3. d

4. b

References

Kumar R, Kalra SK, Vaid VK, et al: Craniovertebral junction anomaly with atlas assimilation and reducible atlantoaxial dislocation: A rare constellation of bony abnormalities, *Pediatr Neurosurg* 44(5):402-405, 2008.

Smith JS, Shaffrey CI, Abel MF, et al: Basilar invagination, *Neurosurgery* 66 (3 Suppl):39-47, 2010.

Smoker WR: MR imaging of the craniovertebral junction, *Magn Reson Imaging Clin N Am* 8(3):635-650, 2000.

Cross-Reference

Neuroradiology: The REQUISITES, 3rd ed, p 300.

Comment

Background

Basilar invagination is a developmental anomaly of the craniovertebral junction in which the odontoid process is located in an abnormally high position because of a decrease in skull base height. The underlying abnormality responsible for basilar invagination in this case is most likely atlantooccipital assimilation. Symptoms in patients with atlantooccipital assimilation usually occur secondary to associated atlantoaxial dislocation, which is typically irreducible. Other common associations include congenital C2-C3 fusion and Chiari I malformation.

Pathophysiology

Components of the craniocervical junction are derived from the last occipital sclerotome or proatlas and from the first three cervical sclerotomes. One of the most common craniocervical anomalies is occipitalization of the atlas, in which there is bony continuity between the atlas and the skull base. This union typically involves the anterior arch and foramen magnum. Union involving the lateral masses or the posterior arch is less common. The embryologic abnormality involves discontinuity between the hypochondral arch of the atlas and the basal plate of the occipital sclerotomes.

Imaging

Basilar invagination is classically defined by plain radiographs. On lateral radiographs, the odontoid process projects too far above Chamberlain's line or McGregor's line and may compress the cervicomedullary junction (Fig. A). CT scan with orthogonal reconstructions can evaluate osseous anatomy better (Figs. B and C). In the case shown, Wackenheim's clivus baseline is also abnormal (see Fig. B). The line is drawn along the dorsal surface of the clivus and extrapolated into the upper cervical canal. Normally, Wackenheim's line forms a tangent with the posterior aspect of the odontoid tip or intersects the posterior one third of the odontoid. Neither of these conditions is met in this case. MRI permits assessment for cord compression and cord signal changes (Fig. D).

Management

Although it is a congenital condition, basilar invagination may remain asymptomatic and unrecognized until adulthood; however, surgical treatment may ultimately be required in a substantial subset of these patients.

Notes

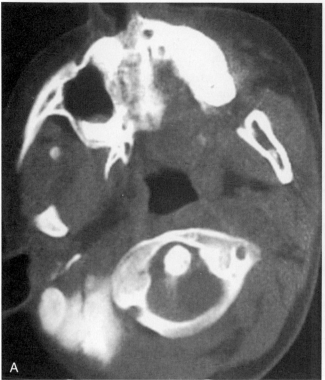 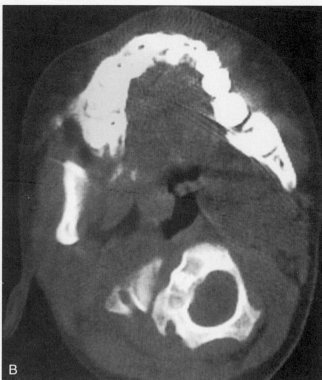

History: A 40-year-old woman presents with neck pain.

1. What should be included in the differential diagnosis? (Choose all that apply.)
   a. Torticollis
   b. Jefferson's fracture
   c. Atlantoaxial dislocation
   d. Atlantoaxial rotatory subluxation
   e. Hangman's fracture

2. Which imaging technique is recommended for establishing the diagnosis of atlantoaxial rotatory fixation?
   a. MRI with head rotation
   b. CT with head rotation
   c. Radiography
   d. Ultrasound

3. All of the following are causes of acquired, nondystonic torticollis *except:*
   a. Atlantoaxial rotatory dislocation
   b. Anterior atlantoaxial subluxation
   c. C2-C3 rotatory dislocation
   d. Cranial settling

4. What is Grisel syndrome?
   a. Atlantoaxial rotatory deformity resulting from trauma
   b. Atlantoaxial rotatory deformity associated with hemi hypertrophy
   c. Atlantoaxial rotatory deformity resulting from infection
   d. Atlantoaxial rotatory deformity and mental retardation

Atlantoaxial Rotatory Deformity

1. a and d

2. b

3. d

4. c

References

Currier BL: Atlantoaxial rotatory deformities. In Levine AM, Eismont FJ, Garfin SR, et al, editors: *Spine trauma*, Philadelphia, 1998, Saunders, pp 249-267.

Fielding JW, Hawkins RJ: Atlanto-axial rotatory fixation. (Fixed rotatory subluxation of the atlanto-axial joint.) *J Bone Joint Surg Am* 59:37-44, 1977.

Kowalski HM, Cohen WA, Cooper P, et al: Pitfalls in the CT diagnosis of atlantoaxial rotary subluxation, *AJR Am J Roentgenol* 149(3):595-600, 1987.

Cross-Reference

Neuroradiology: The REQUISITES, 3rd ed, p 579.

Comment

Background

Atlantoaxial rotatory deformity (Figs. A and B) is a spectrum of disorders. Atlantoaxial rotatory dislocation generally refers to complete dislocation of the C1-C2 facet joints. Rotational deformity of the C1-C2 joints within the physiologic range of motion has been referred to as atlantoaxial rotatory displacement by Fielding and Hawkins, but other authors prefer the term rotary subluxation. In this deformity, the joints are not dislocated. If this condition persists and becomes fixed (refractory to nonoperative management), it is referred to as atlantoaxial rotatory fixation.

Pathophysiology

Rotatory deformity may result from infection, trauma, and other conditions, or it may arise spontaneously (as in this case).

Imaging

Recognizing the importance of transverse ligament integrity in determining the degree of canal compromise accompanying rotational deformities, Fielding and Hawkins described four types of rotatory fixation:

- Type I: Rotatory fixation with no anterior displacement (Figs. A and B). The transverse ligament is intact, and the odontoid acts as the pivot.
- Type II: Rotatory fixation with anterior displacement of 3 to 5 mm. The transverse ligament is mildly deficient or lax, and one facet acts as the pivot.
- Type III: Rotatory fixation with anterior displacement of more than 5 mm. The transverse ligament and alar ligaments are deficient.
- Type IV: Rotatory fixation with posterior displacement. This is rare; the only case reported by Fielding and Hawkins was in an adult with rheumatoid arthritis and absence of the dens because of erosion.

Management

Nonoperative treatment includes a soft collar and anti-inflammatory medications. If subluxation persists, head traction may be required. Operative treatment (posterior C1-C2 fusion) is considered when subluxation persists more than 3 months or if neurologic deficit is present.

Notes

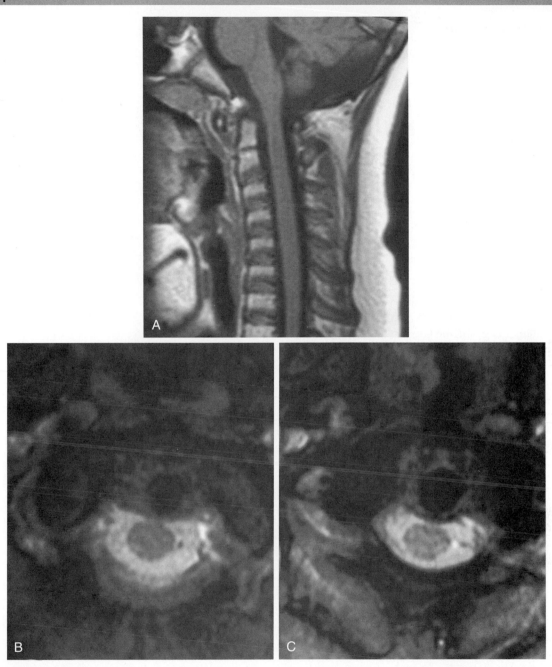

History: An 8-year-old boy was hit by a car while skateboarding.

1. What should be included in the differential diagnosis? (Choose all that apply.)
   a. Torticollis
   b. Hangman's fracture
   c. Atlantoaxial subluxation
   d. Atlantoaxial rotatory deformity
   e. Os odontoideum

2. Which of the following is unlikely in children with cranio-vertebral injury?
   a. Odontoid fracture
   b. Transverse ligament rupture
   c. Atlantoaxial subluxation
   d. Occipital condyle fracture

3. Which of the following statements regarding posttraumatic cervical spinal cord injury in adults and children is true?
   a. Adults tend to have upper cervical cord injuries.
   b. The distribution is the same throughout the cervical spine in children and adults.
   c. Children tend to have upper cervical cord injuries.
   d. Lower cervical cord injuries are more common in both children and adults.

4. Which of the following statements regarding spinal cord injury without radiologic abnormality (SCIWORA) is true?
   a. SCIWORA is more common in adults.
   b. A fracture is usually found.
   c. Myelopathy signs are typically absent.
   d. No evidence of ligamentous instability is found on plain radiographs and CT scan.

Atlantoaxial Subluxation

1. c

2. b

3. c

4. d

Reference

Slack SE, Clancy MJ: Clearing the cervical spine of paediatric trauma patients, *Emerg Med J* 21(2):189-193, 2004.

Cross-Reference

Neuroradiology: The REQUISITES, 3rd ed, p 579.

Comment

Background

Much has been written about the pitfalls in the interpretation of atlantoaxial subluxation and instability in children. The transverse ligament crosses behind the odontoid process and inserts on the inner margin of the C1 ring laterally, restricting the anteroposterior motion of C1 relative to C2. In children, especially those younger than 8 years, ligamentous laxity results in a greater range of motion. The maximum atlantodental distance (distance between the posterior margin of the anterior arch of C1 and the dens) is usually 5 mm in children, versus 2.5 to 3 mm in adults. Ostensibly, greater laxity reduces the frequency of transverse ligament rupture and places the odontoid at greater risk of fracture when a force is applied to the cervicovertebral and upper cervical region.

Imaging

In the present case, both CT scan and conventional radiography, including flexion and extension views, were performed. The atlantodental distance was 5 mm by CT and ranged from 3 mm in extension to 8 mm in flexion on lateral radiographs. No fractures were seen. In addition to the findings on sagittal T1-weighted MRI (Fig. A), axial gradient-echo images (Figs. B and C) demonstrated marked narrowing of the ventral subarachnoid space but no cord compression. No abnormal signal was detected in the spinal cord or in the region of the transverse ligament.

Management

Based on the clinical and imaging results, the neurosurgeon favored a diagnosis of C1-C2 instability secondary to transverse ligament laxity and performed a C1-C2 posterior fusion with cerclage wires and bone graft.

Notes

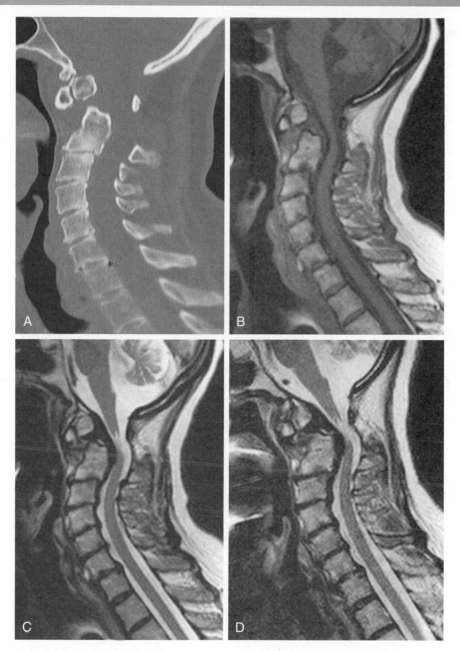

History: A 66-year-old woman presents with a history of neck pain for the past 2 months and a fall 3 years prior.

1. What should be included in the differential diagnosis? (Choose all that apply.)
   a. Klippel-Feil syndrome
   b. Atlantoaxial subluxation
   c. Os odontoideum
   d. Persistent ossiculum terminale
   e. Odontoid nonunion

2. Which of the following is the most common type of odontoid fracture based on the Anderson and D'Alonzo classification?
   a. Type I
   b. Type II
   c. Type III
   d. Type IV

3. Which of the following is a risk factor for odontoid fracture nonunion in adults?
   a. Young age of patient
   b. Adequate halo immobilization
   c. Ability to reduce the fracture
   d. Increased displacement or angulation of fracture fragments

4. Which of the following statements regarding odontoid fracture is true?
   a. Type III fractures are usually stable.
   b. In asymptomatic elderly patients, surgical treatment is recommended.
   c. Type I fractures are the most common.
   d. Nonunion occurs most frequently with type I fractures.

Odontoid Nonunion

1. c and e

2. b

3. d

4. a

References

Blacksin MF, Avagliano P: Computed tomographic and magnetic resonance imaging of chronic odontoid fractures, *Spine (Phila Pa 1976)* 24(2):158-161, 1999.

Koivikko MP, Kiuru MJ, Koskinen SK, et al: Factors associated with nonunion in conservatively-treated type-II fractures of the odontoid process, *J Bone Joint Surg Br* 86(8):1146-1151, 2004.

Cross-Reference

Neuroradiology: The REQUISITES, 3rd ed, p 580.

Comment

Background

Odontoid fractures account for 10% to 15% of all cervical spine fractures. In elderly patients, odontoid fracture can be caused by minimal trauma. The incidence of odontoid fracture nonunion following conservative treatment may be as high as 63%. Nonunion may predispose to a myelopathy secondary to instability of the atlantoaxial joint.

Pathophysiology

The Anderson and D'Alonzo classification of odontoid fractures describes three types: type I, an oblique fracture through the upper portion of the odontoid; type II, a transverse fracture through the base of the odontoid; and type III, a fracture through the body of the axis. The importance of classifying odontoid fractures is that type II fractures, which are most common, may be unstable, whereas type III fractures are usually stable and heal with conservative treatment. Nonunion occurs most frequently with type II fractures. Atlantoaxial subluxation may occur with or without odontoid displacement.

Imaging

Plain radiography assesses atlantoaxial subluxation and stability. CT scan (Fig. A) can provide information about the chronicity of the fracture, the size of the gap between the fracture fragment and the odontoid, and the presence of atlantoaxial subluxation. MRI can evaluate for cord compression, cord signal changes, and the presence or absence of mechanical compression during flexion and extension (Figs. B-D). Posttraumatic fracture fragment and congenital os odontoideum may be indistinguishable if the fracture is old and has smooth, sclerotic margins similar to the ossicle. In patients with os odontoideum, hypoplasia of the dens is almost always present, and there is often a wide gap between the dens and the ossicle. Additional findings that favor the diagnosis of os odontoideum are hypertrophy of the anterior arch of C1, which may be associated with clefting, and absence of the posterior arch of C1.

Management

Odontoid nonunion is a potentially hazardous complication that can lead to neurologic deficits months or years later. In general, odontoid nonunion should be managed surgically.

Notes

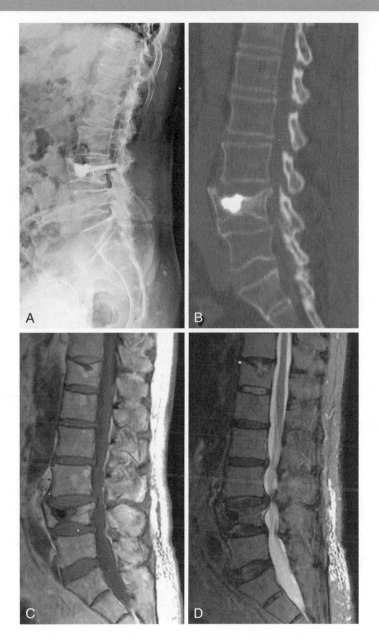

History: A 73-year-old man with a history of a treated compression fracture 1 year ago presents with new back pain.

1. What should be included in the differential diagnosis? (Choose all that apply.)
   a. Compression fracture
   b. Kyphoplasty
   c. Vertebroplasty
   d. Melorheostosis
   e. Sclerotic metastasis

2. All of the following are indications for vertebroplasty *except:*
   a. Osteoporotic compression fracture
   b. Malignant compression fracture
   c. Compression fracture associated with diskitis osteomyelitis
   d. Painful benign lesion such as hemangioma

3. All of the following are immediate complications of the procedure *except:*
   a. Leakage of cement into the epidural space, disk space, or neural foramina
   b. Fracture of an adjacent vertebral body
   c. Rib fracture
   d. Pulmonary embolism

4. Which of the following statements regarding complications of vertebroplasty is true?
   a. The complication rate is higher for osteoporotic fractures than for pathologic fractures.
   b. Leakage into the disk space decreases the risk of a new fracture in the adjacent vertebral body.
   c. Patients frequently experience a temporary increase in pain after vertebroplasty.
   d. The risk of an embolism of cement in the lungs increases with the number of vertebral bodies treated.

Vertebroplasty

1. a, b, and c

2. c

3. b

4. d

References
Galibert P, Deramond H, Rosat P, et al: Preliminary note on the treatment of vertebral angioma by percutaneous acrylic vertebroplasty [article in French], *Neurochirurgie* 33(2):166-168, 1987.

Lin EP, Ekholm S, Hiwatashi A, et al: Vertebroplasty: Cement leakage into the disc increases the risk of new fracture of adjacent vertebral body, *AJNR Am J Neuroradiol* 25(2):175-180, 2004.

Mathis JM: Percutaneous vertebroplasty: Complication avoidance and technique optimization, *AJNR Am J Neuroradiol* 24(8):1697-1706, 2003.

Cross-Reference
Neuroradiology: The REQUISITES, 3rd ed, pp 570-571.

Comment
Background
Deramond and Galibert first performed a percutaneous vertebroplasty in France in 1984 to treat a compression fracture. Since then, the procedure has become a widely accepted alternative for patients with symptomatic compression fractures. Procedural success rates range from 80% to 95%. Back pain after vertebroplasty is common and may be secondary to a new compression fracture at a different vertebral level.

Indications
In the United States, percutaneous vertebroplasty is performed predominantly to treat painful osteoporotic compression fractures that have failed conservative treatment consisting primarily of bed rest. Percutaneous vertebroplasty is also performed to treat pathologic fractures.

Imaging
Radiographs (Fig. A) or CT scan (Fig. B) can be obtained to evaluate for any new fracture or leakage of cement into the disk space or foramina. MRI (Figs. C and D) is needed to establish that there is no new fracture or recurrent fracture of the treated vertebra that would explain the patient's recurrence of symptoms. Imaging findings include progression of height loss in the vertebra or increased marrow edema.

Complications
Complications of vertebroplasty include leakage of cement (polymerizing methylmethacrylate mixed with a radiodense contrast agent) into the epidural space (potentially causing canal compromise and neurologic impairment), the neural foramina, or the disk space. Leakage into the disk space increases the risk of a new fracture in the adjacent vertebral body. Severe complications include leakage of cement into the paravertebral veins, leading to pulmonary embolism.

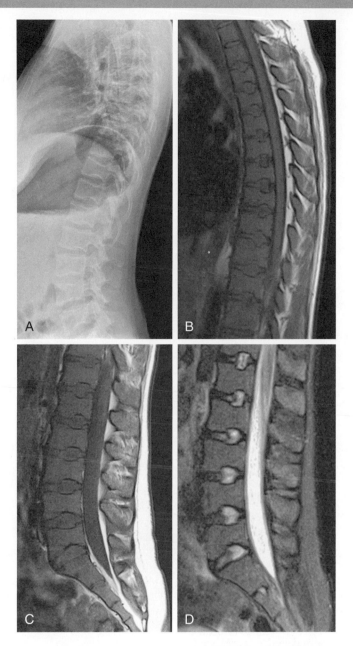

A

B

C

D

History: An 18-year-old woman presents with chronic back pain.

1. What should be included in the differential diagnosis? (Choose all that apply.)
   a. Sickle cell disease
   b. Metastasis
   c. Leukemia
   d. Gaucher disease
   e. Scheuermann's disease

2. The differential diagnosis of H-shaped vertebrae includes all of the following *except:*
   a. Homocystinuria
   b. Thalassemia minor
   c. Hereditary spherocytosis
   d. Sickle cell trait

3. All of the following are potential causes of myelopathy in patients with sickle cell disease *except:*
   a. Spinal cord infarction
   b. Epidural abscess
   c. Vertebral body infarction
   d. Dural arteriovenous fistula

4. Which of the following organisms has the highest tendency to be the infecting agent in osteomyelitis complicating sickle cell disease?
   a. *Salmonella*
   b. *Shigella*
   c. *Escherichia coli*
   d. *Mycobacterium tuberculosis*

Sickle Cell Disease

1. a and d

2. b

3. d

4. a

Reference

Ejindu VC, Hine AL, Mashayekhi M, et al: Musculoskeletal manifestations of sickle cell disease, *Radiographics* 27(4):1005-1021, 2007.

Cross-Reference

Neuroradiology: The REQUISITES, 3rd ed, pp 543-546.

Comment

Background

Sickle cell disease is a hereditary autosomal recessive disorder that causes significant morbidity and mortality. The incidence of sickle cell disease is highest in individuals of African or Mediterranean origin. Patients with sickle cell disease are more susceptible than others to certain infections, including pneumococcal and *Salmonella* infections, as a result of the decreased phagocytic ability of the reticuloendothelial system.

Pathophysiology

Sickle cell disease and its variants are genetic disorders resulting from the presence of a mutated form of hemoglobin: hemoglobin S (HbS). The most common form of sickle cell disease in North America is homozygous HbS disease (HbSS), which is an autosomal recessive disorder. Approximately 50% of these patients experience vaso-occlusive crisis.

Imaging

The skeletal imaging findings in sickle cell disease are due to bone marrow hyperplasia secondary to anemia and bone and marrow ischemia and infarction secondary to sickling episodes. In the spine, the vertebral bodies have been described as having an "H" shape or a smoothly curved end-plate depression (Figs. A-D). This "H" shape has been attributed to a growth disturbance of the central area of the vertebral body secondary to ischemia or infarction. Some authors distinguish this shape from the smoothly curved end-plate depression attributed to osteoporosis secondary to bone marrow hyperplasia. Other authors use the general term "biconcave" to refer to the vertebral end-plate contour abnormalities.

Management

The primary goal of therapy is to reduce the frequency and severity of episodes of sickle cell crisis. Adequate hydration, oxygenation, bone marrow stimulation, and blood transfusion are commonly used to treat sickle cell crisis.

Notes

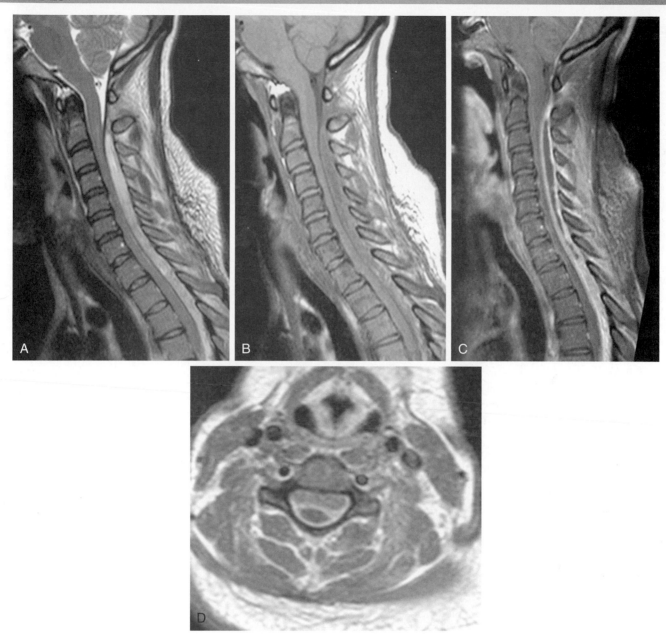

History: A 34-year-old woman presents with fever, headaches, and neck pain for the past 4 days and myelopathy on physical examination.

1. What should be included in the differential diagnosis? (Choose all that apply.)
   a. Epidural abscess
   b. Schwannoma
   c. Ependymoma
   d. Lymphoma
   e. Epidural hematoma

2. What is the next step in the imaging evaluation of this patient?
   a. Gallium scan
   b. CT myelography
   c. MRI of the thoracic and lumbar spine
   d. Radiolabeled leukocyte scan

3. What organism is most likely to cause an epidural abscess?
   a. *Staphylococcus aureus*
   b. *Mycobacterium tuberculosis*
   c. *Escherichia coli*
   d. *Salmonella*

4. Which of the following is not a risk factor for the development of epidural abscess?
   a. Intravenous drug abuse
   b. Alcoholism
   c. Spinal surgery
   d. Disk herniation

Epidural Abscess

1. a, d, and e

2. c

3. a

4. d

References

Chao D, Nanda A: Spinal epidural abscess: A diagnostic challenge, *Am Fam Physician* 65(7):1341-1346, 2002.

Numaguchi Y, Rigamonti D, Rothman MI, et al: Spinal epidural abscess: Evaluation with gadolinium-enhanced MR imaging, *Radiographics* 13(3):545-559, 1993.

Rigamonti D, Liem L, Sampath P, et al: Spinal epidural abscess: Contemporary trends in etiology, evaluation, and management, *Surg Neurol* 52(2):189-196, 1999.

Cross-Reference

Neuroradiology: The REQUISITES, 3rd ed, pp 543-546.

Comment

Background

The peak incidence for spinal epidural abscess is between 60 and 70 years old, and it is most often caused by *S. aureus* infection. The signs and symptoms of epidural abscess are nonspecific and can range from low back pain to frank sepsis. Neurologic dysfunction is often disproportionate to the observed degree of compression of the cord and nerve roots by the extradural mass. This disproportion has been attributed to the effects of edema and inflammation on the epidural venous plexus, compromising circulation and resulting in cord ischemia. Both compressive and ischemic mechanisms may contribute to neurologic dysfunction in such cases.

Pathophysiology

Most epidural abscesses are located posteriorly in the thoracic or lumbar canal and are thought to originate from hematogenous spread from a distant focus, such as a skin infection, pharyngitis, or dental abscess. Anterior epidural abscesses are commonly associated with diskitis osteomyelitis.

Imaging

Epidural abscess is typically hyperintense on T2-weighted images (Fig. A) and isointense to hypointense on T1-weighted images (Fig. B). Enhancement after contrast administration demonstrates one of the following patterns: homogeneous enhancement representing a phlegmon, peripheral enhancement representing a mature abscess (Figs. C and D), or heterogeneous enhancement representing a combination of both. Diffusion imaging shows the same findings reported for pyogenic abscesses in the brain: restricted diffusion and corresponding low apparent diffusion coefficient values.

Management

Treatment consists of both medical and surgical therapy. Empiric antibiotic coverage should include an antibiotic effective against methicillin-resistant *S. aureus,* which was the organism found in this case. Emergency surgical decompression of the spinal cord with drainage of the abscess is the usual surgical treatment.

Notes

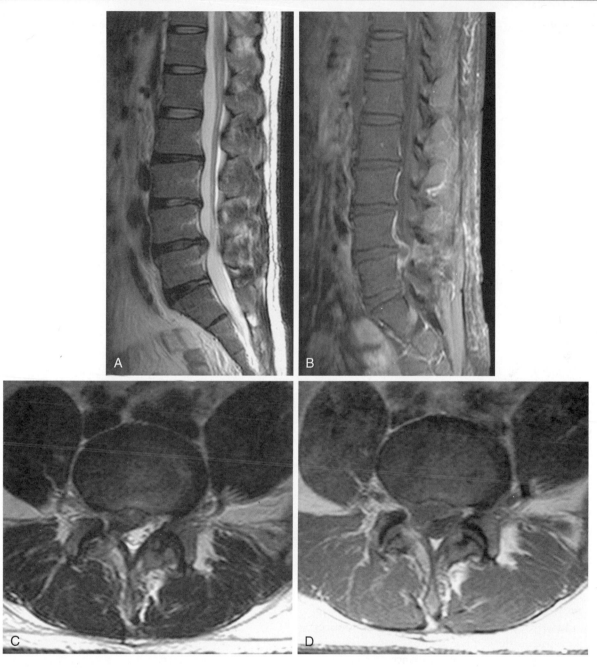

History: A 54-year-old man presents with severe back pain and a history of back surgery 6 months ago.

1. What should be included in the differential diagnosis? (Choose all that apply.)
   a. Disk herniation
   b. Epidural abscess
   c. Meningioma
   d. Lymphoma
   e. Epidural hematoma

2. Which of the following causes of failed back surgery syndrome (FBSS) is most likely in this patient?
   a. Spondylolisthesis
   b. Recurrent disk herniation
   c. Arachnoiditis
   d. Residual bony stenosis

3. Which of the following sequences is better at distinguishing recurrent disk herniation from epidural fibrosis?
   a. Early postcontrast T1-weighted images
   b. Delayed (>30 minutes) postcontrast T1-weighted images
   c. T2-weighted images
   d. T1-weighted images

4. Which of the following statements regarding FBSS is true?
   a. Microdiskectomy has a higher failure rate than spinal fusion.
   b. The surgical success rate increases when the patient undergoes reoperation.
   c. The number of patients with FBSS has increased as rates of spinal surgery have increased.
   d. Advances in technology and surgical techniques have led to decreased rates of FBSS.

Postoperative Recurrent Lumbar Disk Herniation

1. a and e

2. b

3. a

4. c

References

Chan CW, Peng P: Failed back surgery syndrome, *Pain Med* 12(4):577-606, 2011.

Ross JS: MR imaging of the postoperative lumbar spine, *Magn Reson Imaging Clin N Am* 7(3):513-524, 1999.

Cross-Reference

Neuroradiology: The REQUISITES, 3rd ed, pp 537-540.

Comment

Background

FBSS is persistent or recurring low back pain with or without sciatica after one or more spine surgeries. The incidence of FBSS after lumbar spinal surgery with fusion is 30% to 46%. Despite advances in surgical techniques, the rates of FBSS have not changed in the past several decades. However, failure rates are different for the various surgical procedures, with microdiskectomy having the lowest rate (15% to 20%).

Pathophysiology

Multiple factors are likely involved in the development of pain, including patient-related psychological risk factors; intraoperative factors such as inadequate decompression, most frequently in the lateral recess and foramina; and postoperative factors such as recurrent disk herniation, spondylolisthesis, and epidural fibrosis.

Imaging

The reported accuracy of postcontrast MRI in distinguishing between scar and disk (Figs. A-D) at least 6 weeks after surgery is 96% to 100%. Whether the time elapsed since surgery is months or years, scar consistently enhances on images acquired immediately after the injection of contrast material. Because it is avascular, disk does not enhance on these early images (see Figs. C and D). On delayed images (≥30 minutes after injection), disk material may enhance because of the diffusion of contrast material into the disk from adjacent scar, especially when there is a relatively large volume of scar compared with the volume of the herniation. A secondary sign that favors scar over recurrent or persistent disk is retraction of the thecal sac toward the region of the aberrant epidural soft tissue. The presence of mass effect is not helpful because both epidural scar and disk can produce this finding.

Management

Patients should receive interdisciplinary care that includes medications for pain control, psychotherapy, physical therapy, and interventional procedures such as epidural injections. Reoperation is controversial because studies have demonstrated that the overall success rate is low and declines after each additional surgery.

Notes

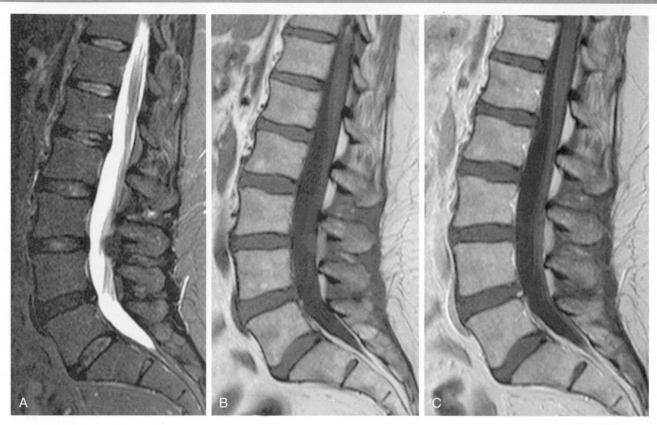

History: A 54-year-old woman presents with lower back pain.

1. What should be included in the differential diagnosis? (Choose all that apply.)
   a. Disk extrusion
   b. Meningioma
   c. Annular fissure (tear)
   d. Diskitis osteomyelitis
   e. Bulging annulus

2. All of the following are types of annular fissure found on postmortem cryomicrotome sections *except:*
   a. Concentric
   b. Radial
   c. Transverse
   d. Bucket-handle

3. Which type of annular fissure is associated with intervertebral disk degeneration?
   a. Concentric
   b. Radial
   c. Transverse
   d. All of the above

4. Which of the following statements regarding annular fissure is true?
   a. Most are symptomatic.
   b. An annular fissure near the dorsal root ganglion is the least likely to be painful.
   c. Diskography can help distinguish partial-thickness versus full-thickness fissure.
   d. Annular fissure is characterized by a region of high T1 signal in the annulus.

Annular Fissure (Tear)

1. c and e

2. d

3. b

4. c

References
Costello RF, Beall DP: Nomenclature and standard reporting terminology of intervertebral disk herniation, *Magn Reson Imaging Clin N Am* 15(2):167-174, 2007.

Pfirrmann CW, Metzdorf A, Zanetti M, et al: Magnetic resonance classification of lumbar intervertebral disc degeneration, *Spine (Phila Pa 1976)* 26(17):1873-1878, 2001.

Cross-Reference
Neuroradiology: The REQUISITES, 3rd ed, pp 525, 526.

Comment
Background
Annular fissure (or tear) is the deficiency of one or more layers that make up the annulus fibrosus. Although very common, most are asymptomatic; however, some may cause pain.

Pathophysiology
The annulus of the disk comprises sheaths of collagen called lamellae. With aging, the annulus loses strength and becomes more susceptible to the development of annular fissures. In some patients, this degenerative process can be accelerated by trauma or a genetic predisposition for annular fissure. Three types of annular fissure have been described: radial, concentric, and transverse. Investigators have shown that the radial fissure is consistently associated with gross anatomic (and MRI) evidence of disk degeneration, including diminished disk height, shrinkage and disorganization of fibrocartilage in the nucleus pulposus, and replacement of the disk by dense fibrous tissue and cystic spaces. The radial fissure, which involves multiple layers of the annulus from the nucleus pulposus to the surface of the disk, allows displacement of the nucleus and disk herniation. Radial annular fissure is a necessary but insufficient condition for herniation. The other two types of annular fissure, concentric and transverse, have been observed in most adult disks examined by cryomicrotome sectioning, and they are considered normal findings.

Imaging
Most annular fissures are not visible on MRI. Fissures that are visible demonstrate a high-intensity zone that is often crescent shaped and is commonly seen in the posterior portion of the disk at L4-5 and L5-S1. Radial fissures represent disruption perpendicular to the axis of the collagen fibers extending from the nucleus pulposus through the annulus fibrosus to the periphery of the disk. Concentric fissures represent a delamination of longitudinal annular fibers. Transverse fissures represent disruption of the insertion of Sharpey fibers into the ring apophysis; they are detected as punctate or linear hyperintense foci adjacent to the periphery of the vertebral end-plates on T2-weighted images (Fig. A). They are typically smaller than radial fissures, which demonstrate a more prominent hyperintense signal and may enhance on postcontrast T1-weighted images; this enhancement is well seen at the L4-5 level in this case (Figs. A-C).

Management
Treatment of annular fissure is conservative and consists of medications to alleviate pain and limited rest to allow the disk to heal.

Notes

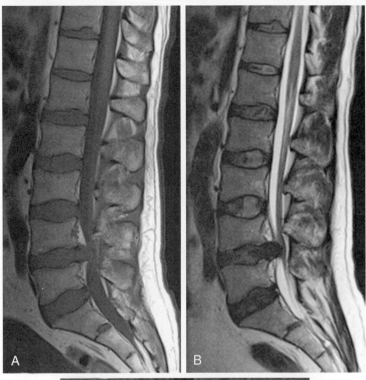

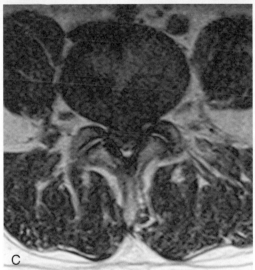

History: A 42-year-old man presents with severe low back pain and bilateral leg weakness.

1. What should be included in the differential diagnosis? (Choose all that apply.)
   a. Meningioma
   b. Lymphoma
   c. Disk herniation
   d. Diskitis osteomyelitis
   e. Ossification of the posterior longitudinal ligament

2. What is the frequency of bulging annulus on MRI in asymptomatic individuals?
   a. Less than 5%
   b. About 25%
   c. About 50%
   d. More than 75%

3. What is the frequency of disk herniation on MRI in individuals with no back pain?
   a. Less than 5%
   b. About 25%
   c. About 50%
   d. More than 75%

4. Which of the following statements best describes an extruded disk?
   a. Disk material has a broad-based neck wider than the edges of the herniated material.
   b. Displacement of disk material involves more than 50% of the disk circumference.
   c. There is radial separation of the annular fibers.
   d. The extruded disk material has a narrow neck and a wider extruded portion, as seen on the axial plane.

Lumbar Disk Extrusion

1. c

2. c

3. b

4. d

References

Brant-Zawadzki MN, Jensen MC, Obuchowski N, et al: Interobserver and intraobserver variability in interpretation of lumbar disc abnormalities: A comparison of two nomenclatures, *Spine (Phila Pa 1976)* 20(11):1257-1263, 1995.

Costello RF, Beall DP: Nomenclature and standard reporting terminology of intervertebral disk herniation, *Magn Reson Imaging Clin N Am* 15(2):167-174, 2007.

Jensen MC, Brant-Zawadzki MN, Obuchowski N, et al: Magnetic resonance imaging of the lumbar spine in people without back pain, *N Engl J Med* 331(2):69-73, 1994.

Cross-Reference

Neuroradiology: The REQUISITES, 3rd ed, pp 525-526.

Comment

Background

Intervertebral disk herniation is a common condition that can be found in both symptomatic and asymptomatic individuals. Generally, there are two nomenclature systems for categorizing degenerative disk pathology as displayed on MRI. In nomenclature I, disks extending beyond the interspace are categorized as bulging (symmetric, with diffuse extension) or herniated (symmetric or asymmetric, with focal extension). In nomenclature II, disks extending beyond the interspace are categorized as bulging (symmetric, with circumferential extension—50% to 100% of the circumference of the disk space), protruded (asymmetric or symmetric, with focal extension, a roughly conical shape pointing posteriorly, and residual low-signal-intensity annular fibers), or extruded (without or with caudad or cephalad extension, with complete rupture of annular fibers). Nomenclature II includes a description of a sequestered disk as an extruded disk with a dissociated fragment ("free fragment"). Nomenclature II, with minor modifications, has been endorsed by the major societies representing clinicians and investigators in the field of spine imaging.

Histopathology

The normal intervertebral disk has an inner nucleus pulposus, which contains hydrophilic glycosaminoglycans with a lattice of collagen fibers, and an outer annulus fibrosus, which contains 15 to 20 collagenous lamellae that are organized obliquely in relation to one another. The intervertebral disk is bordered by the cartilage end-plates. The disk is avascular and obtains its nutrition by diffusion from the adjacent end-plates. The term "herniation" is used to describe the displacement of disk material beyond the normal confines of the disk space.

Imaging

On MRI (Figs. A-C), disk herniation appears as a focal asymmetric protrusion of disk material beyond the confines of the annulus. The herniated portion of the disk is usually hypointense, but it may have a high signal intensity compared with the interspace (parent) portion on T2-weighted images.

Management

Most patients can be managed with conservative treatment, which consists of nonsteroidal anti-inflammatory drugs for pain. Surgery is reserved for severe, debilitating cases.

Notes

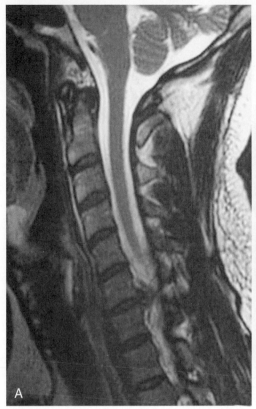

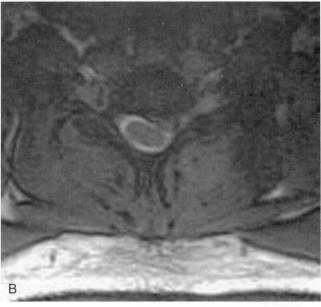

History: A 50-year-old man presents with neck pain and radiculopathy.

1. What should be included in the differential diagnosis? (Choose all that apply.)
   a. Schwannoma
   b. Meningioma
   c. Synovial cyst
   d. Ossification of the posterior longitudinal ligament
   e. Disk herniation

2. What is the most frequent level of nontraumatic cervical disk herniation?
   a. C4-5
   b. C5-6
   c. C6-7
   d. C7-T1

3. Which of the following statements regarding fast-spin-echo (FSE) T2-weighted images compared with gradient-echo T2*-weighted images is true?
   a. Cord signal abnormality is better appreciated on FSE T2-weighted axial images.
   b. FSE T2-weighted images are more sensitive to susceptibility effects.
   c. Fat signal is suppressed on FSE T2-weighted images.
   d. FSE T2-weighted images are more sensitive to cerebrospinal fluid (CSF) pulsation artifacts.

4. What symptom is this patient likely to have?
   a. Left C6 radiculopathy
   b. Left C7 radiculopathy
   c. Myelopathy
   d. Urinary incontinence

Cervical Disk Herniation

1. e

2. c

3. d

4. b

References

Bush K, Chaudhuri R, Hillier S, et al: The pathomorphologic changes that accompany the resolution of cervical radiculopathy: A prospective study with repeat magnetic resonance imaging, *Spine (Phila Pa 1976)* 22(2): 183-186, 1997.

Yousem DM, Atlas SW, Hackney DB: Cervical spine disk herniation: Comparison of CT and 3D FT gradient echo MR scans, *J Comput Assist Tomogr* 16(3):345-351, 1992.

Cross-Reference
Neuroradiology: The REQUISITES, 3rd ed, pp 766-773.

Comment
Background
Cervical disk herniation most commonly occurs at C5-6 and C6-7. It usually develops in individuals 30 to 50 years old. Arm pain is one of the more common presenting symptoms.

Pathophysiology
Cervical disk herniation results from repetitive cervical stress or, rarely, from a single traumatic incident. Cervical radiculopathy results from nerve root compression at the neural foraminal entrance zone; this compression is caused by disk protrusion and uncovertebral osteophytes anteriorly and by superior articulating process, ligamentum flavum, and periradicular fibrous tissue posteriorly. Nerve root irritation may also be caused by proteoglycan-mediated chemical inflammation released from a disk herniation.

Imaging
The sagittal image in this case shows a C6-7 herniated disk (Fig. A). Axial T2*-weighted images (Fig. B) are generally considered more accurate than T1-weighted images in detecting herniated disks because of the high contrast between the nearly isointense disk (mildly hyperintense in this case) and the markedly hyperintense CSF on T2*-weighted images. In addition, a thin, dark line, representing the posterior longitudinal ligament and dura, often separates the extradural herniation from the cord and hyperintense CSF. However, the usefulness of MRI may be limited in differentiating disk herniation (soft cervical disk) from an osteophyte without or with accompanying herniation (hard cervical disk). In such cases, CT may be better at discriminating between these two entities.

Management
Because cervical disk herniations have been shown to regress with time, leading to a resolution of symptoms, conservative approaches to the treatment of cervical radicular pain have been advocated by numerous investigators.

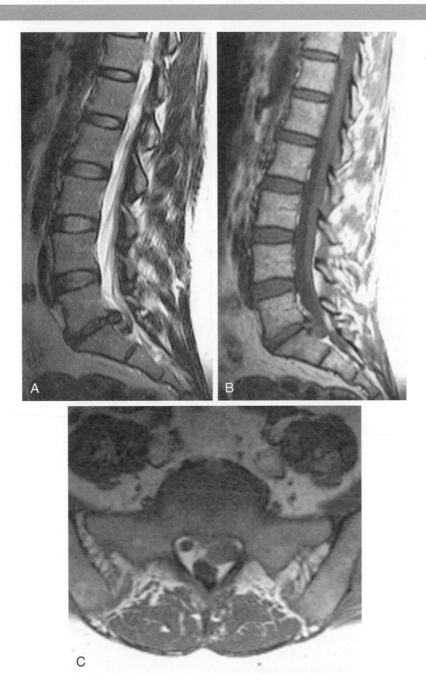

A

B

C

History: A 44-year-old woman presents with a 2-week history of left leg pain and lower extremity weakness.

1. What should be included in the differential diagnosis? (Choose all that apply.)
   a. Herniated disk
   b. Schwannoma
   c. Tarlov cyst
   d. Synovial cyst
   e. Scar tissue

2. Which nerve root is likely affected by this lesion?
   a. Right L5 root
   b. Left L5 root
   c. Right S1 root
   d. Left S1 root

3. Which anatomic structure is considered responsible for confining lumbar disk herniation to either right or left of the midline?
   a. Posterior longitudinal ligament
   b. Anterior longitudinal ligament
   c. Midline septum
   d. Tectorial membrane

4. At what level is lumbar disk herniation most commonly found?
   a. L2-3
   b. L3-4
   c. L4-5
   d. L5-S1

Lumbar Disk Herniation (Sequestration)

1. a

2. d

3. c

4. c

Reference

Schellinger D, Manz HJ, Vidic B, et al: Disk fragment migration, *Radiology* 175(3):831-836, 1990.

Cross-Reference

Neuroradiology: The REQUISITES, 3rd ed, pp 524-526.

Comment

Background

A sequestered disk, or free fragment, is a portion of a herniated disk that perforates the annulus fibrosus and is not in continuity with the parent disk. A sequestered disk (sequestration) is a specific form of an extruded disk (extrusion). Migration of the disk fragment in the cephalad or caudad direction has been observed with approximately equal frequency.

Pathophysiology

Sequestered disk fragments are usually confined to either the left or right anterior epidural space (Fig. C). A collagenous midline sagittal septum divides the anterior epidural space into left and right compartments at the level of the vertebral body. The midline sagittal septum, which is adherent to the vertebral body periosteum and the posterior longitudinal ligament, is most prominent in the lumbar spine.

Imaging

Disk fragments are usually isointense to the parent disk on T1-weighted images (Fig. A) and isointense or hyperintense on T2-weighted images (Fig. B), presumably because hydration of the fragment is maintained. The signal characteristics may mimic extradural or extramedullary intradural tumors such as schwannoma, neurofibroma, or meningioma. The peripheral enhancement pattern helps differentiate a free fragment from these tumors; however, careful technique and interpretation are advised, because disk material may enhance on delayed scans. Fat-saturation pulse sequences help distinguish enhancing granulation tissue from epidural fat on postcontrast images.

Management

Conservative management with rest, physical therapy, and anti-inflammatory medications is the first line of treatment. Selective nerve root injections with corticosteroid may achieve long-term improvement. Surgery is indicated in patients with persistent disabling pain lasting more than 6 weeks who have failed conservative therapy or in patients with progressive and significant weakness and cauda equina syndrome.

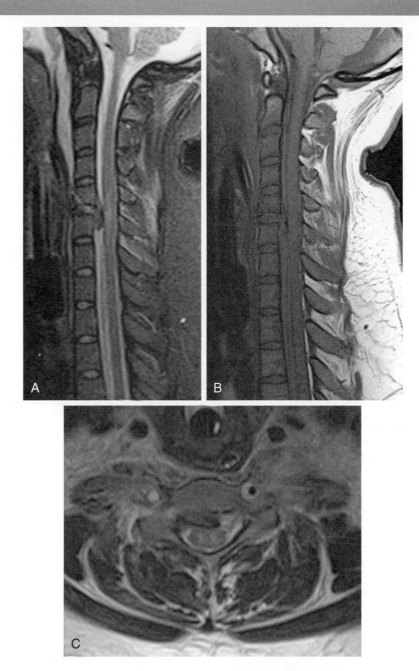

History: A 21-year-old man was involved in a motor vehicle accident.

1. What should be included in the differential diagnosis? (Choose all that apply.)
   a. Epidural hematoma
   b. Cord contusion
   c. Bilateral locked facet
   d. Acute disk herniation
   e. Craniocervical dissociation

2. MRI is likely to be more sensitive than CT scan in the detection of which of the following findings?
   a. Acute fracture
   b. Acute facet subluxation or dislocation
   c. Canal stenosis
   d. Cord contusion

3. What is the most common level of traumatic cervical disk herniation?
   a. C3-4
   b. C4-5
   c. C5-6
   d. C6-7

4. Which of the following statements is true?
   a. Greater than 50% anterior subluxation of the vertebral body above a ruptured disk relative to the vertebral body below the disk favors unilateral facet dislocation.
   b. Rotation of the vertebra above the level of the disk disruption relative to the vertebra below it favors unilateral facet dislocation.
   c. Traumatic cervical disk herniation is more commonly seen in extension injuries.
   d. Myelopathy is the most common presentation in traumatic cervical disk herniation.

Traumatic Cervical Disk Herniation

1. a, b, and d

2. d

3. c

4. b

References

Dai L, Jia L: Central cord injury complicating acute cervical disk herniation in trauma, *Spine (Phila Pa 1976)* 25(3):331-335, 2000.

Flanders AE, Schaefer DM, Doan HT, et al: Acute cervical spine trauma: Correlation of MR imaging findings with degree of neurologic deficit, *Radiology* 177(1):25-33, 1990.

Cross-Reference

Neuroradiology: The REQUISITES, 3rd ed, pp 576-577.

Comment

Background

Cervical disk herniations occur in 20% to 50% of patients with cervical spine trauma. They are more prevalent in men in the fourth decade of life. Disk herniation often complicates acute cervical spine injuries, with or without evidence of fracture or fracture-dislocation.

Pathophysiology

The mechanism of traumatic disk herniation may be acceleration-deceleration injury of the head relative to the trunk or a direct blow to the head or trunk.

Imaging

MRI is the most sensitive imaging modality for the detection of disk herniation and its effect on the spinal cord and nerve roots. MRI can show epidural soft tissue, with signal characteristics similar to those of the disk, extending beyond the posterior cortical margins of the vertebral body (Figs. A-C). MRI allows the detection of intraparenchymal damage (edema, contusion, hemorrhage), which appears as a localized alteration in cord signal intensity. In a retrospective analysis of MRI studies of patients with acute cervical spinal cord injuries, Flanders and colleagues found that subjects with disk herniations were significantly more prone to develop cord edema (65% of cases) than intramedullary hemorrhage (20% of cases).

Management

Recognition of disk herniation is of great importance to the management of cervical spine injury. Recovery of neurologic function in patients with spinal cord compression is more likely with early operation.

Notes

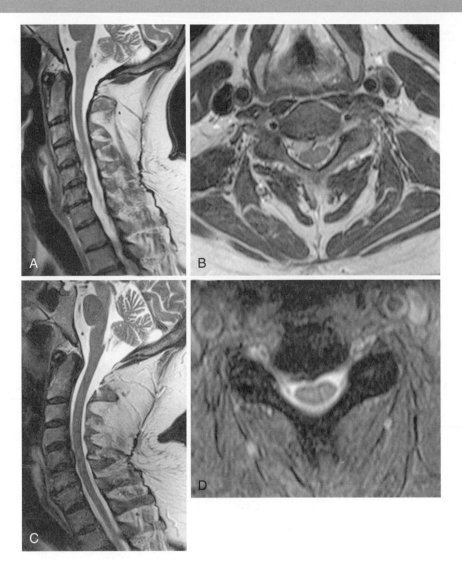

History: A 66-year-old man previously presented with neck pain and radiculopathy; 6-month follow-up MRI was performed.

1. What should be included in the differential diagnosis? (Choose all that apply.)
   a. Spontaneous regression of herniated disk
   b. Surgical treatment of herniated disk
   c. Resolving epidural hematoma
   d. Treated meningioma
   e. Resolving diskitis osteomyelitis

2. Which of the following statements regarding regression of disk herniation is true?
   a. Spontaneous regression is seen less frequently in patients who undergo imaging soon after the onset of symptoms.
   b. Spontaneous regression is more likely in older patients.
   c. Extruded cervical disks are more likely to regress spontaneously compared with protruded disks.
   d. Spontaneous regression of disk herniation is more common with lumbar disk herniation.

3. Which of the following statements regarding regression of disk herniation is true?
   a. Lateral disk herniation is more likely to regress spontaneously.
   b. Central disk herniation is more likely to regress spontaneously.
   c. Foraminal disk herniation is more likely to regress spontaneously.
   d. There is no correlation between the type of disk herniation (lateral, central, foraminal) and the probability of regression.

4. Which of the following statements regarding MRI in patients with spontaneous regression of disk herniation is true?
   a. Herniation with a higher degree of displacement has a slower resorption rate.
   b. Hyperintense T2 signal of the herniated disk is a useful predictive sign of resorption.
   c. Thickness of rim enhancement is a more reliable prognostic indicator of spontaneous resorption than the circumferential extent of rim enhancement.
   d. Rim enhancement around the herniated disk is an unreliable prognostic indicator of spontaneous resorption.

Spontaneous Reduction of Herniated Cervical Disk

1. a and c

2. d

3. d

4. c

References

Komori H, Okawa A, Haro H, et al: Contrast-enhanced magnetic resonance imaging in conservative management of lumbar disc herniation, *Spine (Phila Pa 1976)* 23(1):67-73, 1998.

Pan H, Xiao LW, Hu QF: Spontaneous regression of herniated cervical disc fragments and its clinical significance, *Orthop Surg* 2(1):77-79, 2010.

Vinas FC, Wilner H, Rengachary S: The spontaneous resorption of herniated cervical discs, *J Clin Neurosci* 8(6):542-546, 2001.

Cross-Reference

Neuroradiology: The REQUISITES, 3rd ed, pp 524-526.

Comment

Background

Spontaneous regression of cervical disk herniation without surgical treatment can be regarded as a benign natural course that occurs in some patients with herniated cervical disks.

Pathophysiology

Resorption of the herniated disk is thought to occur secondary to an inflammatory reaction in the outermost layer of the herniation, mainly by macrophages. Many factors related to the resorption process have been recognized, including patient age, size of the disk herniation, penetration of the herniated disk through the posterior longitudinal ligament, and presence of cartilage and annulus fibrosus tissue in the herniated material. Larger disk herniations are more likely to regress than smaller ones because of their tendency to penetrate the annulus fibrosus and posterior longitudinal ligament, exposing the herniated disk material to the systemic circulation in the epidural space.

Imaging

In the present case, fast-spin-echo (FSE) T2-weighted images obtained at presentation showed a superiorly migrated right paracentral disk herniation at C4-5 (Figs. A and B). The patient underwent conservative medical treatment, and follow-up MRI 6 months later demonstrated spontaneous reduction of the disk herniation (Figs. C and D). Herniated disk regression detected on MRI might represent, in part, dehydration of the expanded nucleus pulposus and resorption of hematoma, which can occur after annulus rupture.

MRI is also a useful prognostic tool. Rim enhancement around the herniated disk is thought to be a major determinant of spontaneous resorption. The thickness, rather than the extent, of rim enhancement is a more reliable prognostic indicator of spontaneous resorption. In older patients, the immune response and angiogenesis necessary for disk resorption are weaker, and herniations tend to have less nucleus pulposus and more cartilaginous end-plate material, which can inhibit neovascularization of the herniated disk.

Management

Conservative treatment, including bed rest, heat application, nonsteroidal anti-inflammatory drugs, and muscle relaxants, should be attempted, especially in patients presenting with radiculopathy alone. Patients presenting with myelopathy or those who have failed conservative treatment are candidates for surgical intervention. The most frequent surgical approach is via an anterior diskectomy.

Notes

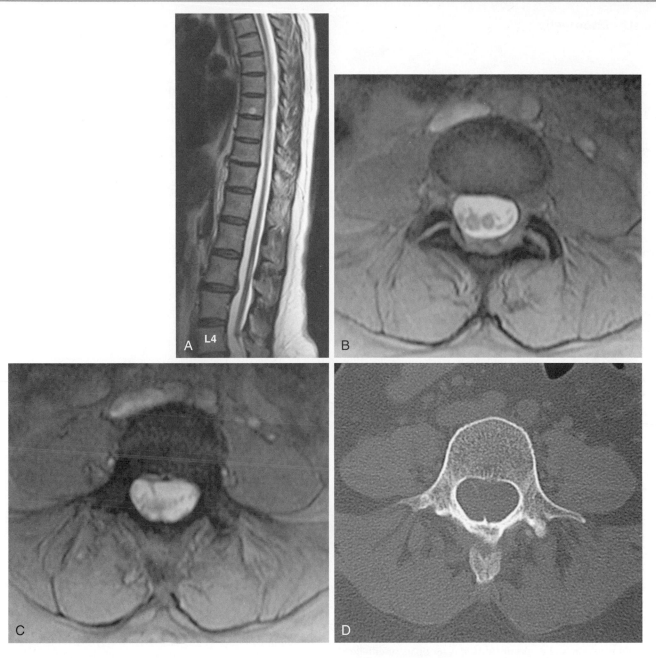

History: A 52-year-old woman presents with intractable low back pain, left leg numbness, and urinary incontinence.

1. What should be included in the differential diagnosis? (Choose all that apply.)
   a. Chronic arachnoiditis
   b. Intradural lipoma
   c. Diplomyelia
   d. Diastematomyelia
   e. Neurofibromatosis

2. Where along the spinal axis is a cleft in the cord most likely to be found?
   a. Upper cervical spine
   b. Upper thoracic spine
   c. Thoracolumbar spine
   d. Lower cervical spine

3. All of the following abnormalities are associated with diastematomyelia *except:*
   a. Spina bifida
   b. Scoliosis
   c. Hemivertebra
   d. Short pedicles

4. Which of the following imaging studies would be least helpful in further evaluating this patient?
   a. Plain radiographs
   b. Bone scan
   c. CT
   d. MRI

Diastematomyelia

1. c and d

2. c

3. d

4. b

References
Lewandrowski KU, Rachlin JR, Glazer PA: Diastematomyelia presenting as progressive weakness in an adult after spinal fusion for adolescent idiopathic scoliosis, *Spine J* 4(1):116-119, 2004.

Pang D, Dias MS, Ahab-Barmada M: Split cord malformation. Part I: A unified theory of embryogenesis for double spinal cord malformations, *Neurosurgery* 31(3):451-480, 1992.

Cross-Reference
Neuroradiology: The REQUISITES, 3rd ed, pp 316-317.

Comment

Background
Diastematomyelia is an uncommon congenital anomaly in which the spinal cord is divided into two hemicords. Females are affected more than males, and the most common location is in the lower thoracic and upper lumbar spine. Most patients present in childhood; presentation in adulthood is highly unusual. Symptoms may range from back pain to progressive neurologic deterioration and signs of spinal cord and cauda equina dysfunction. Patients often have midline cutaneous abnormalities associated with dysraphism, such as dimples and sinus tracts. Vertebral anomalies are present in 85% of cases of diastematomyelia.

Pathophysiology
In diastematomyelia, the spinal cord anatomy may range from a partial ventral or dorsal cleft to nearly complete duplication of the cord. Some authors have proposed that the spectrum of split cord entities be referred to as the *split cord malformation syndrome,* consisting of two types of lesions. Type I lesions have a double dural sac and a double spinal canal, with the two hemicords separated by an extradural bony or partially bony spur. This spur may be strictly anteroposterior in orientation and divide the canal and the cord into two symmetric halves, or it may be slanting in the axial plane and divide the canal asymmetrically (Figs. C and D). Type II lesions have one dural sac, one spinal canal, and two symmetric hemicords, between which there may be an anteroposterior, fibrous intradural septum extending the length of no more than one or two vertebral segments. Type II malformations account for 50% to 60% of all split cord malformations.

Imaging
MRI is the imaging modality of choice for assessing split cord malformations. MRI can demonstrate the conus position and the presence of hydromyelia, and it is very useful in detecting associated spinal abnormalities commonly found in spinal dysraphism (Figs. A-C). CT may demonstrate the bony septum (Fig. D) and is better at showing anomalies of the vertebrae.

Management
Asymptomatic patients do not require treatment. Surgical intervention is warranted in patients who present with a new onset of neurologic signs and symptoms or those with a history of progressive neurologic manifestations. Differentiation between type I and type II split cord malformations has surgical importance: type I lesions are technically more difficult to correct and are associated with greater surgical morbidity than type II lesions, especially if there is an oblique septum dividing the cord asymmetrically.

Notes

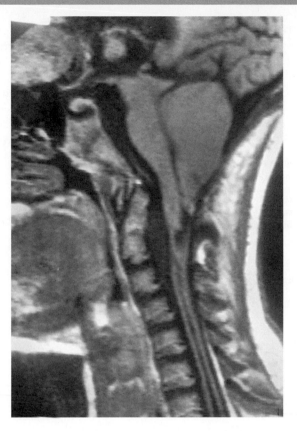

History: A 16-year-old boy presents with nystagmus and spastic quadriparesis.

1. What should be included in the differential diagnosis? (Choose all that apply.)
   a. Chiari I malformation
   b. Chiari II malformation
   c. Intracranial hypotension
   d. Dandy-Walker variant
   e. Joubert syndrome

2. What does the signal change in the cord represent?
   a. Hydromyelia
   b. Syringomyelia
   c. Arachnoid cyst
   d. Myelomalacia

3. What is the peak systolic velocity of the cerebrospinal fluid (CSF) in the foramen magnum in patients with Chiari II malformation compared with that in normal subjects?
   a. Significantly reduced
   b. Significantly elevated
   c. Same as in normal subjects
   d. Mildly reduced

4. Is cervical syrinx more often associated with a Chiari I or a Chiari II malformation?
   a. Chiari I
   b. Chiari II
   c. It is equally frequent in both.
   d. It is infrequent in both.

Chiari II Malformation with Hydromyelia

1. b

2. a

3. b

4. a

References

Haughton VM, Korosec FR, Medow JE, et al: Peak systolic and diastolic CSF velocity in the foramen magnum in adult patients with Chiari I malformations and in normal control participants, *AJNR Am J Neuroradiol* 24(2):169-176, 2003.

Rahman M, Perkins LA, Pincus DW: Aggressive surgical management of patients with Chiari II malformation and brainstem dysfunction, *Pediatr Neurosurg* 45(5):337-344, 2009.

Cross-Reference

Neuroradiology: The REQUISITES, 3rd ed, pp 297-298.

Comment

Background

Chiari II malformation is a congenital malformation of the brain that is nearly always associated with myelomeningocele. It is characterized by caudal displacement of the brainstem and cervicomedullary junction, which results in brainstem compression and hydrocephalus.

Pathophysiology

Chiari II malformation results from a normal-sized cerebellum developing in an abnormally small posterior fossa with a low tentorial attachment. For both Chiari I and II malformations, abnormal CSF flow at the foramen magnum is believed to contribute to the pathogenesis of hydromyelia. Using cardiac-gated, phase-contrast MRI in the axial plane at the foramen magnum, Haughton and colleagues showed that CSF velocities were relatively uniform throughout the subarachnoid space at each cardiac time frame in normal subjects, whereas symptomatic patients with Chiari I malformation had a nonuniform distribution of velocities throughout the subarachnoid space. Peak systolic velocity was significantly higher in patients than in control volunteers. In a subsequent article, these investigators also described several flow abnormalities detected by phase-contrast MRI in pediatric patients with Chiari I malformation; after posterior fossa decompression, the severity of these abnormalities decreased. The same inferences can be made for Chiari II malformation.

Imaging

Chiari II malformation is associated with several infratentorial imaging abnormalities (the key ones are shown in the figure): (1) small posterior fossa; (2) tonsils and medulla herniated through the foramen magnum; (3) fourth ventricle compressed, elongated, and low; (4) beaking of the tectum; (5) enlarged foramen magnum; and (6) low torcular Herophili. In addition to these features, an associated lumbosacral meningocele or a meningomyelocele that tethers the cord is nearly always present.

Syringohydromyelia—or, more specifically, hydromyelia—which represents dilatation of the central canal, may be observed at any cord level but is usually seen in the lower thoracic or lumbar region. In one series of 30 patients (age range, 3 to 32 years) with Chiari II malformation and meningomyelocele, 40% had hydromyelia. In Chiari I malformation, hydromyelia is usually cervical in location. The cystlike, dilated central canal communicates with the fourth ventricle via the obex and has a signal intensity equivalent to CSF.

Management

The treatment of symptomatic brainstem compression is cervical decompression and occipitocervical fusion. Hydrocephalus is treated with ventriculoperitoneal shunt placement.

Notes

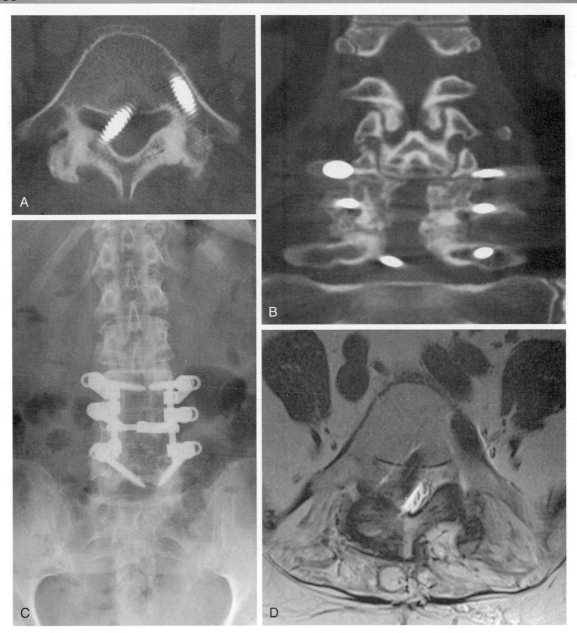

History: A 68-year-old woman presents with loss of motor and sensory function 2 years after undergoing posterior instrumented fusion.

1. What should be included in the differential diagnosis? (Choose all that apply.)
   a. Misplaced pedicle screw
   b. Broken pedicle screw
   c. Loose pedicle screw
   d. Bent pedicle screw
   e. Fracture of pedicle

2. Which of the following is the most common complication of pedicle screw placement?
   a. Screw pullout
   b. Visceral injury
   c. Screw breakage
   d. Screw malpositioning

3. What is the incidence of nerve root or spinal cord injury complicating pedicular screw placement?
   a. Less than 1%
   b. 15%
   c. 25%
   d. 50%

4. Which of the following statements regarding the complications of pedicle screw placement is true?
   a. If a cerebrospinal fluid leak is seen during pedicle screw insertion, it means that the screw is too lateral.
   b. A displacement greater than 2 mm is associated with a high risk of injury to vital structures.
   c. Screw breakage is mainly attributed to metal fatigue.
   d. Pedicle fracture results from loss of metal-bone interface integrity.

Misplaced Pedicle Screws Within the Spinal Canal

1. a

2. d

3. a

4. c

References

Gautschi OP, Schatlo B, Schaller K, et al: Clinically relevant complications related to pedicle screw placement in thoracolumbar surgery and their management: A literature review of 35,630 pedicle screws, *Neurosurg Focus* 31(4):E8, 2011.

Learch TJ, Massie JB, Pathria MN, et al: Assessment of pedicle screw placement utilizing conventional radiography and computed tomography: A proposed systematic approach to improve accuracy of interpretation, *Spine (Phila Pa 1976)* 29(7):767-773, 2004.

Mac-Thiong JM, Parent S, Poitras B, et al: Neurological outcome and management of pedicle screws misplaced totally within the spinal canal, *Spine (Phila Pa 1976)* 38(3):229-237, 2013.

Cross-Reference

Neuroradiology: The REQUISITES, 3rd ed, pp 537-540.

Comment

Background

Pedicle screw placement is a surgical technique commonly performed to achieve fixation and fusion of the thoracic and lumbar spine in patients with degenerative, neoplastic, infectious, and malformative pathologies associated with axial instability. Despite technical advances over the last few decades, pedicle screw insertion is still associated with complications. The most commonly reported complication is screw malpositioning. More serious complications, such as neurologic, visceral, or vascular complications, are very rare, although the prevalence of neurologic complications from misplaced pedicle screws is likely underreported.

Pathophysiology

Neurologic injury after cortical perforation by a pedicle screw is due to the proximity of the pedicle to the neural elements. Neurologic complications may be early or late (up to 2 years).

Imaging

CT scan is the most sensitive modality to demonstrate the location of the screw (Figs. A and B). Ideally, the pedicle screw is completely contained within the pedicle, and the spinal canal is not violated. Pedicle screws that violate the pedicle cortex—specifically, the medial cortex—increase the risk of neurologic injury; however, minor violations of the cortex are common and may be asymptomatic. Detection of screw position on plain films (Fig. C) may be difficult, especially in patients with scoliosis. On MRI, the screw may be seen clearly, as in this case (Fig. D), but in some cases, artifacts may limit MRI evaluation.

Management

The optimal management of misplaced pedicle screws located totally within the spinal canal is unclear, but some authors strongly recommend removal because of the risk of neurologic complications, regardless of the severity of spinal canal intrusion.

Notes

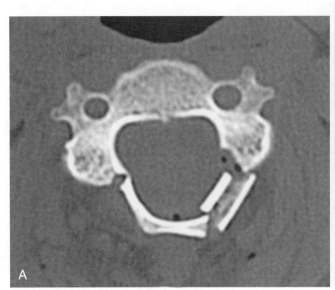

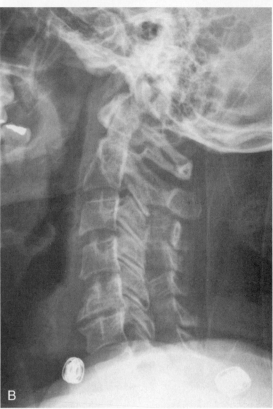

History: A 60-year-old man is treated for cervical myelopathy.

1. What should be included in the differential diagnosis for the imaging findings presented? (Choose all that apply.)
   a. Jefferson fracture
   b. Expansile laminoplasty
   c. Posterior cervical fusion
   d. Klippel-Feil syndrome
   e. Atlantoaxial subluxation

2. Which of the following lines is discontinuous on the lateral radiograph?
   a. Anterior vertebral line
   b. Posterior vertebral line
   c. Spinolaminar line
   d. Posterior spinous line

3. What vertebral structure normally visible in a lateral radiograph is not seen in this patient?
   a. Transverse processes
   b. Anterior arch of C1
   c. End-plates
   d. Spinous processes

4. Which of the following statements regarding open-door laminoplasty is true?
   a. The bone grafts are typically located at every level.
   b. On the "open door" side, there is greater access to the neural foramina.
   c. In most patients, decompression from an open-door cervical laminoplasty is from C2 to C7.
   d. The "hinge" side can be determined on CT scan only.

Open-Door Expansile Cervical Laminoplasty

1. b

2. c

3. d

4. b

References

Lee TT, Manzano GR, Green BA: Modified open-door cervical expansive laminoplasty for spondylotic myelopathy: Operative technique, outcome, and predictors for gait improvement, *J Neurosurg* 86(1):64-68, 1997.

Vitarbo E, Sheth RN, Levi AD: Open-door expansile cervical laminoplasty, *Neurosurgery* 60(1 Suppl 1):S154-S159, 2007.

Cross-Reference

Neuroradiology: The REQUISITES, 3rd ed, pp 531, 533.

Comment

Background

Open-door laminoplasty, which was first described by Hirabayashi in 1977, is a technique used most often to treat multilevel cervical spondylitic myelopathy.

Pathophysiology

In open-door laminoplasty, typically the C3-C7 vertebrae are altered. C2 is left intact because of the attachment of paraspinal muscles necessary for neck stability. There is a step-off in the spinolaminal line between the intact C2 and the altered C3 posterior elements.

Imaging

As shown on the axial CT image at C3 (Fig. A), the left side of the canal is "opened" by resecting most of the ipsilateral lamina; this results in an obvious increase in the cross-sectional area of the canal. Opening of the canal is facilitated by burring through the outer cortex of the bone at the contralateral lamina-facet junction, creating a "hinge." The result is an "open-door" side and a "hinge" side of the altered vertebra. A rib allograft has been used to keep the "door" open. The spinous processes of C3-C6 have been resected, releasing corresponding muscular attachments. The clockwise rotation of the spinolaminar complex, as shown on the CT image, produces the unusual appearance of the postlaminoplasty cervical spine on frontal and lateral radiographs. On the lateral radiograph (Fig. B), the usual smooth junction of the lamina and spinous process for each vertebra is lost, and the lamina of the "hinge" side is seen in profile. The lamina of the "open-door" side is seen on end. The slightly irregular curve produced by the cortices of the lamina seen on end produces a "pseudo-spinolaminar line," which may mislead the radiologist into diagnosing an anterior subluxation of C2 on C3, although there is no offset of the posterior spinal line. The levels of graft placement can often be determined from the lateral radiograph. Careful inspection of the lateral radiograph reveals increased density over the lamina at the levels of graft placement. On the frontal radiograph, the hinged lamina is seen approximately on end and contributes additional density to that side of the canal.

Management

Optimal widening of the anteroposterior diameter of the spinal canal by expansive laminoplasty is considered to be greater than 4 mm.

Notes

Fair Game

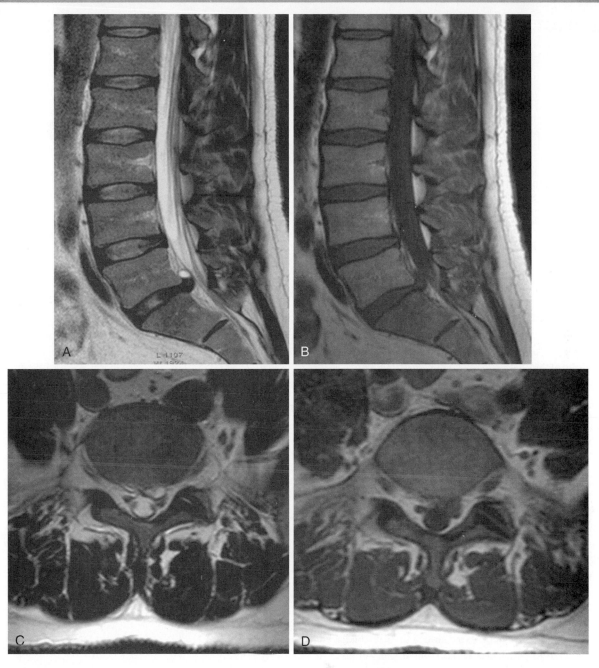

History: A 37-year-old man presents with a 3-month history of low back pain radiating to the left thigh.

1. What should be included in the differential diagnosis? (Choose all that apply.)
   a. Synovial cyst
   b. Diskal cyst
   c. Congenital arachnoid cyst
   d. Tarlov cyst
   e. Ganglion cyst

2. Where is a diskal cyst most commonly found?
   a. L2-3
   b. L3-4
   c. L4-5
   d. L5-S1

3. Which of the following imaging modalities is preferred for imaging diskal cysts?
   a. Plain radiographs
   b. Ultrasound
   c. CT myelography
   d. MRI

4. Which of the following statements regarding diskal cysts is true?
   a. Rim enhancement excludes the diagnosis of a diskal cyst.
   b. There is no communication with a herniated disk on diskography.
   c. Diskal cysts are located in the posterolateral aspect of the spinal canal.
   d. Diskal cysts can cause scalloping of the vertebral body.

Lumbar Diskal Cyst

1. b and e

2. c

3. d

4. d

References

Chiba K, Toyoma Y, Matsumoto M, et al: Intraspinal cyst communicating with the intervertebral disc in the lumbar spine: Discal cyst, *Spine (Phila Pa 1976)* 26(19):2112-2118, 2001.

Kang H, Liu WC, Lee S, et al: Midterm results of percutaneous CT-guided aspiration of symptomatic lumbar discal cysts, *AJR Am J Roentgenol* 190(5):W310-W314, 2008.

Lee HK, Lee DH, Choi CG, et al: Discal cyst of the lumbar spine: MR imaging features, *Clin Imaging* 30(5):326-330, 2006.

Cross-Reference

Neuroradiology: The REQUISITES, 3rd ed, p 531.

Comment

Background

A diskal cyst is a rare companion of a herniated disk that can cause significant lumbar pain and radiculopathy. These cysts are found in a slightly younger age group than typical disk herniation and are most commonly located at L4-5.

Pathogenesis

The cause of lumbar diskal cysts is unknown. Two hypotheses for their pathogenesis have been proposed. One hypothesis suggests that an epidural hematoma forms secondary to disk herniation or disk injury, with impaired hematoma resorption. This theory is supported by the finding of hemorrhagic fluid or hemosiderin in diskal cysts on histopathologic examination. Another theory suggests that spilling of fluid from a herniated disk incites an inflammatory response, leading to reactive pseudomembrane formation and development of a diskal cyst.

Imaging

Characteristic findings on MRI include a well-defined round or oval lesion in the ventrolateral extradural spinal canal adjacent to a herniated disk, which has cerebrospinal fluid–equivalent signal intensity on all pulse sequences (Figs. A-D). Less commonly, diskal cysts can be located in the midline and demonstrate slightly higher T2 signal intensity relative to cerebrospinal fluid. Diskal cysts have been shown to communicate with the intervertebral disk on diskography. Diskal cysts may show rim enhancement and can erode the adjacent vertebral body.

Management

Treatment options for symptomatic patients include conservative treatment with systemic steroids. Other options include epidural transforaminal or translaminar steroid injection, CT-guided percutaneous aspiration of the cyst, and surgical resection.

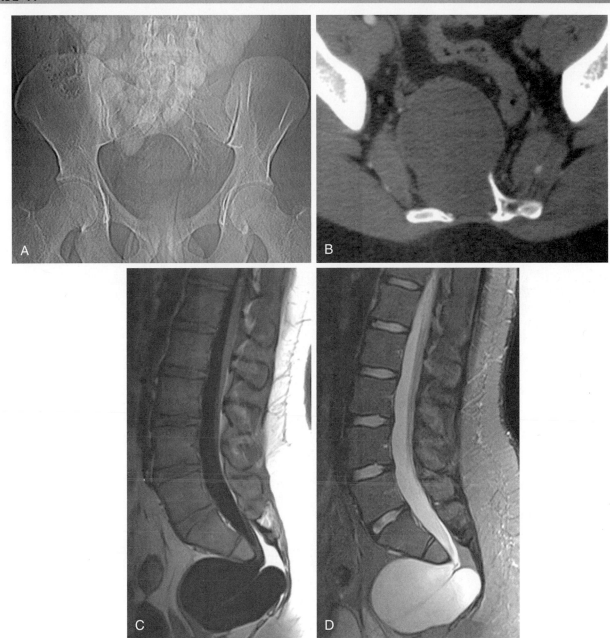

History: A 19-year-old man presents with a 4-month history of back pain and the recent onset of urinary incontinence.

1. What should be included in the differential diagnosis? (Choose all that apply.)
   a. Tarlov cyst
   b. Cystic schwannoma
   c. Chordoma
   d. Anterior sacral meningocele (ASM)
   e. Epidural abscess

2. What sign has been associated with this lesion on plain films?
   a. Honda sign
   b. Scimitar sign
   c. Scottie dog sign
   d. Molar tooth sign

3. Which of the following is the *most dangerous* complication of ASM?
   a. Meningitis
   b. Constipation
   c. Urinary retention
   d. Leg weakness

4. Which of the following has *not* been associated with ASM?
   a. Currarino's triad
   b. Marfan syndrome
   c. Chiari I malformation
   d. Spina bifida

Anterior Sacral Meningocele

1. a, b, and d

2. b

3. a

4. c

References

Kovalcik PJ, Burke JB: Anterior sacral meningocele and the scimitar sign: Report of a case, *Dis Colon Rectum* 31(10):806-807, 1988.

Massimi L, Calisti A, Koutzoglou M, et al: Giant anterior sacral meningocele and posterior sagittal approach, *Childs Nerv Syst* 19(10-11):722-728, 2003.

Cross-Reference

Neuroradiology: The REQUISITES, 3rd ed, pp 313-320.

Comment

Background and Pathophysiology

ASM is a rare congenital malformation. Its real incidence is unknown because it may remain asymptomatic for a long time. When symptomatic, ASMs are usually discovered before the third decade of life. They are usually classified among neurulation defects, based on the neural tube's failure to close. The proposed pathogenetic mechanism is herniation of the arachnoid membrane through a primary dural defect, resulting in pulsatile stresses that erode the bone secondary to cerebrospinal fluid (CSF) pressure oscillations. The sac of an ASM is composed of two layers—an outer dural layer and an inner arachnoid membrane—that contain variable amounts of CSF and occasionally neural roots, benign dysplastic tissue or tumor, or both. The sac may become progressively larger. Partial sacral agenesis is usually found. ASMs usually occur sporadically. Nevertheless, familial cases have been described, which may justify radiologic screening of the relatives of affected subjects.

Clinical Findings

Clinical findings are related mainly to the mass effect exerted by the herniated sac on the pelvic structures. Constipation is the most common symptom of ASM, followed by urinary incontinence and dysmenorrhea. Signs and symptoms of neurologic deficit, such as sensory and motor deficits of the lower limbs and back, are rare. The most frequent and dangerous complication of ASM is spontaneous rupture, which can lead to severe bacterial meningitis.

Imaging

On plain radiographs, the pathognomonic finding in ASM is the scimitar sign, a smooth, sickle-shaped distortion of the sacrum resembling an Arab saber (Fig. A). CT scan (Fig. B) can contribute to the diagnostic workup by showing the dysraphic sacrum. MRI (Figs. C and D) is the technique most frequently used for diagnosis and surgical planning because of its safety, its multiplanar imaging capability, and its effectiveness in discovering associated lesions such as intradural lipoma and tethering of the cord, as seen in this case.

Management

Surgical treatment is mandatory in nearly all cases because ASM does not undergo spontaneous regression and generally increases in size, with a corresponding increase in the risk of complications. The goals of surgery are to obliterate the communication between the ASM and the spinal subarachnoid space, to decompress the pelvis by sac excision, to remove associated tumors, and to untether the spinal cord when necessary.

Notes

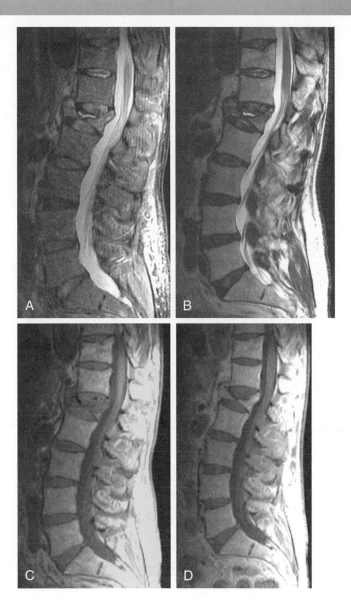

History: A 60-year-old woman presents with the recent onset of severe lower back pain.

1. What should be included in the differential diagnosis? (Choose all that apply.)
   a. Schmorl's node
   b. Pathologic fracture secondary to osseous metastatic disease
   c. Diskitis osteomyelitis
   d. Benign chronic compression fracture

2. Which of the following signs favor benignancy in cases of vertebral collapse?
   a. Posterior cortical bulging
   b. Extraosseous soft tissue mass
   c. Pedicle involvement
   d. Presence of a detectable fracture line

3. Which of the following statements regarding a fluid sign in spine imaging is *false?*
   a. It is a region of cerebrospinal fluid–equivalent signal intensity within a fractured vertebral body.
   b. It is typically located adjacent to a fractured end-plate.

c. Greater than 90% of fractures exhibiting a fluid sign are malignant.
   d. It has a linear appearance, although a triangular or less elongated shape can also be observed.

4. Which of the following statements regarding compression fractures is true?
   a. Currently available diffusion-weighted imaging techniques reliably differentiate benign from malignant compression fractures.
   b. Acute malignant compression fractures enhance after intravenous contrast agent administration, whereas osteoporotic fractures do not.
   c. A patient with a solitary acute compression fracture and no history of malignancy should undergo immediate biopsy.
   d. Statistically, most solitary compression fractures are benign.

Fluid Sign

1. b and d

2. d

3. c

4. d

References

Baur A, Stabler A, Arbogast S, et al: Acute osteoporotic and neoplastic vertebral compression fractures: Fluid sign at MR imaging, *Radiology* 225(3): 730-735, 2002.

Tehranzadeh J, Tao C: Advances in MR imaging of vertebral collapse, *Semin Ultrasound CT MR* 25(6):440-460, 2004.

Cross-Reference

Neuroradiology: The REQUISITES, 3rd ed, p 566.

Comment

Background

Differentiating between malignant (pathologic) and benign vertebral collapse is often problematic. Difficulties in determining the etiology of vertebral collapse arise when there is no history of significant trauma, especially in elderly patients, who are predisposed to benign compression fractures caused by osteoporosis. Even in patients with a known primary malignancy, one third of cases of vertebral collapse are benign. Vertebral collapse is often secondary to osteoporosis, which is more common in postmenopausal women.

Pathophysiology

Baur and colleagues observed a fluid sign in 26% of all fractures that occurred without significant trauma and in 40% of all osteoporotic fractures. Of fractures exhibiting a fluid sign, 94% were benign. These investigators suggested that in acute osteoporotic collapse with bone marrow edema, fluid is pressed into the space of osteonecrosis and causes a fluid sign (Figs. A and B).

Imaging

In osteoporotic collapse, edema and fluid replace the fatty marrow within the vertebral body, appearing hypointense on T1-weighted images and isointense to hyperintense on T2-weighted images; enhancement is seen on images after contrast agent administration (Figs. B-D). The acute signal abnormalities may be diffuse, heterogeneous, or bandlike. Most benign collapses have some amount of normal fatty marrow in the vertebral body on T1-weighted images. The bandlike hypointensity seen adjacent to the preserved marrow on T1-weighted images is considered specific for osteoporotic collapse. In a few cases, there may be complete vertebral body involvement, with no fatty marrow remaining. These cases can be easily confused with malignant collapse. In approximately 19% of cases of benign collapse, there are focal areas of signal abnormality on T1-weighted images in other adjacent vertebrae; most are benign, such as bone impaction or Schmorl's nodes (see Fig. C).

Management

If the findings favor a benign fracture, a follow-up study should be obtained in 2 to 3 months. On the follow-up scan, a benign fracture should show some restoration of normal fatty marrow and less contrast enhancement. If there is a strong suspicion of malignancy, the patient should be evaluated for sources of a primary tumor, and a bone scan can be done to search for additional metastatic foci. Even in patients with vertebral collapse and a known primary tumor, biopsy may be needed for a definitive diagnosis.

Notes

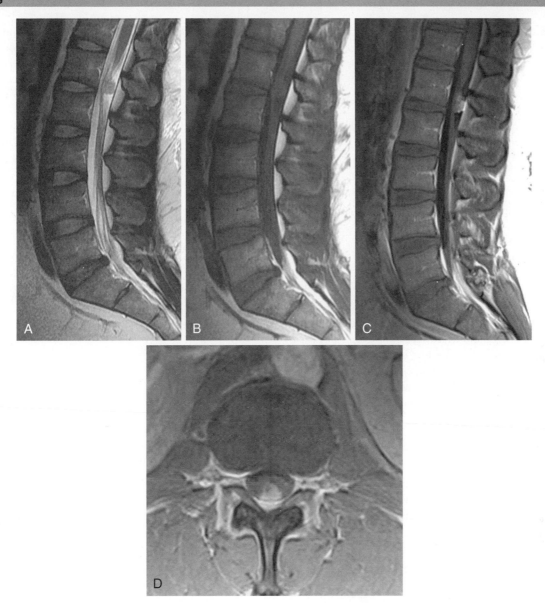

History: A 31-year-old man presents with a 2-year history of intermittent numbness and burning in the left anterior thigh.

1. What should be included in the differential diagnosis? (Choose all that apply.)
   a. Myxopapillary ependymoma
   b. Paraganglioma
   c. Arachnoid cyst
   d. Hemangioblastoma
   e. Schwannoma

2. What is the most common primary tumor involving the filum terminale?
   a. Hemangioblastoma
   b. Dermoid
   c. Ependymoma
   d. Astrocytoma

3. Which of the following statements regarding myxopapillary ependymoma subtype is true?
   a. Overall it accounts for approximately 70% of ependymomas.
   b. It arises almost exclusively from the filum terminale.
   c. It rarely manifests with subarachnoid hemorrhage.
   d. Calcifications are less common in this subtype than in other subtypes.

4. Which of the following best describes the imaging characteristics of myxopapillary ependymoma?
   a. Epidural mass showing hyperintense signal on T1-weighted images and hypointense signal on T2-weighted images and no enhancement
   b. Well-circumscribed mass showing hypointense signal on T1-weighted and T2-weighted images and no enhancement
   c. Well-circumscribed enhancing mass showing isointense to hyperintense T1 signal, hyperintense T2 signal, and enhancement
   d. Well-circumscribed mass with cerebrospinal fluid–equivalent signal on all pulse sequences

Myxopapillary Ependymoma

1. a, b, d, and e

2. c

3. b

4. c

References

Bagley CA, Kothbauer KF, Wilson S, et al: Resection of myxopapillary ependymomas in children, *J Neurosurg* 106(4 Suppl):261-267, 2007.

Wippold FJ II, Smirniotopoulos JG, Moran CJ, et al: MR imaging of myxopapillary ependymoma: Findings and value to determine extent of tumor and its relation to intraspinal structures, *AJR Am J Roentgenol* 165(5):1263-1267, 1995.

Cross-Reference

Neuroradiology: The REQUISITES, 3rd ed, pp 557-558.

Comment

Background and Clinical Findings

Myxopapillary ependymomas of the filum terminale tend to occur in young adults in the fourth decade of life. The most common clinical manifestation is low back pain, which may be accompanied by sciatic pain or other symptoms and signs of lumbosacral radiculopathy. There may be associated lower limb sensory disturbance or urinary sphincter disturbance.

Pathophysiology

Myxopapillary ependymomas are benign, slow-growing gliomas and are classified histologically as World Health Organization grade I. Myxopapillary ependymomas account for most ependymomas that arise in the lumbosacral area; involvement is usually limited to the conus medullaris and filum terminale. Uncommonly, these lesions may invade the nerve roots or sacrum. They are presumed to arise from ependymal cell rests normally present in the filum terminale.

Imaging

MRI is the preferred imaging modality (Figs. A-D). Myxopapillary ependymomas are characteristically well-circumscribed, sausage-shaped tumors causing compression and displacement of the adjacent roots of the cauda equina (see Fig. D). These highly vascular tumors demonstrate mucinous changes that are not present in other histologic subtypes of ependymoma. The mucinous changes are presumed to be responsible for the increased frequency with which hyperintensity relative to cord signal is detected on precontrast T1-weighted images compared with other subtypes. The hypervascularity of these tumors explains the features of intratumoral or subarachnoid hemorrhage (which can result in superficial siderosis) and the marked postcontrast enhancement sometimes observed on MRI. Generally, these tumors are hyperintense on T2-weighted images and isointense to hyperintense on T1-weighted images.

Management

Recognition of these tumors as a distinct entity is of considerable clinical importance because they are more amenable to radical surgical resection than most other variants of ependymoma. The goal of surgical resection, which is the primary mode of therapy, is to achieve complete resection while minimizing postoperative neurologic deficits. The extent of surgical resection is related mainly to tumor encapsulation and involvement of the conus medullaris and cauda equina.

Notes

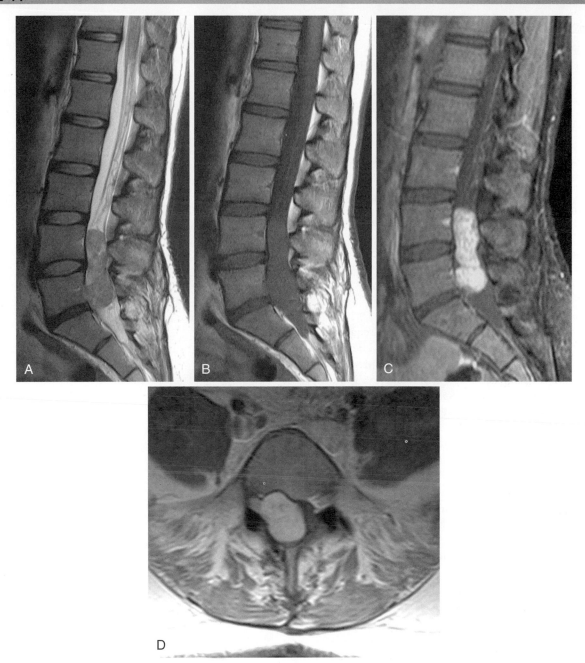

A

B

C

D

History: A 30-year-old woman presents with back pain and cauda equina syndrome.

1. What should be included in the differential diagnosis? (Choose all that apply.)
   a. Myxopapillary ependymoma
   b. Paraganglioma
   c. Arachnoid cyst
   d. Hemangioblastoma
   e. Schwannoma

2. What is the most common location of spinal schwannomas?
   a. Extradural or dumbbell
   b. Intradural extramedullary
   c. Intramedullary
   d. Intradural with an extradural component

3. Which of the following statements regarding spinal schwannomas is true?
   a. Necrosis and cyst formation are much more frequent in spinal schwannomas than in intracranial and peripheral nerve schwannomas.
   b. Schwannomas frequently originate from the motor root, assuming an anterior location within the spinal canal.
   c. Tumor heterogeneity indicates malignant change.
   d. The histologic features of spinal schwannomas correlate with their MRI appearance.

4. Hypointense regions on T2-weighted images may result from all of the following *except:*
   a. Hemorrhage
   b. Dense cellularity
   c. Collagen deposition
   d. Cyst formation

Lumbar Schwannoma

1. a, b, d, and e

2. b

3. a

4. d

References

Conti P, Pansini G, Mouchaty H, et al: Spinal neurinomas: Retrospective analysis and long-term outcome of 179 consecutively operated cases and review of the literature, *Surg Neurol* 61(1):34-43, 2004.

Friedman DP, Tartaglino LM, Flanders AE: Intradural schwannomas of the spine: MR findings with emphasis on contrast-enhancement characteristics, *AJR Am J Roentgenol* 158(6):1347-1350, 1992.

Cross-Reference

Neuroradiology: The REQUISITES, 3rd ed, pp 561-563.

Comment

Background

Schwannomas and neurofibromas are the most frequent primary tumors of the spine. There is no significant difference in prevalence between males and females. The age at presentation is around the fourth decade. The site of the lesion is mostly intradural extramedullary. These lesions have a higher incidence in the lumbosacral spine, with a spike between L1 and L3.

Histopathology and Clinical Presentation

Schwannomas are encapsulated tumors composed of spindle-shaped neoplastic Schwann cells. Histologically, the tumor comprises densely cellular areas, known as Antoni A areas, composed of sheets of uniform spindle cells, some of which form palisades called Verocay bodies. A second histologic pattern, Antoni B, is composed of less cellular and more randomly arranged spindle cells in a loose myxomatous stroma. Tumor growth is usually very slow, and the mean duration of symptoms is 2 to 3 years. The first symptom is pain; other deficits manifest later.

Imaging

MRI allows an early diagnosis. Spinal schwannomas are typically capsulated, sometimes cystic, regularly shaped, smooth, and occasionally bumpy in appearance (Figs. A and B). They frequently originate from the sensory root, assuming a posterior or posterolateral location. Intradural schwannomas tend to have a signal intensity equal to or less than that of the spinal cord on T1-weighted images (see Fig. B); they have mild to marked hyperintensity on T2-weighted images (see Fig. A) and show intense and fairly homogeneous enhancement (Fig. C). Large schwannomas may exhibit vertebral body scalloping (Fig. D). The hyperintense, nonenhancing regions within the tumor often correspond pathologically to areas of cyst formation and necrosis; however, these regions may also represent areas of diminished vascularity or increased tumor compactness. No correlation has been established between signal characteristics or enhancement patterns and the prevalence of Antoni type A or type B tissue within intradural schwannomas. Caution should be exercised when attempting to distinguish filum ependymomas from cauda equine schwannomas on the basis of MRI findings because they may have a similar appearance.

Management

Total surgical removal of the tumor is often an attainable goal and helps avoid eventual recurrence.

Notes

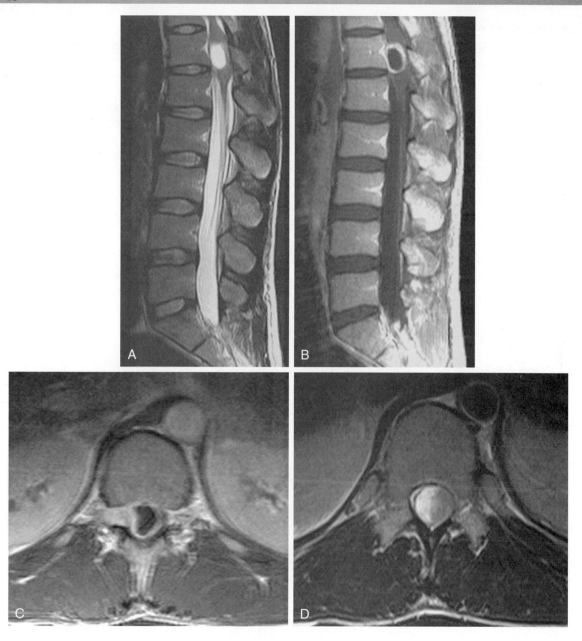

History: A 33-year old man with a 6-month history of back pain, progressive weakness of the lower extremities, constipation, and bladder dysfunction presents to the emergency department with a recent worsening of symptoms.

1. What should be included in the differential diagnosis? (Choose all that apply.)
   a. Myxopapillary ependymoma
   b. Cystic meningioma
   c. Cystic schwannoma
   d. Teratoma
   e. Congenital arachnoid cyst

2. Where is the lesion located?
   a. Intradural extramedullary
   b. Extradural
   c. Intramedullary
   d. Epidural

3. Which of the following cystic lesions should *not* be included in the differential diagnosis of the lesion shown?
   a. Enterogenous (neurenteric) cyst
   b. Epidermoid
   c. Tarlov cyst
   d. Arachnoid cyst

4. Intraspinal schwannomas are more frequently observed in patients with which of the following conditions?
   a. Neurofibromatosis type 1
   b. Neurofibromatosis type 2
   c. von Hippel-Lindau disease
   d. Chiari I malformation

Cystic Schwannoma of the Conus Medullaris Region

1. a, b, c, and d

2. a

3. c

4. b

References

Borges G, Bonilha L, Proa M Jr, et al: Imaging features and treatment of an intradural lumbar cystic schwannoma, *Arq Neuropsiquiatr* 63(3A):681-684, 2005.

Jaiswal A, Shetty AP, Rajasekaran S: Giant cystic intradural schwannoma in the lumbosacral region: A case report, *J Orthop Surg (Hong Kong)* 16(1):102-106, 2008.

Cross-Reference

Neuroradiology: The REQUISITES, 3rd ed, pp 561-563.

Comment

Background

Intraspinal schwannomas are most frequently seen in the lumbar region, with a predilection for the thoracolumbar junction. Spinal schwannomas may be well circumscribed, intradural or extradural, or combined intradural-extradural. The percentage of purely intradural nerve sheath tumors increases from 8% in the upper cervical region to 80% in the thoracolumbar region. This increase may be explained by the anatomic features of the spinal nerve roots, which have a longer intradural component in the caudal portion of the spinal axis.

Clinical Presentation

Back pain is the most common symptom of lumbar schwannomas. In schwannomas of the conus region, features of cauda equina and conus compression, including progressive pain, neurologic deficits, and bladder dysfunction, may be observed. These features help differentiate tumor from mechanical causes of back pain. A delayed presentation is common because these tumors are slow growing, and the affected patients are young and otherwise healthy.

Imaging

MRI is the preferred imaging modality (Figs. A-D). Peripheral contrast enhancement is a feature of intradural schwannomas that may help differentiate these lesions from neurofibromas, which tend to have more homogeneous, solid enhancement (see Figs. B and C). This pattern of peripheral enhancement has been observed when patients are scanned immediately after contrast agent injection. Delayed scans may or may not reveal this pattern. The hyperintense, nonenhancing regions within the tumor on T2-weighted images (see Figs. A and D) often correspond pathologically to areas of cyst formation and necrosis; however, these regions may also represent areas of diminished vascularity or increased tumor compactness. No correlation has been established between signal characteristics or enhancement patterns and the prevalence of Antoni type A or type B tissue within intradural schwannomas.

Management

Cystic schwannomas behave in a similar fashion to solid schwannomas and should be treated with surgical excision. This can be difficult, however, because of the tumor capsule's adhesion to surrounding structures, a fragile tumor capsule, and problems identifying the arachnoidal planes. Complete excision without resultant neurologic deficits is feasible, provided there is no entrapment of nerve roots. Prognosis is usually excellent, with the exception of the melanotic variant, malignant forms, and cases of neurofibromatosis.

Notes

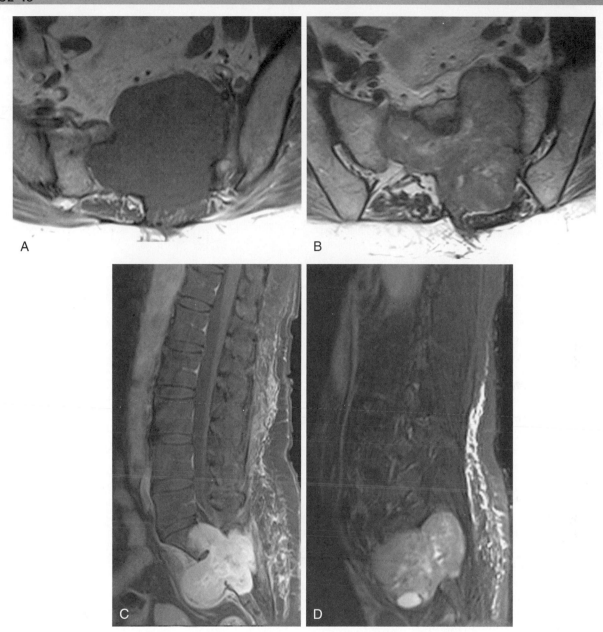

History: A 58-year-old woman presents with a 1-year history of back pain, left lower extremity pain, and numbness in the left foot.

1. What should be included in the differential diagnosis? (Choose all that apply.)
   a. Chordoma
   b. Nerve sheath tumor
   c. Osteoblastoma
   d. Dural ectasia
   e. Metastatic disease

2. What percentage of spinal schwannomas occurs in the sacrum?
   a. Less than 5%
   b. 25%
   c. 50%
   d. Greater than 90%

3. The compression of which of the following structures can account for the patient's symptoms?
   a. Sacral bone
   b. Sacroiliac joint
   c. Iliac vessels
   d. Sacral plexus

4. Which of the following imaging features suggests malignant transformation?
   a. Well-defined, smooth margins
   b. Foraminal scalloping
   c. Invasion of adjacent muscle
   d. Mixed cystic and solid components

Sacral Schwannoma

1. a, b, and e

2. a

3. d

4. c

References

Dominguez J, Lobato RD, Ramos A, et al: Giant intrasacral schwannomas: Report of six cases, *Acta Neurochir (Wien)* 139(10):954-959, 1997.

Takeyama M, Koshino T, Nakazawa A, et al: Giant intrasacral cellular schwannoma treated with high sacral amputation, *Spine (Phila Pa 1976)* 26(10):E216-E219, 2001.

Cross-Reference

Neuroradiology: The REQUISITES, 3rd ed, pp 561-563.

Comments

Background

Spinal schwannomas are uncommon, and less than 1% to 5% occur in the sacrum. They typically do not compromise motor function but may cause paresthesias or pain owing to pressure.

Histopathology and Pathophysiology

Schwannomas are encapsulated tumors composed of spindle-shaped neoplastic Schwann cells. Histologically, the tumor comprises densely cellular areas, known as Antoni A areas, composed of sheets of uniform spindle cells, some of which form palisades called Verocay bodies. A second histologic pattern, Antoni B, consists of less cellular and more randomly arranged spindle cells in a loose myxomatous stroma. Sacral schwannomas are often designated "giant" because of their enormous size; they may destroy the sacrum and expand into the pelvis and spinal canal (Figs. A-C) as well as the dorsal muscles and fat (Fig. A).

Imaging and Differential Diagnosis

MRI is helpful in detecting the specific characteristics of the tumor. It provides information about the tumor's size, exact location, and invasion of and relationship to other organs (Figs. A-D). Typically, a schwannoma is well encapsulated and solid when it is small, but it may manifest cystic (Fig. D) and necrotic changes when it is large. The overall imaging features in this case are not those of a malignant lesion, and the signal characteristics of the myxoid matrix found in chordoma and chondrosarcoma are lacking. Benign bone lesions such as giant cell tumor, aneurysmal bone cyst, and osteoblastoma occur infrequently in the sacrum, and the latter two typically involve posterior elements. Rarely, sacrococcygeal teratoma and myxopapillary ependymoma occur in the presacral area.

Management

The goal of treatment is the same as for schwannomas located elsewhere: complete resection. This is often difficult because of their size, robust blood supply, and proximity to neurologic and abdominal structures. The surgical approach may be anterior, posterior, or combined, depending on the degree of intrasacral and retroperitoneal extension.

Notes

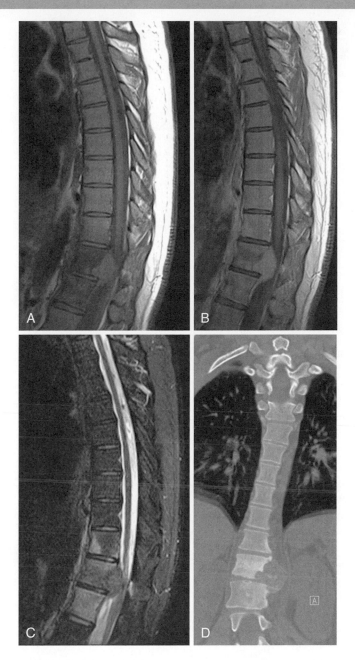

History: A 26-year-old man presents with a 7-month history of left-sided lower back pain.

1. What should be included in the differential diagnosis? (Choose all that apply.)
   a. Giant cell tumor
   b. Lymphoma
   c. Osteoid osteoma
   d. Osteoblastoma
   e. Osteosarcoma

2. What is the distribution of occurrence along the spinal axis?
   a. Cervical spine
   b. Thoracic spine
   c. Lumbosacral spine
   d. Equal throughout the spine

3. Which of the following statements regarding osteoblastoma and osteoid osteoma is true?
   a. Reactive bone changes are more common in osteoblastoma than in osteoid osteoma.
   b. Spinal lesions causing painful scoliosis are more common with osteoblastomas than with osteoid osteomas.
   c. The nidus of an osteoblastoma is smaller than the nidus of an osteoid osteoma.
   d. In contrast to the pain associated with osteoid osteoma, the pain of an osteoblastoma is usually less intense, is usually not worse at night, and is not relieved readily with salicylates.

4. Which finding is used to differentiate osteoid osteoma from osteoblastoma?
   a. Size of the lesion
   b. Age of the patient
   c. Involvement of the posterior elements
   d. Presence of edema

Thoracic Osteoblastoma

1. a, b, d, and e

2. c

3. d

4. a

References

Kan P, Schmidt MH: Osteoid osteoma and osteoblastoma of the spine, *Neurosurg Clin N Am* 19(1):65-70, 2008.

Murphey MD, Andrews CL, Flemming DJ, et al: From the archives of the AFIP. Primary tumors of the spine: Radiologic pathologic correlation, *Radiographics* 16(5):1131-1158, 1996.

Sherazi Z, Saifuddin A, Shaikh MI, et al: Unusual imaging findings in association with spinal osteoblastoma, *Clin Radiol* 51(9):644-648, 1996.

Cross-Reference

Neuroradiology: The REQUISITES, 3rd ed, pp 568-569.

Comment

Background

Osteoblastoma is a rare primary neoplasm of bone. It is categorized as a benign bone tumor, but an aggressive type of osteoblastoma has been described that has characteristics similar to osteosarcoma. Approximately 25% to 50% of osteoblastomas are found in the spine. The most common location for spinal osteoblastoma (and the smaller osteoid osteoma) is the transverse process or posterior elements. Osteoblastoma most commonly occurs during the first 3 decades of life.

Histopathology and Clinical Presentation

Osteoblastoma is defined by numerous osteoblasts that produce osteoid and woven bone and often cause bony expansion. Aggressive osteoblastomas may have features similar to those of malignancy, such as cortical destruction and extraosseous soft tissue extension. The primary symptom is pain. Patients may also present with neurologic symptoms as a result of spinal cord or nerve root compression. Associated aneurysmal bone cysts may be seen in 10% of osteoblastomas.

Imaging and Differential Diagnosis

Osteoblastomas may have a lucent or ossified center. They are usually differentiated from osteoid osteomas by size, with osteoblastomas generally being greater than 1.5 to 2 cm. The overall appearance is a densely calcified mass or an expansile soft tissue mass with margins that are often, but not always, well defined (Figs. A-D). CT scan may demonstrate a predominantly osteolytic and expansile lesion, with or without central mineralization (see Fig. D). Diffuse sclerosis of the vertebral body may result (see Fig. D), producing a radiographic "ivory vertebra." Reactive sclerosis at multiple levels has also been reported. On MRI (see Figs. A-C), a typical osteoblastoma has decreased signal intensity on T1-weighted images (see Fig. A); the signal intensity on T2-weighted images is variable. MRI aids in the detection of nonspecific reactive marrow and soft tissue edema (see Fig. C) and is best at defining soft tissue extension, although this finding is not typical of osteoblastoma.

Management

Treatment is complete excision of the lesion.

Notes

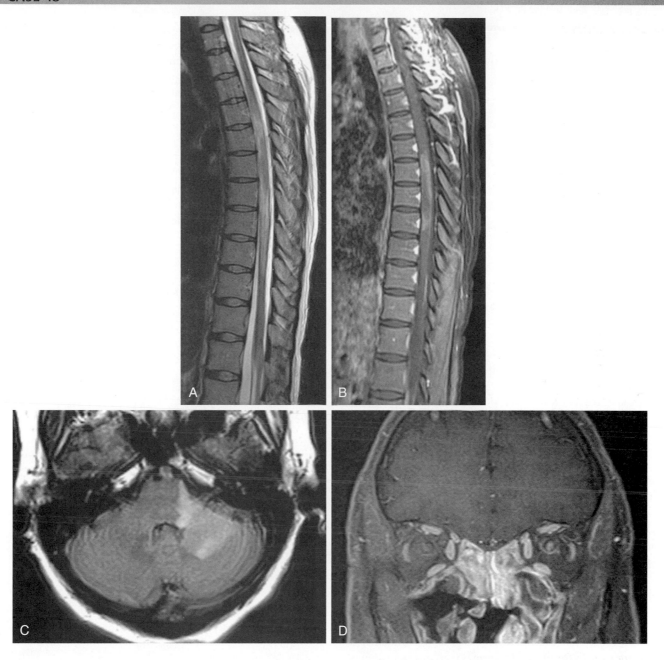

History: A 52-year-old woman presents with shooting pain and numbness in the legs followed by loss of vision in her left eye.

1. What should be included in the differential diagnosis? (Choose all that apply.)
   a. Neuromyelitis optica (NMO)
   b. Systemic lupus erythematosus
   c. Sarcoid
   d. Acute disseminated encephalomyelitis
   e. Multiple sclerosis

2. Which of the following statements regarding NMO is true?
   a. The symptoms in NMO are less profound than in multiple sclerosis.
   b. Most patients are NMO-IgG seropositive.
   c. NMO is monophasic in most cases.
   d. Brain lesions on MRI exclude the diagnosis of NMO.

3. All of the following findings favor NMO over typical multiple sclerosis *except:*
   a. Spinal cord lesion at a single level
   b. Severe cord atrophy
   c. Cord necrosis
   d. Hypointense spinal cord lesions on T1-weighted images

4. All of the following are characteristic brain lesions found in NMO *except:*
   a. Lesions in the dorsal medulla
   b. Hypothalamic lesions
   c. Lesions involving the posterior limb of the internal capsule
   d. Ovoid periventricular or corpus callosum signal abnormality extending in a Dawson finger configuration

Neuromyelitis Optica (Devic's Disease)

1. a, b, c, and e

2. b

3. a

4. d

References

Cabrera-Gomez JA, Kister I: Conventional brain MRI in neuromyelitis optica, *Eur J Neurol* 19(6):812-819, 2012.

Kim W, Kim SH, Kim HJ: New insights into neuromyelitis optica, *J Clin Neurol* 7(3):115-127, 2011.

Cross-Reference

Neuroradiology: The REQUISITES, 3rd ed, p 347.

Comment

Background

NMO is an idiopathic inflammatory disorder of the central nervous system that preferentially affects the optic nerves and spinal cord. A monophasic course of acute transverse myelitis with simultaneous optic neuritis is classic; however, more than 90% of patients experience a relapsing course. Optic neuritis can be separated from transverse myelitis by months or years and tends to relapse, resulting in significant disability.

Pathophysiology and Diagnostic Criteria

Recent clinical, pathologic, immunologic, and imaging studies have suggested that NMO is distinct from multiple sclerosis. A disease-specific autoantibody, NMO-IgG, has been identified in the serum of patients with NMO and incorporated into new diagnostic criteria. The autoantibody targets aquaporin-4 (AQP4), the most abundant water channel in the central nervous system, localized on astrocytic end-feet. The NMO-IgG autoantibody, found in most patients with NMO, binds to AQP4 and, in conjunction with complement, causes the lysis of astrocytes. NMO is occasionally associated with other autoimmune diseases, such as Sjögren's syndrome, systemic lupus erythematosus, rheumatoid arthritis, and mixed connective tissue disorders.

An international task force recently recommended new diagnostic criteria for NMO. Three major criteria are required for a diagnosis of NMO but may be separated by an unspecified time interval: optic neuritis, transverse myelitis with a spinal cord lesion extending over three spinal segments, and no other disease present. In addition, at least one minor criterion must be present: positive NMO-IgG in the serum or cerebrospinal fluid; normal brain MRI or nonspecific brain T2 signal (this does not satisfy the Barkhof criteria as outlined in the McDonald criteria); lesions in the dorsal medulla, hypothalamus, or brainstem; or linear periventricular white matter signal abnormalities.

Imaging

MRI typically shows a lesion that extends longitudinally over three or more vertebral segments; it has a sensitivity of 98% and a specificity of 83% (Figs. A-D). MRI of the orbit often reveals gadolinium enhancement of the optic nerve during an acute attack of optic neuritis. Patients with NMO are frequently found to have symptomatic or asymptomatic brain lesions. These lesions characteristically occur in the hypothalamus and periventricular areas, which correspond to brain regions with high levels of AQP4 expression.

Management

The optimal treatment for NMO has not been established. High-dose corticosteroids have been used to treat acute attacks. Therapeutic plasmapheresis should be considered in patients who fail to improve with high-dose corticosteroid therapy. Other treatment options include immunosuppressants.

Notes

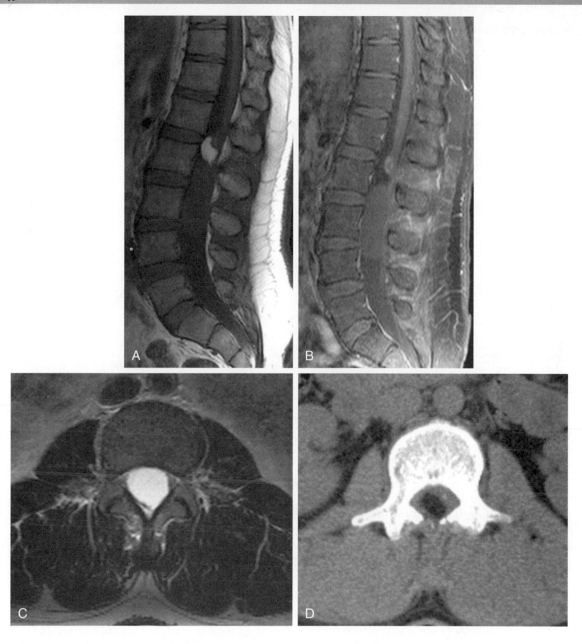

History: A 38-year-old man presents with a long-standing history of progressive urinary and bowel incontinence, erectile dysfunction, and neurogenic bladder.

1. What should be included in the differential diagnosis? (Choose all that apply.)
   a. Teratoma
   b. Lymphoma
   c. Intradural lipoma
   d. Nerve sheath tumor
   e. Dermoid

2. Which of the following findings on MRI or CT would not favor teratoma over lipoma?
   a. Cystic or gelatinous components
   b. Presence of coarse calcifications
   c. Presence of cord tethering
   d. Presence of teeth

3. Which of following is *not* associated with intradural spinal teratomas?
   a. Spina bifida
   b. Tethered cord
   c. Diastematomyelia
   d. Chiari I malformation

4. What is the "gold standard" diagnostic imaging technique in the diagnosis of spinal teratomas?
   a. Plain radiographs
   b. CT scan
   c. MRI
   d. Octreotide scan

Lumbar Intradural Mature Cystic Teratoma

1. a and e

2. c

3. d

4. c

References

Stevens QE, Kattner KA, Chen YH, et al: Intradural extramedullary mature cystic teratoma: Not only a childhood disease, *J Spinal Disord Tech* 19(3): 213-216, 2006.

Sung KS, Sung SK, Choi HJ, et al: Spinal intradural extramedullary mature cystic teratoma in an adult, *J Korean Neurosurg Soc* 44(5):334-337, 2008.

Cross-Reference

Neuroradiology: The REQUISITES, 3rd ed, pp 564-565.

Comment

Embryology

With the exception of sacrococcygeal teratomas, which occur relatively frequently, teratomas within the spinal canal are far less common than their cranial counterparts and constitute less than 1% of primary spinal tumors. Although the pathogenesis of spinal teratomas is still unclear, the most widely accepted embryogenetic theory is that primordial germ cells are displaced into the dorsal midline during their normal migration from primitive yolk sac to gonadal ridges.

Histopathology

Histologically, a mature teratoma is composed of derivatives of the three primitive germ cell layers (ectoderm, mesoderm, and endoderm) and may have fully differentiated tissue elements, such as epidermal, dermal, adipose, vascular, cartilaginous, neural, and muscular. Immature teratomas include more primitive elements derived from these germ cell layers. By comparison, dermoids are unilocular or multilocular cystic masses lined by simple or stratified squamous epithelium with an underlying layer similar to dermis; this layer may contain hair follicles, sweat glands, and sebaceous glands.

Imaging

Spinal teratomas may be extradural, intradural, or intramedullary and may be associated with spinal dysraphisms such as spina bifida and diastematomyelia, particularly in the first decade. The MRI images in this case (Figs. A-C) show an elongated mass of mixed consistency between L1 and L4, with a solid component emanating from the conus tip (this contained neural elements on pathology), an adjacent area isointense to fat at L1-2, and a more inferior large cystic component extending to the L4 level. The CT scan (Fig. D) shows that the area at L1-2 has lipid density.

Management

Optimal management relies on a correct diagnosis at an early stage and total surgical resection whenever possible. In spinal teratomas, total resection is often impossible owing to their extensive adherence to the surrounding roots of the cauda equina and adjacent spinal cord. Additional surgery is sometimes needed for tumor recurrence or progression. Adjuvant chemotherapy or radiotherapy may be required in malignant immature forms.

Notes

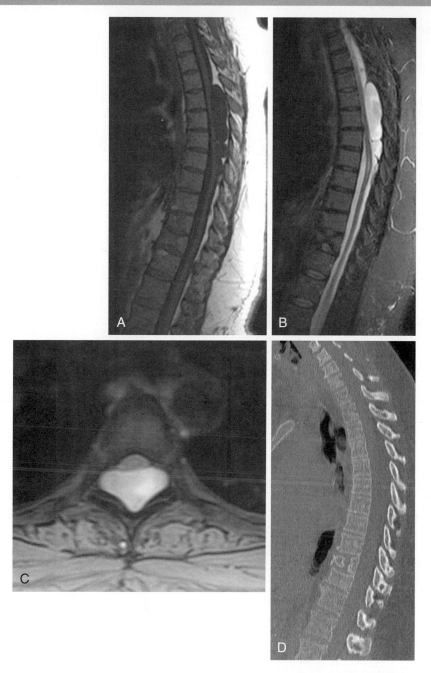

History: A 45-year-old man presents with back pain and progressive paraparesis.

1. What should be included in the differential diagnosis? (Choose all that apply.)
   a. Cystic schwannoma
   b. Congenital arachnoid cyst
   c. Infectious cyst
   d. Posttraumatic pseudomeningocele
   e. Primary epidural lymphoma

2. What is the location of the lesion?
   a. Intramedullary
   b. Intradural extramedullary
   c. Extradural
   d. Paraspinal

3. All of the following radiologic findings may be associated with this lesion *except:*
   a. Foraminal expansion
   b. Canal expansion
   c. Erosion of the adjacent vertebral body
   d. Short pedicles

4. What additional study may help narrow the differential diagnosis?
   a. Ultrasound
   b. CT scan without contrast
   c. CT myelography
   d. Plain radiographs

Congenital Arachnoid Cyst

1. b, c, and d

2. c

3. d

4. c

References

Nabors MW, Pait TG, Byrd EB, et al: Updated assessment and current classification of spinal meningeal cysts, *J Neurosurg* 68(3):366-377, 1988.

Netra R, Min L, Shao Hui M, et al: Spinal extradural meningeal cysts: An MRI evaluation of a case series and literature review, *J Spinal Disord Tech* 24(2):132-136, 2011.

Cross-Reference

Neuroradiology: The REQUISITES, 3rd ed, pp 551-552.

Comment

Background

Spinal extradural meningeal cysts are a rare type of spinal meningeal cyst that occurs most commonly in the middle or lower thoracic spine. They usually appear in the third to fifth decades of life and are found predominantly in men.

Histopathology and Clinical Findings

Congenital arachnoid cysts correspond to type I meningeal cysts in the classification of Nabors and colleagues. The term *arachnoid cyst* may be a misnomer because arachnoid cells are not always present at histopathologic examination. Type I cysts are subdivided into types IA and IB. Type IA cysts almost always occur within the dorsal aspect of the canal and have a strong thoracic predilection. Neither type IA nor type IB has nerve root fibers within the cyst wall. This determination is made at the time of surgery and by histopathology. A ball-valve mechanism has been proposed to explain the development of these cysts. Symptoms may include spasticity and sensory levels.

Imaging

The epidural location of the cyst in this case is easily determined from a sagittal T1-weighted image that shows a "cap" of epidural fat along the cyst margin (Fig. A) and from axial and sagittal T2-weighted images that reveal a hypointense line separating the cyst from the thecal sac (Figs. B and C). Without a history of trauma, detection of an extradural nonenhancing cystic lesion raises the possibility of a postinfectious cyst, such as occurs in neurocysticercosis. This possibility is considered unlikely, however, if CT myelography shows iodinated contrast flowing from the subarachnoid space into the cyst. Delayed images may be necessary to demonstrate filling of the cyst. CT may demonstrate associated vertebral body anomalies (Fig. D).

Management

Treatment involves complete surgical resection. At the time of surgery, the cyst pedicle is identified and sutured. The pedicle is almost always located near the entrance of a dorsal nerve root.

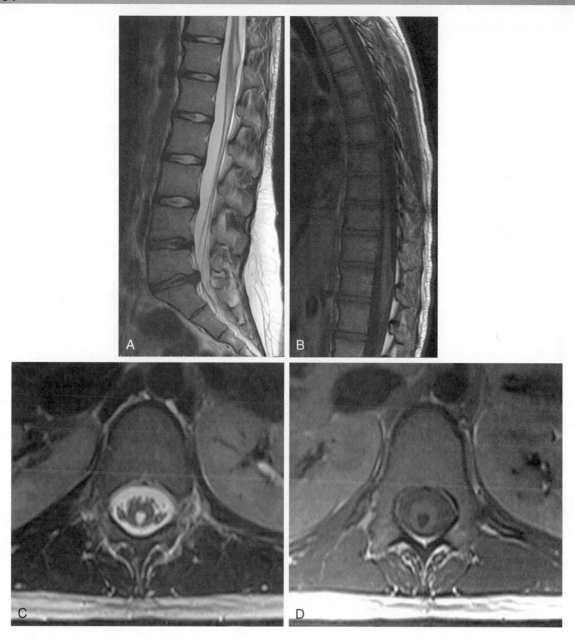

History: An 18-year-old woman presents with lower back pain and numbness in the left sciatic region.

1. What should be included in the differential diagnosis? (Choose all that apply.)
   a. Persistent terminal ventricle (ventriculus terminalis)
   b. Syringomyelia
   c. Hydromyelia
   d. Ependymoma
   e. Dermoid cyst

2. Ventriculus terminalis may be associated with all of the following malformations of the central nervous system *except:*
   a. Chiari malformation
   b. Myelomeningocele
   c. Diastematomyelia
   d. Spinal bifida

3. Which of the following MRI findings does *not* suggest a diagnosis of ventriculus terminalis?
   a. Hypointense T1 signal
   b. Hyperintense T2 signal
   c. Rim enhancement after contrast agent administration
   d. Well-defined margins

4. All of the following embryologic structures give rise to ventriculus terminalis *except:*
   a. Lamina terminalis
   b. Notochord
   c. Neural tube
   d. Caudal cell mass

Ventriculus Terminalis (Persistent Terminal Ventricle)

1. a, b, and c

2. c

3. c

4. a

References

Coleman LT, Zimmerman RA, Rorke LB: Ventriculus terminalis of the conus medullaris: MR findings in children, *AJNR Am J Neuroradiol* 16(7):1421-1426, 1995.

Liccardo G, Ruggeri F, De Cerchio L, et al: Fifth ventricle: An unusual cystic lesion of the conus medullaris, *Spinal Cord* 43(6):381-384, 2005.

Cross-Reference

Neuroradiology: The REQUISITES, 3rd ed, pp 318-319.

Comment

Background

Persistent terminal ventricle, also called ventriculus terminalis or "fifth ventricle," is a small ependyma-lined cavity within the conus medullaris. The persistent terminal ventricle is generally asymptomatic, although low back pain, sciatica, and bladder disorders have been reported. Enlargement of the terminal ventricle with cyst formation may be a developmental variant or may result from pathologic changes leading to obstruction.

Embryology and Histopathology

The ventriculus terminalis is formed during fetal development. In the normal development of the spinal cord, different stages are recognized: neurulation, canalization, and retrogressive differentiation. During neurulation, the neural plate closes to form the neural tube. At about 4 to 5 weeks of gestation, the caudal end of the neural tube and the notochord combine to become an aggregate of undifferentiated cells, termed the *caudal cell mass;* this cell mass canalizes and forms an ependyma-lined tube that usually fuses with the most rostral central canals. This cavity is the ventriculus terminalis. Most authors believe that isolated cystic dilatation of the ventriculus terminalis is due to the persistence of this lesion in adulthood and to abnormal closure of the communication between the ventriculus terminalis and the central canal by ependyma.

Imaging

Ventricular dilatation appears on MRI as a small, rounded cavity with well-defined borders; this cavity is filled with fluid of the same intensity as cerebrospinal fluid on both T1 and T2 sequences, without enhancement, after injection of a contrast agent (Figs. A-D). Differential diagnoses include hydromyelia, syringomyelia, and tumors of the conus. Differentiation with hydromyelia is based on a location immediately above the filum terminale; in terminal syringomyelia, there is no ependymal lining, and in tumors of the conus, there is marked enhancement of the cyst wall. MRI makes it possible to identify isolated forms of fifth ventricle by ruling out any association with other malformations.

Management

Conservative treatment, including periodic follow-up examinations to monitor the lesion and assess its temporal evolution, is recommended for asymptomatic patients and those with mild symptoms. Surgical treatment should be considered only in patients who present with severe clinical symptoms and signs.

Notes

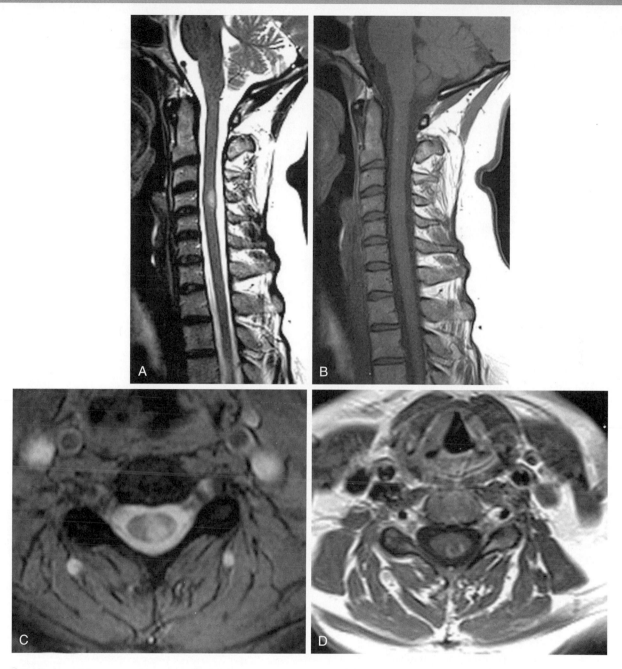

History: A 45-year-old woman presents with left upper extremity numbness and tingling and mild weakness of the hand for 5 days.

1. What should be included in the differential diagnosis? (Choose all that apply.)
   a. Multiple sclerosis (MS)
   b. Cord infarct
   c. Acute disseminated encephalomyelitis
   d. Vasculitis
   e. Sarcoid

2. Where is the epicenter of MS plaques most commonly located?
   a. Central cord
   b. Anterior or anterolateral cord periphery
   c. Posterior or posterolateral cord periphery
   d. Equally distributed throughout the cord

3. Where are most spinal cord MS plaques detected?
   a. Cervical cord
   b. Thoracic cord
   c. Conus region
   d. Equally in the cervical and thoracic cord

4. Which of the following findings favors the diagnosis of a demyelinating over a neoplastic process?
   a. Cord enlargement
   b. Avid solid lesion enhancement
   c. Diffuse cord T2 hyperintensity
   d. Scattered hyperintense white matter lesions oriented perpendicular to the ventricles on brain MRI

Multiple Sclerosis of the Cervical Spine

1. a, c, d, and e

2. c

3. a

4. d

References

Bot JC, Barkhof F, Polman CH, et al: Spinal cord abnormalities in recently diagnosed MS patients: Added value of spinal MRI examination, *Neurology* 62(2):226-233, 2004.

Klawiter EC, Benzinger T, Roy A, et al: Spinal cord ring enhancement in multiple sclerosis, *Arch Neurol* 67(11):1395-1398, 2010.

Lycklama a Nijeholt GJ, Barkhof F, Scheltens P, et al: MR of the spinal cord in multiple sclerosis: Relation to clinical subtype and disability, *AJNR Am J Neuroradiol* 18(6):1041-1048, 1997.

Cross-Reference

Neuroradiology: The REQUISITES, 3rd ed, pp 232-233, 548-549.

Comment

Background

MS is a demyelinating disease affecting the brain and spinal cord. It is the most common neurologic disorder in young white adults, affecting predominantly women and usually beginning in the second or third decade of life. Approximately 55% to 75% of patients have spinal cord lesions at some point during the course of the disease. Greater than 58% of patients with cord plaques have multiple plaques. Among patients with spinal cord lesions, only 20% do not have brain lesions. About 14% of spinal cord lesions enhance.

Pathophysiology

MS is an inflammatory, demyelinating disease of the central nervous system. In pathologic specimens, the demyelinating lesions of MS, called *plaques,* appear as indurated areas—hence the term *sclerosis.* The cause of MS is unknown, but it is likely that multiple factors act in concert to trigger or perpetuate the disease.

Imaging and Differential Diagnosis

On T2-weighted images, typical MS plaques (i.e., plaques less than two spinal segments in length and less than half the cross-sectional area of the cord) have a posterior or posterolateral cord location, where they involve the posterior or lateral columns (Fig. A). The posterior location of the enhancing nodule in the patient in this case should raise the suspicion that it is an acute MS plaque rather than a neoplastic or infectious process (Figs. A-D). Tumoral and nontumoral cyst formation is lacking in this case.

Ring enhancement, particularly the incomplete ring sign, is a frequently observed pattern on MRI of the brain. Spinal cord ring enhancement can also be seen in MS, and the ring is often incomplete (Fig. D). Spinal cord ring enhancement should prompt further workup for demyelinating diseases, including MRI of the brain and cerebrospinal fluid analysis. Additional imaging evidence supporting the diagnosis of MS might preclude the need for spinal cord biopsy in patients in whom other diagnoses are suspected. In addition to MS, the differential diagnosis for spinal cord ring enhancement includes neoplasm, abscess, and granulomatous disease.

Management

Treatment consists of immunomodulatory therapy and management of symptoms.

Notes

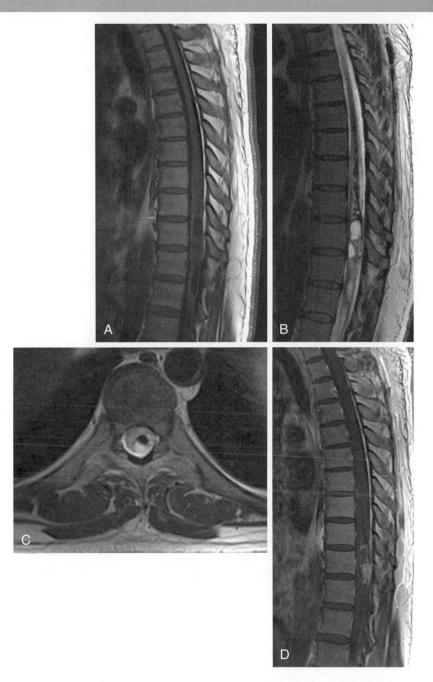

History: A 43-year-old man presents with burning pain in the left flank and numbness in the left leg for 1 year.

1. What should be included in the differential diagnosis? (Choose all that apply.)
   a. Astrocytoma
   b. Hemangioblastoma
   c. Ependymoma
   d. Arteriovenous malformation
   e. Meningioma

2. What is the location of the lesion?
   a. Intradural extramedullary
   b. Epidural
   c. Intramedullary
   d. Extraspinal

3. What is the most common intramedullary tumor in adults?
   a. Astrocytoma
   b. Ependymoma
   c. Metastasis
   d. Schwannoma

4. All of the following intramedullary lesions have been shown to cause superficial siderosis of the central nervous system *except:*
   a. Arteriovenous malformation
   b. Ependymoma
   c. Hemangioblastoma
   d. Sarcoid

Thoracic Ependymoma

1. a, b, and c

2. c

3. b

4. d

References
Kahan H, Sklar EM, Post MJ, et al: MR characteristics of histopathologic subtypes of spinal ependymoma, *AJNR Am J Neuroradiol* 17(1):143-150, 1996.

Sun B, Wang C, Wang J, et al: MRI features of intramedullary spinal cord ependymomas, *J Neuroimaging* 13(4):346-351, 2003.

Cross-Reference
Neuroradiology: The REQUISITES, 3rd ed, pp 557-558.

Comment

Background

Spinal ependymomas are the most common intramedullary neoplasm in adults and are most often found in the cervical cord, followed by the thoracic cord and conus. They occur most frequently in men in the fourth decade of life. The clinical presentation can include neck or back pain and, less often, numbness or paresthesias. Given the slow growth and relatively well-defined margins of these tumors, symptoms generally progress slowly, and patients may have a long history of clinical symptoms before diagnosis.

Histopathology

Ependymomas arise from ependymal cells lining the central canal and expand centrally. The World Health Organization (WHO) classification of ependymal cell tumors includes four types, based on histologic appearance: subependymoma (WHO grade I); myxopapillary ependymoma (WHO grade I); ependymoma (WHO grade II), which includes the cellular, papillary, and clear cell variants; and anaplastic ependymoma (WHO grade III). These masses are well-circumscribed, noninfiltrating, benign tumors that are generally more sharply demarcated than astrocytomas. They have a propensity for intratumoral hemorrhage and may produce subarachnoid hemorrhage with leptomeningeal deposition of hemosiderin (superficial siderosis). Cystic degeneration of the tumor (as shown in this case) and extensive cyst formation rostral or caudal to the tumor may be observed.

Imaging

On T1-weighted images, ependymomas generally appear isointense relative to the normal cord signal intensity (Fig. A). Less often, they are hypointense. Heterogeneous signal and regions of hyperintensity on T1-weighted images are usually the result of hemorrhagic tumor components. On T2-weighted images, ependymomas are generally hyperintense relative to the normal cord, although hemorrhage can result in central or peripheral hypointensity owing to susceptibility effects associated with hemosiderin deposition (Figs. B and C). This hypointensity is usually better shown on gradient-echo images than on fast-spin-echo T2-weighted images. About one third of ependymomas show the "cap" sign—a rim of hypointensity (hemosiderin) seen at the poles of the tumor on T2-weighted images (see Fig. B). This finding is thought to be due to hemorrhage, which is common in ependymomas and in other highly vascular tumors. The contrast enhancement pattern is variable (Fig. D), with homogeneous, heterogeneous, rimlike, minimal, or no enhancement observed.

Management

Complete surgical resection is the treatment of choice.

Notes

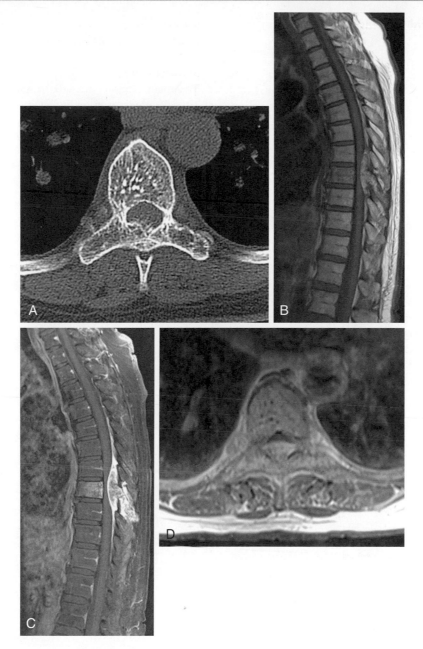

History: A 61-year-old woman presents with progressive difficulty walking and bladder and bowel incontinence.

1. What should be included in the differential diagnosis? (Choose all that apply.)
   a. Metastasis
   b. Plasmacytoma
   c. Osteomyelitis
   d. Lymphoma
   e. Aggressive vertebral hemangioma

2. What is the location of the lesion?
   a. Intramedullary
   b. Intradural extramedullary
   c. Extradural
   d. Subdural

3. What are the typical signal characteristics of a vertebral hemangioma on MRI?
   a. Hyperintense on T1-weighted images and hyperintense on T2-weighted images
   b. Hyperintense on T1-weighted images and hypointense on T2-weighted images
   c. Hypointense on T1-weighted images and hyperintense on T2-weighted images
   d. Hypointense on T1-weighted images and hypointense on T2-weighted images

4. All of the following imaging features may be seen in aggressive vertebral hemangiomas *except:*
   a. Extension into the neural arch
   b. Cord invasion
   c. Lytic areas
   d. Poorly defined cortical margins

111

Aggressive Vertebral Hemangioma

1. a, b, and e

2. c

3. a

4. b

References

Alexander J, Meir A, Vrodos N, et al: Vertebral hemangioma: An important differential in the evaluation of locally aggressive spinal lesions, *Spine* 35:E917-E920, 2010.

Cross JJ, Antoun NM, Laing RJ, et al: Imaging of compressive vertebral hemangiomas, *Eur Radiol* 10:997-1002, 2000.

Cross-Reference

Neuroradiology: The REQUISITES, 3rd ed, p 567.

Comment

Background

Vertebral hemangiomas have been found in approximately 10% of spines at autopsy. The most common location is the thoracic spine, followed by the lumbar spine. Aggressive hemangiomas are markedly hypervascular. About 1% of vertebral hemangiomas produce symptoms as a result of vertebral collapse, cord compression, or nerve root compression.

Pathophysiology

Vertebral hemangiomas are considered benign vascular lesions of bone. They are composed of multiple thin-walled vessels surrounded by fat infiltrating the medullary cavity between bony trabeculae.

Imaging

Generally, solitary vertebral hemangiomas can be categorized as indolent or aggressive. All are composed of a stroma within an osseous network that is responsible for the vertical striation seen on plain radiographs and the coarse trabecular pattern seen on CT scan (Fig. A). Indolent and aggressive hemangiomas differ in their stromal content, although some overlap exists. In indolent hemangiomas, the stroma is predominantly fatty and appears markedly hypodense (lipid attenuation values) on CT scan and hyperintense on T1-weighted MRI. In aggressive hemangiomas, the stroma is predominantly angiomatous and consists of conglomerates of thin-walled, dilated vessels packed with red blood cells (the cavernous type of hemangioma). This stroma has soft tissue density on CT scan. On MRI, it is hypointense on T1-weighted images (Fig. B) and hyperintense on T2-weighted images; it enhances after contrast agent administration (Fig. C). The observation of intraosseous signal voids on MRI may be an important finding that suggests vertebral hemangioma (Fig. D). In a review, Cross and colleagues showed that the characteristic findings associated with vertebral hemangiomas were absent in 35% of plain films, 20% of CT scans, and 48% of MRI scans of aggressive lesions, resulting in an inability to make an accurate diagnosis. Many more recent reviews recommend the routine use of angiography

whenever vertebral hemangioma is suspected or the diagnosis of a locally aggressive spinal lesion is unclear.

Management

Treatment options include surgical decompression, transarterial embolization, radiotherapy, ethanol sclerotherapy, or a combination of these methods.

Notes

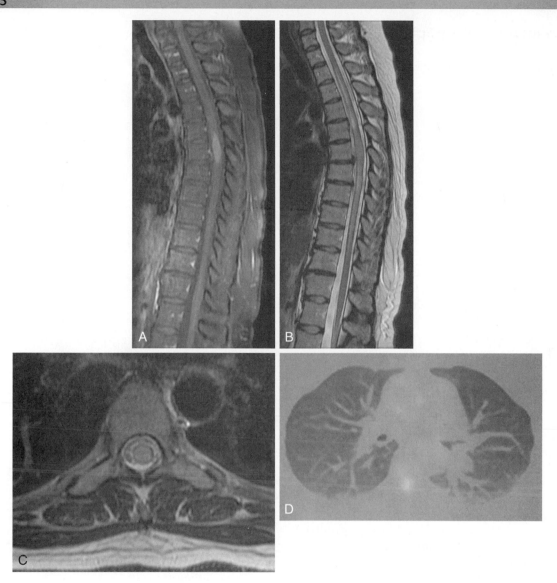

History: A 37-year-old woman presents with right lower extremity numbness, weakness, and tingling in the midabdomen.

1. What should be included in the differential diagnosis? (Choose all that apply.)
   a. Ependymoma
   b. Tuberculoma
   c. Sarcoid
   d. Lymphoma
   e. Spinal cord metastasis

2. Which MRI signal characteristic would *not* be expected in secondary intramedullary spinal cord involvement of non-Hodgkin's lymphoma (NHL)?
   a. Hyperintense T1 signal relative to cord
   b. Isointense T1 signal relative to cord
   c. Isointense T2 signal relative to cord
   d. Avid contrast enhancement

3. Which of the following imaging features would help differentiate intramedullary lymphoma from other causes of intramedullary lesions?
   a. Persistent gadolinium enhancement
   b. Fluorodeoxyglucose avidity
   c. Location within the thoracic cord
   d. Cauda equina enhancement

4. Which of the following statements comparing solid organ intramedullary spinal cord metastases and secondary intramedullary NHL is *false?*
   a. Widespread dissemination of cancer is more common than active systemic NHL outside the central nervous system in patients with intramedullary spinal cord involvement.
   b. Secondary intramedullary NHL involvement is more common than intramedullary metastases from solid organ cancers.
   c. Secondary intramedullary NHL involvement manifests earlier in the disease course compared with intramedullary metastases from solid organ cancers.
   d. Survival for patients with secondary intramedullary NHL is longer than that for patients with intramedullary metastases secondary to solid tumors.

Secondary Intramedullary Spinal Cord Lymphoma

1. a, b, c, d, and e

2. a

3. c

4. b

Reference
Flanagan EP, O'Neill BP, Habermann TM, et al: Secondary intramedullary spinal cord non-Hodgkin's lymphoma, *J Neurooncol* 107(3):575-580, 2012.

Cross-Reference
Neuroradiology: The REQUISITES, 3rd ed, pp 565-566.

Comment

Background

This patient was previously diagnosed with diffuse large B-cell lymphoma, which is an aggressive type of NHL. It accounts for approximately 40% of lymphomas in adults. The median age at diagnosis is 70 years, but it also occurs in children and young adults. As with most NHLs, there is a male predominance.

Clinical Presentation

Secondary intramedullary spinal cord involvement of NHL is rare and usually occurs early in the course of NHL. The median time from diagnosis of systemic NHL to central nervous system involvement is 6 months (as in this case). The most common clinical presentation is Brown-Séquard syndrome.

Imaging

Typical MRI findings in secondary intramedullary spinal cord involvement of NHL are focal, expansile gadolinium-enhancing lesions in the cervical or thoracic spine, with spinal cord enlargement and hypermetabolism on 18F-FDG PET scan (Figs. A-D). Brain MRI is helpful diagnostically because two thirds of patients have brain lesions in addition to symptomatic intramedullary spinal cord involvement. Radiation myelopathy may result in changes similar to those of secondary intramedullary spinal cord involvement of NHL, with gadolinium enhancement and FDG-avidity. It is therefore important to obtain a detailed treatment history.

Management

Pathologic confirmation of lymphoma can be achieved by cerebrospinal fluid (CSF) examination. In patients without CSF malignant cells, characteristic MRI features, evidence of systemic NHL, and intramedullary spinal cord FDG-avidity aid in the diagnosis (see Fig. D). Treatment includes systemic or intrathecal chemotherapy, radiation treatment, and possibly autologous peripheral blood stem cell transplantation. Because of the relative sensitivity of lymphoma to treatment, survival is longer compared with solid organ metastases.

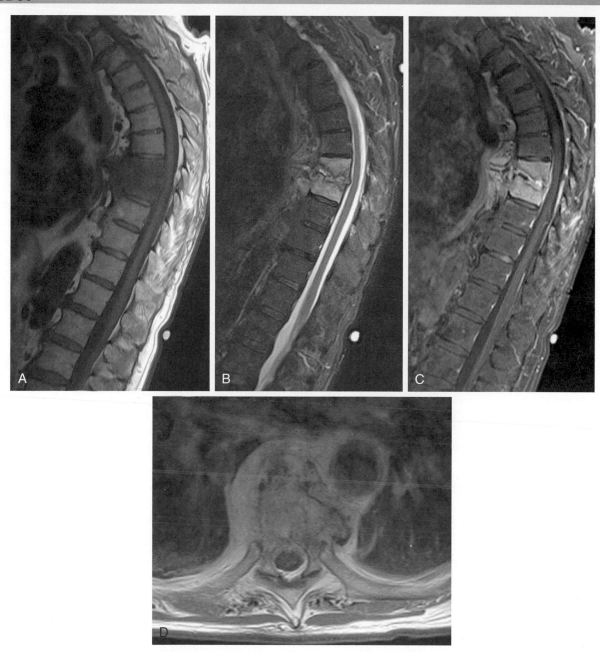

History: A 78-year-old man presents with a 3-month history of pain in the midback.

1. What should be included in the differential diagnosis? (Choose all that apply.)
   a. Primary spinal tumor
   b. Diskitis osteomyelitis
   c. Neuropathic spine
   d. Metastatic disease
   e. Degenerative disk disease

2. Which of the following is *not* considered a "typical" finding of diskitis osteomyelitis on MRI?
   a. Loss of end-plate definition on T1-weighted images
   b. Decreased vertebral body signal on T1-weighted images
   c. Increased vertebral body signal on T2-weighted images
   d. Increased disk signal intensity on T2-weighted images

3. In what percentage of patients are "typical" findings of diskitis osteomyelitis observed?
   a. 5%
   b. 35%
   c. 75%
   d. 95%

4. Which of the following organisms most commonly causes diskitis osteomyelitis?
   a. *Mycobacterium tuberculosis*
   b. *Staphylococcus aureus*
   c. Gram-negative organisms
   d. *Escherichia coli*

Thoracic Diskitis Osteomyelitis

1. b and c

2. d

3. d

4. b

Reference

Dagirmanjian A, Schils J, McHenry M, et al: MR imaging of vertebral osteomyelitis revisited, *AJR Am J Roentgenol* 167(6):1539-1543, 1996.

Cross-Reference

Neuroradiology: The REQUISITES, 3rd ed, p 543.

Comment

Background

Vertebral osteomyelitis occurs primarily in adults, with most affected patients older than 50 years. The lumbar region is most commonly affected, followed by the cervical spine and thoracic spine. In adults, diskitis osteomyelitis has a slow, insidious onset, which may cause a delay in diagnosis. Pain with localized tenderness is the initial presenting symptom.

Pathophysiology

Diskitis and vertebral osteomyelitis are almost always present together and share much of the same pathophysiology. In most cases, the infection does not originate in the vertebra or disk space but rather spreads to the involved intervertebral disk hematogenously from a systemic infection (urinary tract infections, pneumonia, and soft tissue infections are the most common sources).

Imaging

In this case, MRI shows the findings that are considered "typical" of diskitis osteomyelitis: decreased vertebral body signal on T1-weighted images (Fig. A), loss of end-plate definition on T1-weighted images, increased disk signal intensity on T2-weighted images (Fig. B), and contrast enhancement of the disk and adjacent vertebral bodies (Fig. C). Modic and colleagues reported that each of these findings was observed with a frequency of approximately 95%. In comparison, increased vertebral body signal on T2-weighted images was observed in only 56% of spinal levels affected by diskitis osteomyelitis. The absence of this finding should not dissuade the clinician from making an MRI diagnosis of diskitis osteomyelitis when the above-described typical findings are present (as in this case). The variation in signal intensity of the involved vertebral bodies on T2-weighted images has been attributed in part to variability in the ratio of sclerotic bone (as seen on standard radiographs) to edematous marrow.

The typical contrast enhancement pattern of the involved disk can vary from thick, patchy enhancement to linear enhancement to a ringlike peripheral enhancement that may be either thick (see Fig. C) or thin and either continuous or discontinuous. The intensity of vertebral body enhancement is variable. Enhancement of epidural and paraspinal associated soft tissue masses provides additional evidence of infection (Fig. D). Homogeneous enhancement favors phlegmon, and ring enhancement favors mature abscess.

Management

Elevated erythrocyte sedimentation rate and C-reactive protein are the most consistent laboratory abnormalities seen in cases of diskitis, whereas leukocytosis is frequently absent. Blood cultures are positive in 50% to 70% of patients and should be obtained for any patient suspected of having diskitis osteomyelitis. Treatment includes antibiotics and immobilization to allow the vertebral bodies to fuse in an anatomically aligned position. Indications for surgery include neurologic deficit and spinal deformity.

Notes

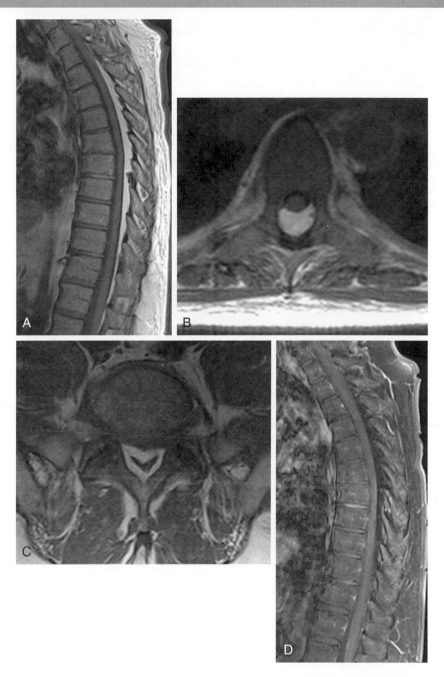

History: A 66-year-old man presents with back pain and lower extremity numbness.

1. What should be included in the differential diagnosis? (Choose all that apply.)
   a. Lipoma
   b. Meningioma
   c. Angiolipoma
   d. Spinal epidural lipomatosis (SEL)
   e. Lymphoma

2. What finding on axial images has been described as pathognomonic of this abnormality when it involves the lumbar spine?
   a. "Y" sign
   b. "Shiny corner" sign
   c. "Empty sac" sign
   d. "Dural tail" sign

3. Which of the following statements regarding SEL is true?
   a. Involvement of the cervical spine is rare.
   b. Idiopathic SEL typically favors the thoracic spine.
   c. Males are affected more than females.
   d. SEL causing neurologic deficits occurs more frequently in the thoracic spine than in the lumbar spine.

4. Which of the following is *not* a cause of SEL?
   a. Cushing's syndrome
   b. Exogenous steroid use
   c. Idiopathic
   d. Addison's syndrome

Spinal Epidural Lipomatosis

1. d

2. a

3. c

4. d

References

Al-Khawaja D, Seex K, Eslick GD: Spinal epidural lipomatosis—a brief review, *J Clin Neurosci* 15(12):1323-1326, 2008.

Lee SB, Park HK, Chang JC, et al: Idiopathic thoracic epidural lipomatosis with chest pain, *J Korean Neurosurg Soc* 50(2):130-133, 2011.

Cross-Reference

Neuroradiology: The REQUISITES, 3rd ed, p 570.

Comment

Background

SEL is a rare disorder defined as a pathologic overgrowth of normal extradural fat. It is most often associated with the administration of exogenous steroids and conditions of endocrine dysfunction, such as Cushing's disease and hypothyroidism. Obesity is the second most common association. Cervical spine involvement is extremely rare. Several authors assert that the term *idiopathic* should be used solely to characterize cases of SEL that develop in nonobese patients who were not receiving corticosteroid therapy and do not have any other underlying SEL-related disease.

Pathophysiology

The main mechanism of SEL-induced neurologic symptoms is direct compression of the adjacent nervous structures and epidural blood vessels, resulting in venous engorgement; this contributes to the evolution of myelopathic and radicular symptoms. Back pain and weakness are the most frequent presenting complaints.

Imaging

MRI is the diagnostic test of choice. The normal thickness of epidural fat in the sagittal plane ranges from 3 to 6 mm, whereas a thickness of 7 to 15 mm has been reported in patients with symptomatic SEL (Figs. A and B). The thecal sac may be completely effaced, resulting in the typical Mercedes-Benz sign on axial images (Fig. C). The most commonly involved levels in the thoracic and lumbar spine are T6-T8 and L4-L5. Epidural lipomatosis should be differentiated from other extradural mass lesions, such as lipoma and angiolipoma. Lipomatosis consists of unencapsulated, diffuse fatty tissue derived from preexisting epidural fat by hypertrophy, whereas lipoma and angiolipoma are typically well-encapsulated, circumscribed masses. Angiolipoma may also show enhancement, which was not seen in this case (Fig. D).

Management

Surgical decompression is the treatment of choice when patients present with abnormal neurologic signs. Weight reduction may be beneficial in patients who present with mild symptoms.

Notes

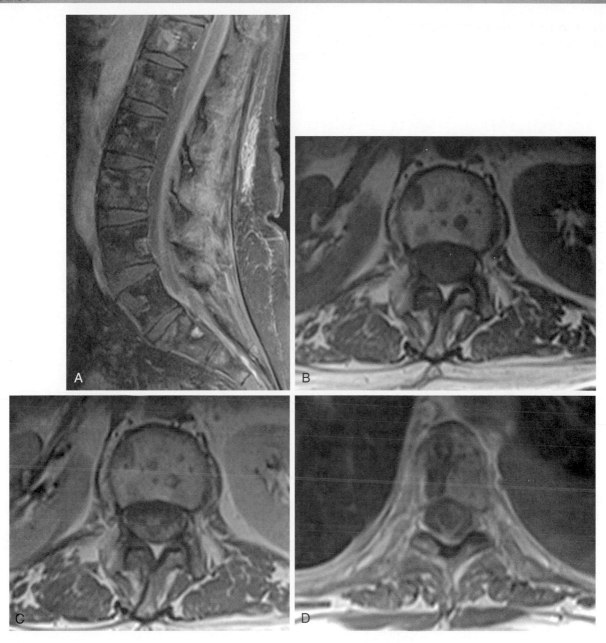

History: A 32-year-old woman presents to the emergency department with lower back pain, weakness, and numbness of the lower extremities.

1. What should be included in the differential diagnosis? (Choose all that apply.)
   a. Multiple myeloma
   b. Leptomeningeal metastases
   c. Sarcoid
   d. Tuberculous meningitis
   e. Lymphoma

2. All of the following tumors are common causes of intradural (leptomeningeal) metastases *except:*
   a. Breast cancer
   b. Lung cancer
   c. Colon cancer
   d. Melanoma

3. Where along the spinal axis are leptomeningeal metastases most likely to be found?
   a. Cervical cord
   b. Thoracic cord
   c. Lumbar canal
   d. Sacral canal

4. In what percentage of patients with positive initial cerebrospinal fluid cytology does contrast-enhanced MRI detect spinal leptomeningeal metastases?
   a. 10%
   b. 25%
   c. 60%
   d. 90%

Leptomeningeal Carcinomatosis (Breast Carcinoma)

1. a, b, c, d, and e

2. c

3. c

4. d

References

Gomori JM, Heching N, Siegal T: Leptomeningeal metastases: Evaluation by gadolinium enhanced spinal magnetic resonance imaging, *J Neurooncol* 36(1):55-60, 1998.

Holtz AJ: The sugarcoating sign, *Radiology* 208(1):143-144, 1998.

Cross-Reference

Neuroradiology: The REQUISITES, 3rd ed, pp 559-560.

Comment

Background

Infiltration of the leptomeninges by malignant cells is a common complication of cancer and is called carcinomatous meningitis or leptomeningeal carcinomatosis. Leptomeningeal carcinomatosis arises from either solid tumors or hematologic malignancies. Overall, neoplastic meningitis occurs in 5% to 8% of patients with cancer. The most common associated malignancies are breast and lung cancer, melanoma, lymphomas, and leukemias.

Histopathology

The two most common pathways by which cancer cells can reach the leptomeninges are hematogenous spread and intrathecal cerebrospinal fluid spread (drop metastases) of malignant cells. The primary central nervous system neoplasms that have a propensity for drop metastases are glioblastoma multiforme, medulloblastoma, ependymoma, and choroid plexus carcinoma.

Imaging

MRI is the imaging technique of choice for the detection of leptomeningeal disease. The findings on contrast-enhanced T1-weighted images, as illustrated in this case (Figs. A-D), are linear and nodular regions of enhancement along the conus and cauda equina roots (see Figs. A and C), which appear thickened (see Fig. C). Linear enhancement on the surface of the cord has been called the "sugarcoating" or "frosting" sign (see Fig. D).

Management

Therapeutic management of leptomeningeal carcinomatosis includes intrathecal administration of chemotherapy and radiotherapy. Treatment remains controversial, and no straightforward guidelines exist in the literature.

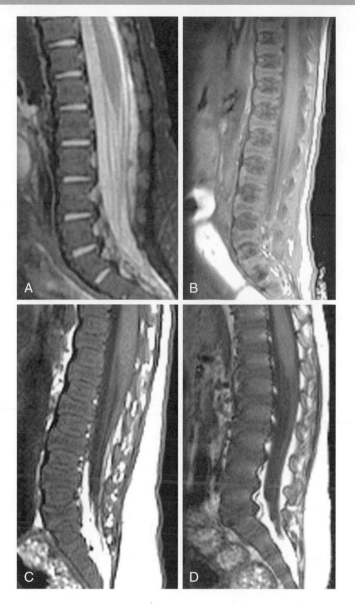

History: Sacral dimples in four children of different ages are evaluated.

1. What should be included in the differential diagnosis? (Choose all that apply.)
   a. Acute myelocytic leukemia
   b. Sacral lipomeningocele
   c. Low-lying conus with cord tethering
   d. Normal spine MRI for patient's age
   e. Sacrococcygeal teratoma

2. All of the following statements regarding the MRI appearance of the normal spine in infants are true *except:*
   a. Three stages are characterized on MRI.
   b. Stage I is from birth to 1 month.
   c. In stage I, the ossification center is markedly hyperintense on T1-weighted images.
   d. The disk is markedly hyperintense on T2-weighted images in all stages.

3. Which lumbar spine structures enhance prominently in children younger than 18 months of age?
   a. Anterior and posterior longitudinal ligaments
   b. Cartilaginous end-plate and ossification center
   c. Cauda equina nerve roots
   d. Intervertebral disk

4. Which of the following statements regarding a "pseudodisk" appearance is true?
   a. The hyperintense ossification center appears as a "pseudodisk."
   b. The true disk and ossification center are isointense on T1-weighted images, appearing as one thick "pseudodisk."
   c. T2-weighted images rarely help distinguish the structures constituting a "pseudodisk."
   d. This appearance is noted only on MRI scanners that are 0.5 tesla in strength.

Pediatric Spine—Normal MRI Signal Intensities

1. d

2. c

3. b

4. a

Reference

Sze G, Baierl P, Bravo S: Evolution of the infant spinal column: Evaluation with MR imaging, *Radiology* 181(3):819-827, 1991.

Cross-Reference

Neuroradiology: The REQUISITES, 3rd ed, p 524.

Comment

Background

The growth of the spine starts long before birth and continues through infancy and childhood until the end of adolescence. The most striking differences between the pediatric spine and the adult spine are the significantly higher cartilage component and the greater degree of overall water content in the nucleus pulposus of the pediatric spine (Fig. A).

Pathophysiology

The cartilage of the vertebral end-plate contributes to the overall growth in height. The vertebral end-plate contains the physeal cartilage adjacent to the bony vertebral body. At birth, the vertebral end-plate is entirely cartilage. By age 5 years, ossification islands start to appear in the thickened margins of the upper and lower cartilaginous plates and gradually fuse to form an annular ring apophysis.

Imaging

The MRI appearance of the normal spine in infants and children proceeds through three stages, as described by Sze and colleagues. The signal intensities of the vertebral ossification center, adjacent cartilage, and disk are characterized relative to the signal intensity of muscle on T1- and T2-weighted images.

On T1-weighted images, the stages are as follows:
- Stage I (birth to 1 month): ovoid vertebral body with markedly hypointense ossification center (except for a thin central hyperintense band), markedly hyperintense cartilage, and isointense disk (Fig. B).
- Stage II (1 to 6 months): ovoid vertebral body with increasingly hyperintense superior and inferior aspects of the ossification center (inferior aspect is more hyperintense), hyperintense cartilage, and isointense disk (Fig. C).
- Stage III (7 months to 2 years): rectangular vertebral body with rounded corners (by 2 years of age), hyperintense ossification center, isointense cartilage, and isointense disk (Fig. D).

On T2-weighted images, the stages are as follows:
- Stage I: markedly hypointense ossification center, mildly hyperintense cartilage, and markedly hyperintense disk.
- Stage II: isointense to mildly hyperintense superior and inferior aspects of the ossification center, with a variably less intense central portion, isointense to mildly hyperintense cartilage, and markedly hyperintense disk. The similar intensity of the vertebral bodies and cartilage in this 4-month-old infant results in their appearance as single rectangular units.
- Stage III: mildly hyperintense ossification center, isointense to mildly hyperintense cartilage, and markedly hyperintense disk.

Management

Because the appearance of the developing spine at different ages may vary significantly, knowledge of the normal evolution is necessary to identify pathologic changes.

Notes

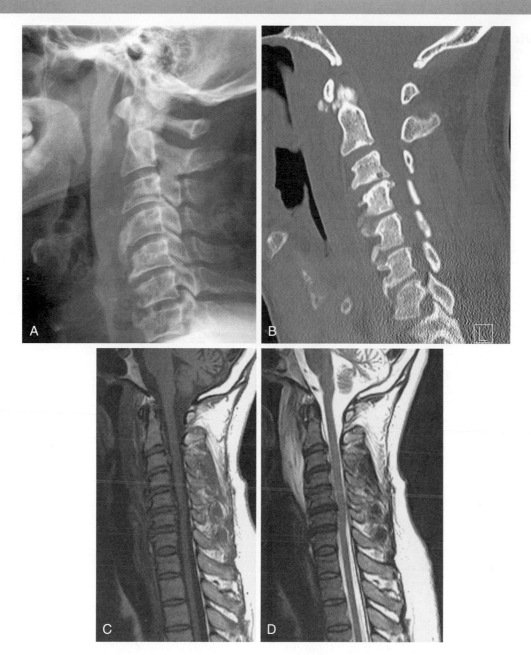

History: A 49-year-old man presents with acute worsening of neck pain for 3 days.

1. What should be included in the differential diagnosis for the imaging findings presented? (Choose all that apply.)
   a. Prevertebral phlegmon
   b. Postradiation edema
   c. Acute calcific prevertebral tendinitis
   d. C2 fracture with prevertebral soft tissue edema
   e. Diskitis osteomyelitis with prevertebral phlegmon

2. Which one of the following findings supports the diagnosis of calcific tendinitis of the longus colli muscle?
   a. Peripheral enhancement of the prevertebral effusion
   b. Necrotic retropharyngeal nodes
   c. Amorphous calcifications inferior to the anterior arch of C1
   d. Bone destruction

3. Which of the following structures is *not* a boundary of the retropharyngeal space?
   a. Deep layer of the deep cervical fascia
   b. Sagittal partition
   c. Middle layer of the deep cervical fascia
   d. Superficial layer of the deep cervical fascia

4. What is the preferred treatment of this condition?
   a. Steroids
   b. Antibiotic
   c. Nonsteroidal anti-inflammatory drugs (NSAIDs)
   d. Percutaneous drainage

Acute Calcific Tendinitis of the Longus Colli Muscle

1. a, b, and c

2. c

3. d

4. c

Reference
Razon RV, Nasir A, Wu GS, et al: Retropharyngeal calcific tendonitis: Report of two cases, *J Am Board Fam Med* 22(1):84-88, 2009.

Cross-Reference
Neuroradiology: The REQUISITES, 3rd ed, p 533.

Comment
Background
Calcific tendinitis of the longus colli muscle is an uncommon condition that affects adults 30 to 60 years old. The clinical history is sudden onset of odynophagia, dysphagia, and neck pain with limited range of motion. Some patients develop a low-grade fever, mild leukocytosis, and an elevated sedimentation rate. This constellation of findings may mimic those of a retropharyngeal space infection.

Pathophysiology
The longus colli muscles are paired neck flexors that extend from the anterior arch of C1 to the anterior tubercle of T3. Calcific tendinitis of the longus colli muscle refers to an inflammatory condition of the longus colli tendon secondary to the deposition of calcium hydroxyapatite crystals. Classically, calcification affects the superior oblique portion of the muscle at C1-C2. These superolateral fibers originate on the anterior tubercles of the transverse processes of the third to fifth cervical vertebrae and insert on the anterior tubercle of the atlas.

Imaging
Calcifications may be seen on radiographs (Fig. A), but the definitive diagnosis is made by CT. On CT scan, amorphous calcifications are seen in the superior fibers of the longus colli muscle tendons at the C1-C2 level (Fig. B). Retropharyngeal effusion and edema of the adjacent prevertebral soft tissues may also be seen. MRI shows the edema (Figs. C and D) but is not as sensitive as CT in detecting calcifications. Keys to the diagnosis are (1) the presence of calcification in the longus colli muscle, usually from C1 to C4; (2) lack of an enhancing wall surrounding the fluid collection; and (3) the absence of necrotic nodes within the retropharyngeal space.

Management
Symptoms typically resolve within days after initiation of treatment with NSAIDs.

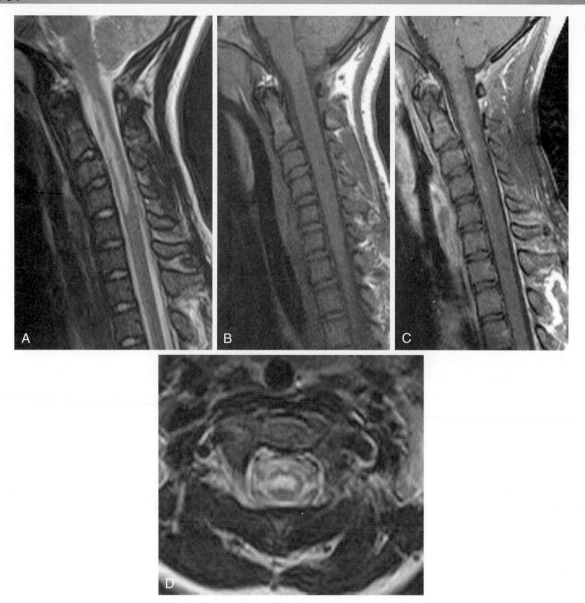

History: A 14-year-old girl develops acute paralysis and respiratory failure.

1. What should be included in the differential diagnosis? (Choose all that apply.)
   a. Acute disseminated encephalomyelitis (ADEM)
   b. Systemic lupus erythematosus
   c. Spinal vascular malformation
   d. Neuromyelitis optica
   e. Astrocytoma

2. All of the following statements regarding acute transverse myelitis (ATM) are true *except:*
   a. Diagnosis is made on spinal cord biopsy.
   b. ATM is clinically characterized by the development of motor sensory and autonomic dysfunction.
   c. MRI is the imaging modality of choice in the evaluation of ATM.
   d. ATM can be the presenting feature of multiple sclerosis (MS).

3. Which of the following statements regarding ADEM is *false?*
   a. Antibodies to myelin oligodendrocyte glycoprotein are found in children with ADEM.
   b. Children are more affected than adults.
   c. One third of patients have relapses.
   d. Cerebrospinal fluid analysis typically reveals oligoclonal bands.

4. All of the following MRI findings may help differentiate ADEM from MS *except:*
   a. Spinal cord lesion extending over a longer segment
   b. Spinal cord lesion showing ringlike enhancement
   c. Spinal cord lesion with poorly defined margins
   d. Spinal cord lesion affecting the thoracic cord

Acute Disseminated Encephalomyelitis

1. a, b, and d

2. d

3. d

4. b

References

Callen DJ, Shroff MM, Branson HM, et al: Role of MRI in the differentiation of ADEM from MS in children, *Neurology* 72(11):968-973, 2009.

Pröbstel AK, Dornmair K, Bittner R, et al: Antibodies to MOG are transient in childhood acute disseminated encephalomyelitis, *Neurology* 77(6):580-588, 2011.

Rossi A: Imaging of acute disseminated encephalomyelitis, *Neuroimaging Clin N Am* 18(1):149-161, 2008.

Cross-Reference

Neuroradiology: The REQUISITES, 3rd ed, pp 236-237.

Comment

Background and Clinical Presentation

ADEM is a monophasic demyelinating disease of the central nervous system that occurs in most cases following a viral illness, vaccination, or nonspecific respiratory infection. ADEM most commonly affects young children and adolescents. It typically affects the gray matter and white matter of the brain and spinal cord (30% of cases). Symptoms include fever, headache, ataxia, and seizures. Symptoms may progress for 2 weeks. Although ADEM is classically considered to be a monophasic disorder, one third of patients experience relapses. ADEM relapses occurring within 3 months of the inciting ADEM episode are considered part of the same acute event. At least 18% of all children ultimately diagnosed with MS experience a first demyelinating event that is clinically indistinguishable from typical ADEM.

Histopathology

The pathogenesis of ADEM is unclear; however, it is thought to be an immune-mediated disorder resulting from an autoimmune reaction to myelin. In the acute stages, ADEM is characterized histologically by perivenous edema, demyelination, and infiltration with macrophages and lymphocytes, with relative axonal sparing. The late stage of the disease is characterized by perivascular gliosis.

Imaging

Although the MRI features of ADEM and MS cannot be reliably distinguished, large lesions, or longitudinally extensive lesions involving the spinal cord (Figs. A-C), are associated with ADEM and with neuromyelitis optica. In contrast, the spinal lesions in MS tend be small (one to two spinal segments in length). Lesions may involve the gray matter or white matter (Fig. D) and may or may not enhance (see Fig. C).

Management

Cerebrospinal fluid analysis typically reveals lymphocytes and mildly increased protein. Treatment includes the early use of high-dose intravenous steroids. Severe cases may be treated with a combination of intravenous corticosteroids and intravenous immunoglobulin, immunosuppressants, or plasmapheresis. The prognosis is favorable, with complete recovery within 6 months.

Notes

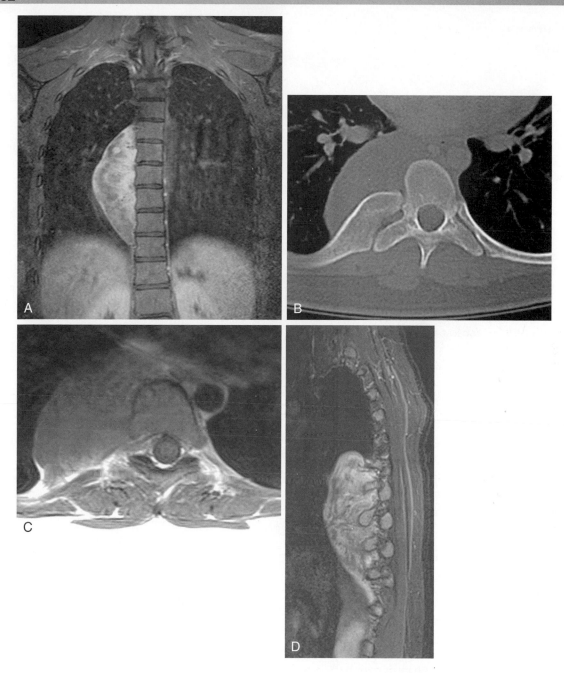

History: A 22-year-old woman is incidentally found to have a mediastinal mass on a chest x-ray done for a positive purified protein derivative (PPD) test.

1. What should be included in the differential diagnosis? (Choose all that apply.)
   a. Ganglioneuroma
   b. Schwannoma
   c. Chordoma
   d. Lymphoma
   e. Meningioma

2. In what region are the organs of Zuckerkandl located?
   a. Mediastinal, at approximately the T5 level
   b. Retroperitoneal, at approximately the L3 level
   c. Intraperitoneal, at approximately the L1 level
   d. Presacral

3. What is the most specific nuclear medicine test for tumors of the sympathetic nervous system?
   a. Octreoscan
   b. Positron emission tomography with fluorodeoxyglucose (18F-FDG PET)
   c. Gallium scan
   d. Meta-iodobenzylguanidine (MIBG) scan

4. Which of the following features supports the diagnosis of ganglioneuroma when attempting to differentiate ganglioneuroma from more aggressive ganglioneuroblastoma and neuroblastoma?
   a. Presence of bone metastases
   b. Coarse calcifications on CT scan
   c. Occurrence in older patients
   d. Encasement of the aorta

Ganglioneuroma

1. a, b, c, and d

2. b

3. d

4. c

References

Lonergan GJ, Schwab CM, Suarez ES: Neuroblastoma, ganglioneuroblastoma and ganglioneuroma: Radiologic-pathologic correlation, *Radiographics* 22(4):911-934, 2002.

Tanaka O, Kiryu T, Hirose Y, et al: Neurogenic tumors of the mediastinum and chest wall: MR imaging appearance, *J Thorac Imaging* 20(4):316-320, 2005.

Cross-Reference

Neuroradiology: The REQUISITES, 3rd ed, pp 566-567.

Comment

Background

Ganglioneuromas account for less than 1% of all soft tissue neoplasms. They are usually found in children (5 to 8 years old) or adolescents but may manifest in adulthood. There is a slight female predominance. Although slow growing, these tumors may cause pressure erosion of bone.

Histopathology

Ganglioneuromas are benign tumors of the sympathetic nervous system that originate from the neural crest. They are composed of nerve fibers and mature ganglion cells. Along with neuroblastomas, ganglioneuromas and ganglioneuroblastomas are collectively termed *neurogenic tumors*. These tumors can grow wherever sympathetic nervous tissue is found. The most common locations for neurogenic tumors are the adrenal gland, paraspinal sympathetic chain (especially thoracic and lumbar), head, and neck.

Imaging

Ganglioneuromas appear radiologically as well-defined, smooth or lobulated, oblong masses located anterior and lateral to the spine. They typically span three to five vertebral levels (Fig. A). On CT scan (Fig. B), these tumors may be homogeneous or heterogeneous, with low to intermediate density. Calcifications are found in approximately 20% of cases and are usually punctate (in contrast to the coarse calcifications seen with ganglioneuroblastomas and neuroblastomas). MRI is the modality of choice for evaluating the extension of these tumors. Ganglioneuromas appear homogeneous on MRI and have low to intermediate signal intensity on T1-weighted images (Fig. C). On T2-weighted images (Fig. D), the signal intensity is usually heterogeneous and either intermediate to high or markedly high. Tumors with intermediate to high signal intensity on T2-weighted images have a small myxoid stroma component, a higher degree of cellularity, and a greater amount of collagen, whereas markedly high T2 signal intensity signifies a large myxoid stroma component. Ganglioneuromas

have characteristic curvilinear bands of low signal intensity on T2-weighted images, resulting in a whorled pattern (Fig. D). These bands comprise collagen fibers and intertwined bundles of Schwann cells. Enhancement varies from mild to moderate and may be heterogeneous (see Fig. A).

Management

Treatment is complete surgical resection. Recurrence has been reported; routine surveillance is also necessary.

Notes

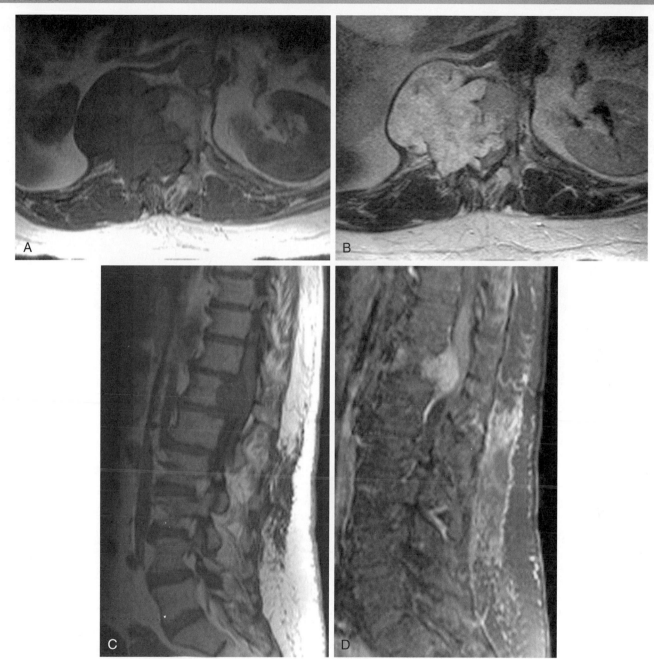

History: A 63-year-old woman presents with urinary incontinence, progressive perineal numbness, and difficulty walking for the past 6 months.

1. What should be included in the differential diagnosis? (Choose all that apply.)
   a. Diskitis osteomyelitis
   b. Chordoma
   c. Metastasis
   d. Plasmacytoma
   e. Lymphoma

2. What is the embryologic origin of this lesion?
   a. Neural crest
   b. Mesoderm
   c. Endoderm
   d. Notochord remnants

3. What findings on MRI suggest the diagnosis?
   a. Sparing of the disk space
   b. Epidural involvement
   c. Pattern of hyperintense lobules separated by hypointense septations on T2-weighted images
   d. Involvement of the vertebral bodies

4. What percentage of chordomas originates in the vertebral bodies?
   a. 5%
   b. 15%
   c. 50%
   d. 90%

Thoracic Chordoma

1. b, c, d, and e

2. d

3. c

4. b

References
Casali PG, Stacchiotti S, Sangalli C, et al: Chordoma, *Curr Opin Oncol* 19(4): 367-370, 2007.
Smolders D, Wang X, Drevelengas A, et al: Value of MRI in the diagnosis of non-clival, non-sacral chordoma, *Skeletal Radiol* 32(6):343-350, 2003.

Cross-Reference
Neuroradiology: The REQUISITES, 3rd ed, pp 567, 568.

Comment
Background
Chordomas account for less than 5% of primary malignant bone tumors. In order of decreasing frequency, the reported locations of chordoma are sacrococcygeal (50% to 60%), skull base (25% to 35%), and cervicothoracolumbar vertebral bodies (approximately 15%). The cervical spine is the most common site, with predominance in the C2 vertebra; the thoracic and lumbar spine is involved less frequently.

Histopathology
Chordomas arise from intraosseous notochordal remnants and are slow growing and lobulated. Two types are distinguished histopathologically: typical chordomas, which have a watery, gelatinous matrix; and chondroid chordomas, in which this matrix is replaced by cartilaginous foci.

Imaging
Chordomas are primarily paravertebral (Figs. A and B), which may be the result of tumor extension from the most frequent site of involvement: the vertebral body. Alternatively, the paravertebral location may represent growth originating from one of the extraosseous notochordal rests (ecchordoses) known to exist in this region. On CT scan, chordomas appear homogeneous and isodense to muscle. CT is useful for detecting calcifications (occurring in 30% to 70% of cases) and vertebral osteosclerosis. On MRI, chordomas are usually inhomogeneous on T1-weighted images because of a combination of cystic and solid components; however, they may occasionally have relatively low signal intensity compared with muscle (Figs. A and C). On T2-weighted images (Fig. B), chordomas are heterogeneously hyperintense and have a lobular contour, with hypointense septations separating the lobules. This appearance is characteristic of chordomas, in which fibrous strands (accounting for the hypointense septations) create lobules of either mucin-containing physaliphorous cells or purely cystic mucinous pools (accounting for the lobular hyperintensities). This feature may help differentiate chordomas from the more common paraspinal and spinal masses.

Enhancement of chordomas after contrast agent administration is variable (Fig. D).

Management
Surgery and adjuvant radiation therapy in cases of incomplete resection are the mainstays of treatment. Imatinib, a platelet-derived growth factor receptor inhibitor, was shown to be active in a phase II trial, with symptomatic and radiologic responses.

Notes

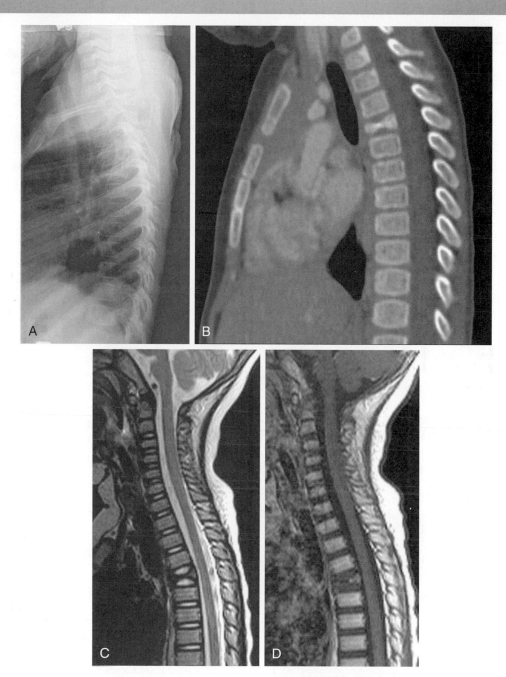

History: A 2-year-old girl presents with weakness and decreased appetite.

1. What should be included in the differential diagnosis? (Choose all that apply.)
   a. Ewing's sarcoma
   b. Langerhans cell histiocytosis
   c. Osteomyelitis
   d. Giant cell tumor
   e. Lymphoma

2. What is the most common skeletal site of involvement in patients with this disorder?
   a. Spine
   b. Skull
   c. Pelvis
   d. Ribs

3. What would be the most likely treatment in this case?
   a. Surgery
   b. Radiotherapy
   c. Conservative treatment
   d. Vertebroplasty

4. Which of the following is *not* a cause of vertebra plana in adults?
   a. Trauma
   b. Osteopoikilosis
   c. Metastatic disease
   d. Multiple myeloma

Langerhans Cell Histiocytosis with Vertebra Plana

1. a, b, c, and e

2. b

3. c

4. b

Reference

Azouz EM, Saigal G, Rodriguez MM, et al: Langerhans' cell histiocytosis: Pathology, imaging and treatment of skeletal involvement, *Pediatr Radiol* 35(2):103-115, 2005.

Cross-Reference

Neuroradiology: The REQUISITES, 3rd ed, p 569.

Comment

Background

Vertebra plana is marked flattening of a vertebral body with preserved intervertebral disk space and lack of kyphosis. Langerhans cell histiocytosis is the most common cause of vertebra plana in children. Other causes of vertebra plana include multiple myeloma, metastatic disease, Ewing's sarcoma, lymphoma, leukemia, Gaucher disease, aneurysmal bone cyst, trauma, and infection. Langerhans cell histiocytosis is predominantly a disease of childhood, with more than 50% of cases diagnosed between ages 1 and 15 years. Boys are affected slightly more often than girls. The disease may be focal or systemic. The most frequent site of skeletal lesions is the skull. Other sites include the pelvis, spine, mandible, ribs, and tubular bones. In the spine, Langerhans cell histiocytosis involves mainly the vertebral bodies, with a predilection for the thoracic spine, followed by the lumbar and cervical spine. Involvement of posterior elements is less common. Involvement of the vertebral body may result in anterior wedging or, more commonly, near collapse, with marked flattening of the vertebral body—the characteristic "vertebra plana" appearance.

Histopathology

Langerhans cell histiocytosis encompasses a set of clinico-pathologic entities (previously called histiocytosis X) that result from abnormal clonal proliferation of Langerhans cells. Eosinophilic granuloma is the unifocal clinical variant.

Imaging

When a clinical diagnosis of Langerhans cell histiocytosis is suspected, a radiographic skeletal survey or bone scintigraphy should be performed to detect other bony lesions; however, lesions may be missed on both bone scans and radiographs. Rib, spine, and pelvic lesions are more easily missed on radiographs (Fig. A). On CT scan, Langerhans cell histiocytosis initially manifests as a lytic area with poorly defined margins. The body of the vertebra is usually involved, with bony destruction leading to a pathologic fracture and a characteristic vertebra plana deformity. CT three-dimensional sagittal reconstructions help identify the vertebra plana and its surrounding anatomy. Preservation of the disk space above and below the vertebral body collapse (Fig. B) helps differentiate this lesion from vertebral osteomyelitis.

MRI on initial presentation usually shows a lesion that is hyperintense on T2-weighted images and hypointense on T1-weighted images and exhibits enhancement (relative to unaffected vertebrae) after contrast agent administration. Later, the involved vertebral body becomes isointense on T1-weighted images and isointense to hypointense on T2-weighted images (Fig. C), shows no enhancement (Fig. D), and appears as a thin plane of collapsed bone separating the two adjacent, intact intervertebral disks. The adjacent disks are similar in stature and intensity to normal nonadjacent disks (see Figs. C and D). The posterior portion of the vertebra plana may be displaced into the canal, resulting in an epidural mass. Some authors have suggested that the variations in signal intensity in the collapsed vertebral body over time are manifestations of a healing stage.

Management

Partial or almost complete height reconstitution is the usual healing pattern observed in vertebra plana lesions. Neurologic deficits usually resolve as osseous healing progresses. Because most lesions spontaneously regress, vertebra plana is often treated conservatively. Surgery is rarely indicated for spinal lesions in these patients unless they have symptoms secondary to compression of the spinal cord by the collapsed vertebra.

Notes

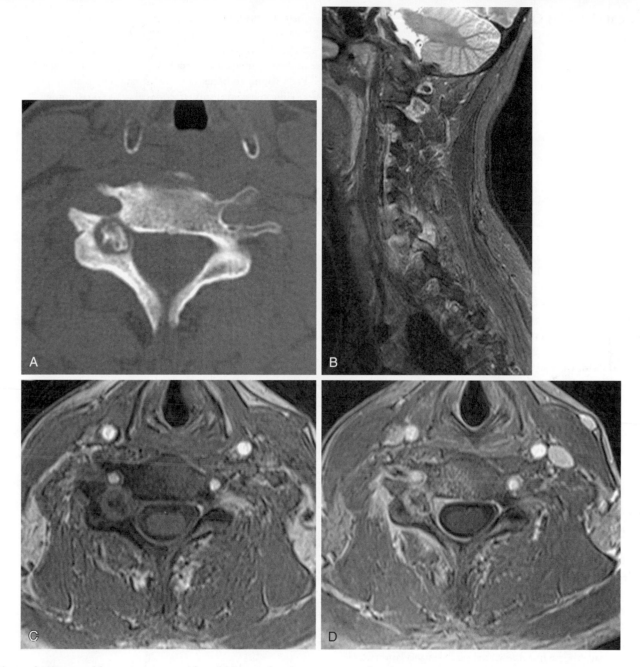

History: A 40-year-old man presents with stabbing neck pain radiating to the right arm and scapula for the past 5 years, relieved by naproxen.

1. What should be included in the differential diagnosis? (Choose all that apply.)
   a. Osteoid osteoma
   b. Osteoblastoma
   c. Lymphoma
   d. Stress fracture
   e. Atypical infection

2. Which part of the vertebra does osteoid osteoma most commonly affect?
   a. Vertebral body
   b. Pedicle

   c. Lamina
   d. Articular facet

3. What is the most common symptom in patients with osteoid osteoma?
   a. Local pain
   b. Radicular pain
   c. Fever
   d. Lower extremity weakness

4. Which imaging technique is the study of choice for the detection and characterization of suspected osteoid osteoma?
   a. MRI
   b. Plain film
   c. CT
   d. Bone scan

Cervical Osteoid Osteoma

1. a and e

2. c

3. a

4. c

References

Laus M, Albisinni U, Alfonso C, et al: Osteoid osteoma of the cervical spine: Surgical treatment or percutaneous radiofrequency coagulation? *Eur Spine J* 16(12):2078-2082, 2007.

Liu PT, Chivers FS, Roberts CC, et al: Imaging of osteoid osteoma with dynamic gadolinium-enhanced MR imaging, *Radiology* 227(3):691-700, 2003.

Spouge AR, Thain LM: Osteoid osteoma: MR imaging revisited, *Clin Imaging* 24(1):19-27, 2000.

Cross-Reference

Neuroradiology: The REQUISITES, 3rd ed, pp 568-569.

Comment

Background

Osteoid osteoma is a benign bone neoplasm of unknown etiology. The tumor is usually smaller than 1.5 cm in diameter. In about two thirds of cases, the appendicular skeleton is involved, with the lumbar region most commonly affected, followed by the cervical spine. The posterior elements are involved in 75% of cases, and the vertebral body is involved in only 7%. Affected patients are usually 10 to 30 years old and are predominantly male. The classic manifestation is focal bone pain at the site of the tumor. The pain worsens at night and is relieved by salicylates or nonsteroidal anti-inflammatory drugs.

Histopathology

Osteoid osteoma consists of a small nidus of vascular connective tissue with a surrounding osteoid matrix. The extent of the sclerotic bony reaction around the nidus is variable and may include the entire vertebral body and the adjacent vertebrae.

Imaging

CT scan is the study of choice for the detection and precise localization of the nidus. CT is particularly effective in areas with complex anatomy, such as the spinal pedicles and laminae. The classic finding is a small (<1.5 cm), rounded area of low attenuation, with or without central calcification, surrounded by a variable zone of sclerosis (Fig. A). MRI findings (Figs. B-D) are less characteristic and may simulate a malignant tumor or osteomyelitis, owing to the marrow and soft tissue edema (see Fig. B). MRI alone may lead to misdiagnosis. Lesions are typically low to intermediate signal on spin-echo T1-weighted images (see Fig. C). Signal intensity on T2-weighted sequences is variable. Marrow edema is most conspicuous on inversion-recovery or fat-suppressed fast-spin-echo T2-weighted sequences (see Fig. B). Enhancement of the nidus may be variable (see Fig. D) and is more prominent in lesions that have less mineralization. Dynamic contrast-enhanced MRI can depict osteoid osteomas with greater conspicuity.

Management

Osteoid osteoma can be treated by percutaneous ablation using radiofrequency, ethanol, laser, or thermocoagulation under CT guidance. Percutaneous radiofrequency ablation has been found to be as effective as surgery with respect to controlling the symptoms of cervical osteoid osteoma.

Notes

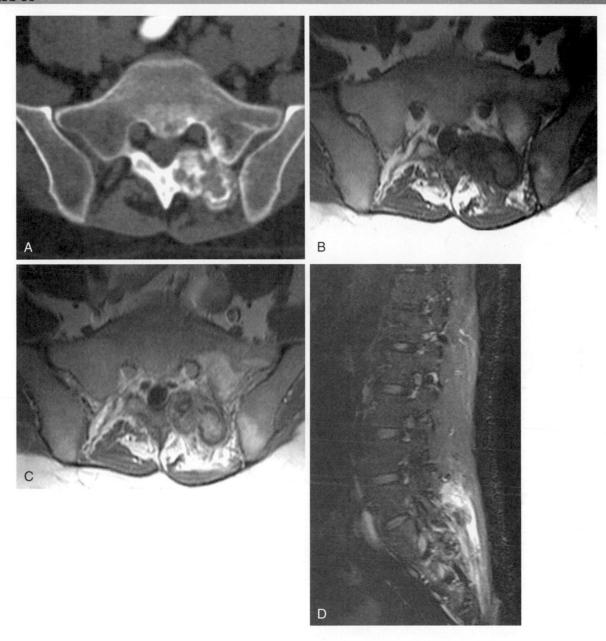

History: A 35-year-old man presents with left lower back and buttock pain for the past 6 months. The pain is worse at night; oral medications provide minimal relief.

1. What should be included in the differential diagnosis? (Choose all that apply.)
   a. Giant cell tumor
   b. Lymphoma
   c. Osteoblastoma
   d. Metastasis
   e. Chordoma

2. What percentage of spinal osteoblastomas are found in the sacrum?
   a. 3%
   b. About 20%
   c. More than 50%
   d. 75%

3. What is the "flare phenomenon"?
   a. Redness in the skin overlying the tumor
   b. Rapid tumor growth after radiation therapy
   c. Peritumoral edema in bone and soft tissue
   d. Facial flushing seen in patients with osteoblastoma

4. All of the following statements regarding osteoblastoma are true *except:*
   a. Affected patients are usually young men.
   b. The diagnosis is often delayed when the lesion involves the sacrum.
   c. Calcifications are usually multiple.
   d. The recurrence rate after intralesional excision is high.

Osteoblastoma of the Sacrum

1. a, b, c, d, and e

2. b

3. c

4. d

References

Llauger J, Palmer J, Amores S, et al: Primary tumors of the sacrum: Diagnostic imaging, *AJR Am J Roentgenol* 174(2):417-424, 2000.

Whittingham-Jones P, Hughes R, Fajinmi M, et al: Osteoblastoma crossing the sacro-iliac joint, *Skeletal Radiol* 36(3):249-252, 2007.

Cross-Reference

Neuroradiology: The REQUISITES, 3rd ed, pp 568-569.

Comment

Background

Osteoblastomas are rare lesions, constituting 1% to 2% of all primary bone tumors. Approximately 40% of all osteoblastomas are located in the spine; 17% of spinal osteoblastomas are found in the sacrum. The mean age of patients at presentation is 20 years, with a slight male preponderance. Pain, scoliosis, and neurologic deficits are the most common presenting symptoms.

Histopathology

Osteoblastomas comprise numerous osteoblasts that produce osteoid and woven bone. Spinal osteoblastomas most frequently involve the posterior vertebral elements.

Imaging

The typical osteoblastoma shows a lytic defect larger than 1.5 cm in diameter, surrounded by a sclerotic ring. Calcifications, when present, are usually multiple (Fig. A). In some patients, osteoblastomas showing cortical destruction and extension into adjacent soft tissue have an aggressive appearance. On MRI (Figs. B-D), signal intensity patterns are usually nonspecific. Peritumoral edema in marrow and in soft tissue (flare phenomenon), representing an inflammatory response to the lesion, is a characteristic finding (see Fig. D).

Management

Treatment consists of extensive intralesional curettage or wide excision in more aggressive lesions.

Notes

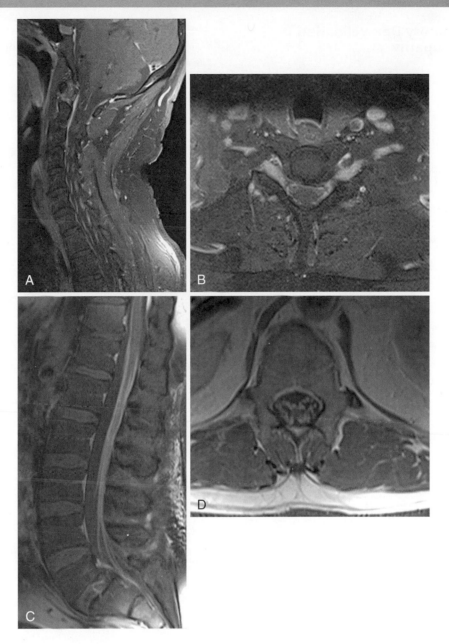

History: A 50-year-old patient presents with progressive numbness and weakness in the upper and lower extremities for the past 4 months.

1. What should be included in the differential diagnosis? (Choose all that apply.)
   a. Guillain-Barré syndrome (GBS)
   b. Chronic inflammatory demyelinating polyradiculoneuropathy (CIDP)
   c. Sarcoidosis
   d. Cytomegalovirus (CMV) infection
   e. Acute disseminated encephalomyelitis

2. Which of the following features is *least* helpful in differentiating CIDP from GBS?
   a. Illness develops and progresses over months
   b. Patient improves and then deteriorates a year later
   c. Motor involvement
   d. Intrathecal nerve root enlargement and enhancement

3. Which of the following statements regarding enhancement of the nerve roots is *false?*
   a. Nerve root enhancement is often seen in patients with Charcot-Marie-Tooth disease.
   b. Radiculopathy secondary to focal disk herniation may show nerve root enhancement.
   c. Nerve root enhancement in the neural foramina is a common finding with no significance.
   d. Leptomeningeal carcinomatosis may cause enlargement and enhancement of the nerve roots.

4. Which of the following entities is *not* a cause of spinal nerve root enhancement?
   a. Radiation-induced polyradiculopathy
   b. Lymphoma
   c. CMV polyradiculitis
   d. Diabetic amyotrophy

Chronic Inflammatory Demyelinating Polyradiculoneuropathy

1. a, b, c, and d

2. c

3. a

4. d

References

Midroni G, de Tilly LN, Gray B, et al: MRI of the cauda equina in CIDP: Clinical correlations, *J Neurol Sci* 170(1):36-44, 1999.

Toyka KV, Gold R: The pathogenesis of CIDP: Rationale for treatment with immunomodulatory agents, *Neurology* 60(8 Suppl):S2-S7, 2003.

Cross-Reference

Neuroradiology: The REQUISITES, 3rd ed, p 564.

Comment

Background

CIDP is an acquired, immune-mediated demyelinating disorder of the peripheral nervous system characterized by either a relapsing and remitting course or a progressive course. It is characterized by progressive motor weakness, sensory dysfunction, or both in more than one limb, with loss or reduction of reflexes. Diagnostic criteria are based on clinical features, electrodiagnostic findings, cerebrospinal fluid results, and nerve biopsy findings, although they have been modified over the years to include imaging characteristics as supportive diagnostic criteria for CIDP.

Histopathology

The immunopathogenesis of CIDP is not fully understood. Breakdown of the blood-nerve barrier likely plays a cardinal role, allowing macrophages and T cells to enter the endoneurium and initiate an immune reaction involving antimyelin antibodies and other elements that cause demyelination and axonal loss. Biopsy of the sural nerve may demonstrate evidence of segmental demyelination and remyelination with occasional "onion bulb" formation, particularly in relapsing cases.

Imaging

Enlargement and enhancement of the spinal nerve roots (Figs. A and B), cauda equina (Figs. C and D), brachial and lumbosacral plexus, cranial nerves, and sciatic nerve are well documented in CIDP, central canal stenosis, spinal cord compression, and spinal cord atrophy secondary to nerve root hypertrophy. Nerve root enhancement as shown in this case (Figs. A-D) may be observed in GBS, sarcoidosis, postradiation injury, and CMV infection and, less commonly, in hereditary motor and sensory neuropathy, infectious (pyogenic or granulomatous) disease, and neoplastic disease involving the leptomeninges (carcinomatosis, lymphoma, leukemia).

Management

Corticosteroids, intravenous immunoglobulin, and plasmapheresis provide clinical improvement in most patients with CIDP.

Notes

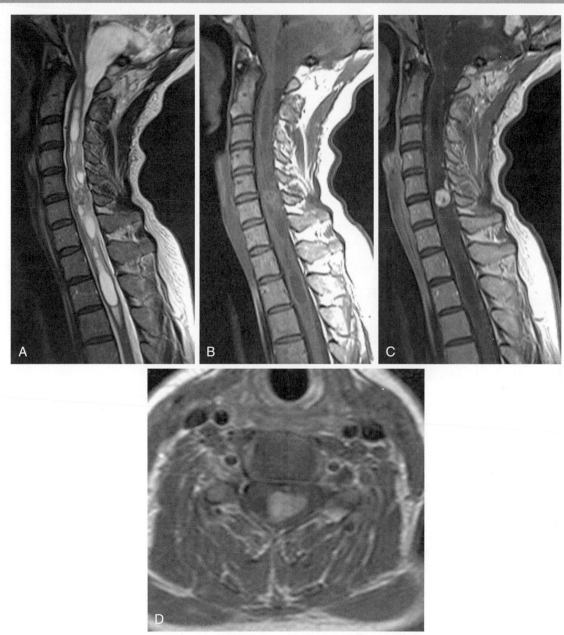

History: A 49-year-old woman with a history of resection of a posterior fossa tumor 17 years ago now presents with numbness in the fingers.

1. What should be included in the differential diagnosis? (Choose all that apply.)
   a. Arteriovenous malformation
   b. Hemangioblastoma
   c. Ependymoma
   d. Meningioma
   e. Vascular metastasis

2. Which of the following neurocutaneous syndromes is associated with multiple hemangioblastomas?
   a. von Hippel-Lindau (VHL) disease
   b. Neurofibromatosis type 1
   c. Neurofibromatosis type 2
   d. Tuberous sclerosis

3. Which of the following studies would be *least* appropriate in the workup of this patient?
   a. Abdominal ultrasound
   b. MRI of the brain
   c. MRI of the brachial plexus
   d. Ophthalmoscopic evaluation

4. Which of the following temporal bone lesions is reportedly associated with VHL disease?
   a. Cholesteatoma
   b. Cholesterol granuloma
   c. Squamous cell carcinoma
   d. Endolymphatic sac tumor

Cervical Hemangioblastoma

1. a, b, c, and e

2. a

3. c

4. d

Reference

Chu BC, Terae S, Hida K, et al: MR findings in spinal hemangioblastoma: Correlation with symptoms and with angiographic and surgical findings, *AJNR Am J Neuroradiol* 22(1):206-217, 2001.

Cross-Reference

Neuroradiology: The REQUISITES, 3rd ed, pp 558-559.

Comment

Background

Hemangioblastomas are vascular tumors that can be found throughout the neuraxis, primarily in the cerebellum and spinal cord. These tumors occur more commonly as sporadic, isolated lesions; however, approximately one third of patients with spinal hemangioblastomas have VHL disease, which means that a workup for VHL disease and its various clinically significant manifestations should be undertaken if a spinal hemangioblastoma is found.

Imaging

Spinal hemangioblastoma is usually intramedullary but may have an exophytic component (Figs. A-D). It involves the thoracic (51% of cases) or cervical (38% of cases) cord. Intramedullary hemangioblastoma is typically located in the posterior half of the spinal cord, supplied by the posterior spinal arteries. The tumor consists of a hypervascular nodular mass, usually with an associated cyst or syrinx and a variable degree of surrounding edema (see Fig. C). An associated cyst is present in 43% of all spinal hemangioblastomas; if only intramedullary hemangioblastomas are considered, 67% have an associated cyst. The cyst may contain hemorrhagic components. Although a cyst or syrinx is not specific to spinal hemangioblastomas, a small, superficially located intramedullary tumor with a large cyst is considered characteristic. No individual vessels are recognized within the nodular mass angiographically, although a rapid shunt through the tumor nodule and into a distended venous structure or structures has been described. As shown in this case, diffuse cord enlargement often extends over several segments, with heterogeneous signal intensity on T1- and T2-weighted images.

Foci of low signal intensity within the cord or on its surface can be due to flowing blood or the magnetic susceptibility effects of hemosiderin. Magnetic resonance angiography (MRA) with contrast agent administration is useful to establish these "signal voids" as blood flow within normal-sized or enlarged vessels and to show that some of the vessels are contiguous with the enhancing tumor nodule.

Management

Although considered histologically benign, hemangioblastomas may cause significant neurologic deficits, depending on their location. Advances in imaging and microsurgery have markedly improved the treatment of these intraspinal lesions.

Notes

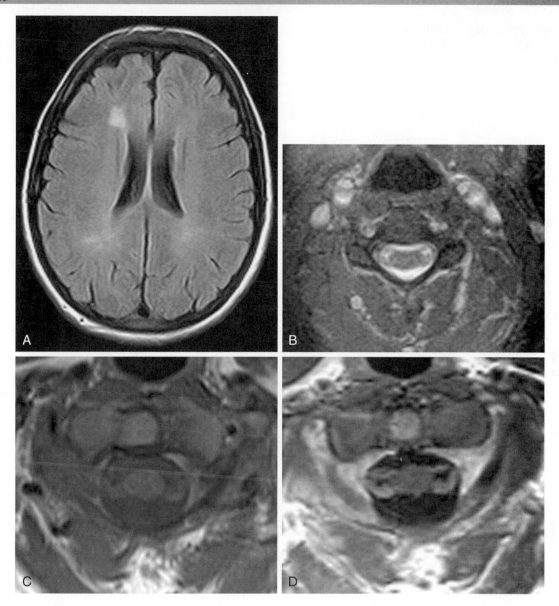

History: A 30-year-old woman with a history of long-standing multiple sclerosis presents with multiple episodes of numbness and weakness in the upper and lower extremities for the past 7 years.

1. What should be included in the differential diagnosis? (Choose all that apply.)
   a. Charcot-Marie-Tooth disease
   b. Chronic inflammatory demyelinating polyradiculo-neuropathy (CIDP)
   c. Neurofibromatosis
   d. Systemic lupus erythematosus

2. All of the statements regarding the criteria used in the diagnosis of CIDP are true *except:*
   a. CIDP should be considered in any patient with relapsing and remitting progressive polyradiculoneuropathy.
   b. Electrodiagnostic tests are mandatory.
   c. Increased cerebrospinal fluid (CSF) protein and normal CSF white blood cell count are typical.
   d. The final diagnosis of CIDP is made with nerve biopsy.

3. All of the following findings support acute-onset CIDP in a patient initially diagnosed as having Guillain-Barré syndrome *except:*
   a. Deterioration continues for more than 2 months after onset.
   b. Isolated enhancement of the anterior spinal roots of the cauda equina is seen on MRI.
   c. More than three treatment-related fluctuations occur.
   d. Initial presentation includes prominent sensory symptoms and signs.

4. Which of the following nerves is *unlikely* to be involved with CIDP?
   a. Sciatic nerve
   b. Brachial plexus
   c. Olfactory nerve
   d. Trigeminal nerve

Chronic Inflammatory Demyelinating Polyradiculoneuropathy Associated with Multiple Sclerosis

1. b

2. d

3. b

4. c

References

Beydoun SR, Muir J, Apelian RG, et al: Clinical and imaging findings in three patients with advanced inflammatory demyelinating polyradiculoneuropathy associated with nerve root hypertrophy, *J Clin Neuromuscul Dis* 13(3):105-112, 2012.

Joint Task Force of the EFNS and the PNS: European Federation of Neurological Societies/Peripheral Nerve Society guideline on management of chronic inflammatory demyelinating polyradiculoneuropathy: Report of a Joint Task Force of the European Federation of Neurological Societies and the Peripheral Nerve Society—first revision, *J Peripher Nerv Syst* 15(1):1-9, 2010.

Sharma KR, Saadia D, Facca AG, et al: Chronic inflammatory demyelinating polyradiculoneuropathy associated with multiple sclerosis, *J Clin Neuromuscul Dis* 9(4):385-396, 2008.

Cross-Reference

Neuroradiology: The REQUISITES, 3rd ed, p 564.

Comment

Clinical Findings

CIDP should be considered in any patient with a progressive symmetric or asymmetric polyradiculoneuropathy in whom the clinical course is relapsing and remitting or progresses for more than 2 months. CIDP has been reported in patients with central nervous system demyelinating diseases such as multiple sclerosis (Fig. A), suggesting that there may be common antigenic targets in the central and peripheral nervous systems in this subset of patients. Although most patients with CIDP have a chronic onset, some have an acute onset resembling Guillain-Barré syndrome.

Diagnostic Criteria

The diagnosis of CIDP rests on a combination of clinical, electrodiagnostic, and laboratory features that excludes or eliminates other disorders that may appear similar to CIDP. CSF examination, MRI, and a trial of immunotherapy may assist the diagnosis. Nerve biopsy can provide supportive evidence for the diagnosis of CIDP; however, positive findings are not specific, and negative findings do not exclude the diagnosis. The nerve selected for biopsy should be clinically and electrophysiologically affected; usually the sural nerve is chosen.

Imaging

The characteristic findings on MRI are diffuse, marked enlargement of peripheral nerves and spinal roots (Figs. B-D) and plexus hypertrophy, with nerve root enhancement and minimal enhancement of the trunks.

Management

Treatment is with intravenous immunoglobulins or corticosteroids. Plasma exchange is also effective but may be less tolerated.

Notes

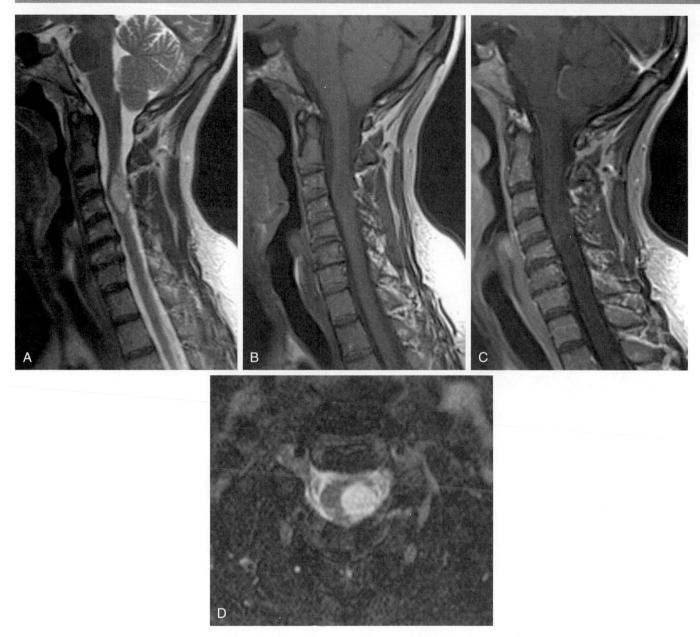

History: A 45-year-old woman presents with neck pain radiating to the scapula and left arm pain, numbness, and tingling for the past 9 months.

1. What should be included in the differential diagnosis? (Choose all that apply.)
   a. Ependymoma
   b. Subependymoma
   c. Neurenteric cyst
   d. Meningioma
   e. Cavernoma

2. All of the following imaging features favor the diagnosis of subependymoma over ependymoma *except:*
   a. Eccentric location within the cord
   b. Exophytic component
   c. Lack of enhancement
   d. Presence of edema

3. All of the following are typical imaging features of subependymoma *except:*
   a. Sharply demarcated tumor margins
   b. Hypointense T1 signal
   c. Hypointense T2 signal
   d. Minimal enhancement

4. What is the most common site of spinal subependymomas?
   a. Cervical region
   b. Cervicothoracic junction
   c. Thoracic region
   d. Lumbar region

Cervical Subependymoma

1. a, b, and c

2. d

3. c

4. a

References

Jang WY, Lee JK, Lee JH, et al: Intramedullary subependymoma of the thoracic spinal cord, *J Clin Neurosci* 16(6):851-853, 2009.

Zenmyo M, Ishido Y, Terahara M, et al: Intramedullary subependymoma of the cervical spinal cord: A case report with immunohistochemical study, *Int J Neurosci* 120(10):676-679, 2010.

Cross-Reference

Neuroradiology: The REQUISITES, 3rd ed, pp 557-558.

Comment

Background

Spinal subependymomas are rare, accounting for less than 2% of all spinal cord tumors. They are more common in men, and the mean age at presentation is 42 years. Although spinal subependymomas occur much less frequently than subependymomas in intracranial locations, they become symptomatic early. Most subependymomas are intramedullary lesions occurring in the cervical and cervicothoracic regions. Because these lesions grow slowly, an acute onset of symptoms is unlikely.

Histopathology

Subependymomas are histologically characterized by sparse cellularity, with clusters of glial cells in a fibrillary stroma that typically contains prominent vascular structures and microcystic changes. In contrast to astrocytomas and ependymomas, subependymomas tend to grow eccentrically within the cord or have an exophytic component.

Imaging

Spinal subependymomas are difficult to distinguish from other intramedullary spinal tumors based on imaging findings; however, the possibility of subependymoma should be kept in mind when an eccentric, well-demarcated intramedullary tumor is identified in an adult. MRI usually reveals segmental, fusiform dilatation of the cord (Figs. A-C), with isointense or low T1 signal (Fig. B) and high T2 signal (Figs. A and D) intensities. Contrast enhancement is minimal or absent (Fig. C).

Management

Total removal of the tumor is usually curative and results in improved function. Subtotal removal should be considered when the tumor is poorly demarcated from the spinal cord, to avoid postoperative neurologic deficits.

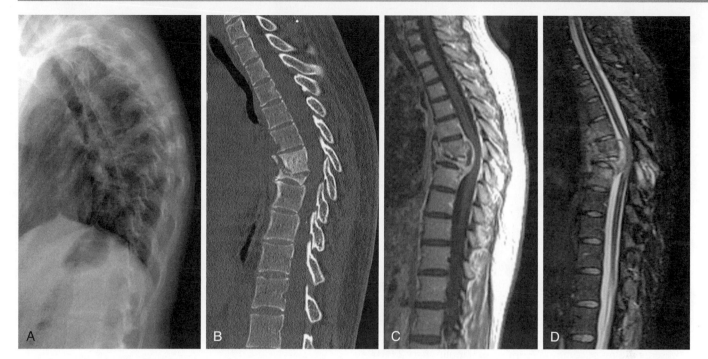

A | B | C | D

History: A 29-year-old woman who recently emigrated from India presents with a long-standing history of back pain between the shoulder blades, which has worsened over the last month, and numbness below the level of her breasts for the past few days.

1. What should be included in the differential diagnosis? (Choose all that apply.)
   a. Pyogenic diskitis osteomyelitis
   b. Tuberculous spondylitis
   c. Paget's disease
   d. Metastasis
   e. Neuropathic spondyloarthropathy

2. All of the following findings favor tuberculous spondylitis over pyogenic spondylitis *except:*
   a. Involvement of several contiguous segments
   b. Body collapse with kyphotic deformity
   c. Rapid progression with early destruction of the disk space
   d. Paraspinal abscesses containing calcifications

3. Which spinal segment is most commonly involved in tuberculous spondylitis?
   a. Cervical spine
   b. Thoracic spine
   c. Lumbar spine
   d. Sacrum

4. Which of the following statements regarding tuberculous spondylitis is *false?*
   a. Involvement of the posterior elements is highly suggestive of tuberculosis (TB).
   b. Involvement of the spine occurs by direct spread from a paraspinal infection.
   c. Isolated involvement of the vertebral arch is more commonly found in patients with AIDS.
   d. Early disk destruction is not typical.

Tuberculous Spondylitis (Pott's Disease)

1. a, b, d, and e

2. c

3. b

4. b

References

Rivas-Garcia A, Sarria-Estrada S, Torrents-Odin C, et al: Imaging findings of Pott's disease, *Eur Spine J* 4:567-578, 2013.

Shikhare SN, Singh DR, Shimpi TR, et al: Tuberculous osteomyelitis and spondylodiscitis, *Semin Musculoskelet Radiol* 15(5):446-458, 2011.

Cross-Reference

Neuroradiology: The REQUISITES, 3rd ed, pp 543-546.

Comment

Background

Musculoskeletal involvement with TB is uncommon; however, more than 50% of cases of skeletal TB affect the vertebral column. Tuberculous spondylitis, also known as Pott's disease, represents the most common form of extrapulmonary TB. It is most prevalent in adults, with no sex predominance.

Pathophysiology

Involvement of the spine usually occurs by hematogenous spread via the paravertebral vascular plexus and, rarely, by direct extension. Because the mycobacterium does not produce proteolytic enzymes, early disk destruction is not typical.

Imaging

Radiographic changes are often present at the time of the initial study (Fig. A), and plain films are the initial screening modality when infectious spondylitis is suspected. CT better evaluates vertebral body destruction (Fig. B) and reliably detects calcifications in paraspinal soft tissue masses, a finding highly suggestive of TB. MRI is the modality of choice for early detection of the disease and evaluation of the canal.

Four different MRI patterns of disease are found in vertebral TB: paradiskal, anterior, central, and posterior lesions. Paradiskal infection begins in the vertebral metaphysis, eroding the end-plate and leading to disk involvement; this results in decreased T1 and increased T2 and short tau inversion recovery (STIR) signals in the vertebral bodies. In the anterior pattern, the infection starts in the corner of the vertebral body and spreads to the adjacent vertebrae underneath the anterior longitudinal ligament, leading to anterolateral scalloping of the vertebral body and anterior vertebral collapse. MRI findings in this pattern consist of a subligamentous abscess with contrast enhancement, preservation of the disks, and abnormal signal involving multiple vertebral segments (Figs. C and D). In central lesions, the infection affects a single vertebral body. If the infection progresses, the whole vertebral body collapses, and this can be confused with malignancy. MRI shows hypointense T1-weighted signal in the one affected vertebra and vertebral collapse with disk preservation. Posterior arch involvement (Fig. D) is found in 5% of patients and may be difficult to differentiate from metastasis, especially when the disk is preserved. Advanced stages of the disease are characterized by sclerosis, ankylosis, and anterior body collapse, leading to progressive kyphosis and gibbous deformity.

Management

Treatment is with anti-TB drugs. The minimum duration of treatment is 6 to 9 months.

Notes

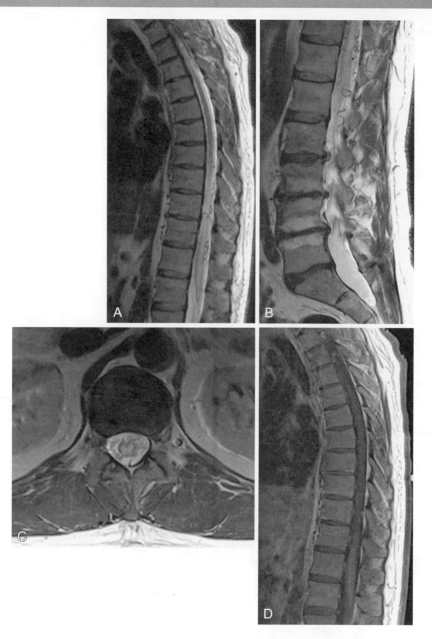

History: A 57-year-old man with a 2-year history of back pain and progressive lower extremity numbness for the past 8 months presents with recent episodes of imbalance and urinary incontinence.

1. What should be included in the differential diagnosis? (Choose all that apply.)
   a. Arteriovenous malformation (AVM)
   b. Dural arteriovenous fistula (DAVF)
   c. Perimedullary fistula
   d. Hemangioblastoma
   e. Paraganglioma

2. Which of the following spinal vascular lesions is most common in the general population?
   a. DAVF
   b. Intramedullary glomus AVM
   c. Juvenile-type AVM
   d. Perimedullary fistula

3. Which MRI finding is most frequently observed in DAVF?
   a. Cord hyperintensity on T2-weighted images
   b. Cord enlargement
   c. Cord enhancement
   d. Abnormal intradural (subarachnoid) vessels

4. What is the cause of spinal cord enhancement on the T1-weighted image?
   a. Arterial cord infarct
   b. Capillary leak
   c. Venous congestion
   d. Neoplastic metaplasia

Dural Arteriovenous Fistula

1. b and c

2. a

3. a

4. c

References

Krings T, Geibprasert S: Spinal dural arteriovenous fistulas, *AJNR Am J Neuroradiol* 30(4):639-648, 2009.

Saraf-Lavi E, Bowen BC, Quencer RM, et al: Detection of spinal dural arteriovenous fistulae with MRI and contrast-enhanced MR angiography: Sensitivity, specificity, and prediction of vertebral level, *AJNR Am J Neuroradiol* 23(5):858-867, 2002.

Cross-Reference

Neuroradiology: The REQUISITES, 3rd ed, pp 572-574.

Comment

Background

Spinal DAVFs are uncommon vascular malformations that are underdiagnosed. Delayed treatment can lead to considerable morbidity. Men are affected five times more often than women, and the mean age at diagnosis is 55 to 60 years.

Pathophysiology

Most fistulas are solitary lesions and are found in the thoracolumbar spine between T6 and L2. It is thought that spinal DAVF is an acquired disease. The arteriovenous shunt is located inside the dura mater close to the spinal nerve root, where the arterial blood flow from the radiculomedullary artery directly connects with the vein at the dorsal surface of the dural root sleeve in the neural foramen. The increased pressure in the vein leads to decreased drainage and venous congestion, with intramedullary edema and progressive myelopathy.

Imaging

The findings of cord signal abnormality and enhancement are nonspecific and may result from neoplastic, inflammatory, or vascular conditions. Cord enlargement usually favors neoplasm, although any intramedullary process that produces edema and breakdown of the blood-cord barrier can mimic neoplasm. The finding of multiple "flow voids" is the key to narrowing the differential diagnosis. The presence of flow voids and serpentine enhancement extending over at least three contiguous vertebral segments in the intradural space, as well as increased number, size, and tortuosity of these vessels, is strongly associated with the presence of DAVF. In this case (Figs. A-D), no intramedullary tangle of vessels (nidus) was identified. An intramedullary AVM causing the perimedullary flow voids was considered less likely than a DAVF. Other causes of enlargement of the intradural veins include craniospinal hypotension and collateral venous drainage secondary to inferior vena cava occlusion.

Management

Treatment is either surgical interruption of the draining medullary vein or endovascular therapy with glue to occlude the fistula permanently.

Notes

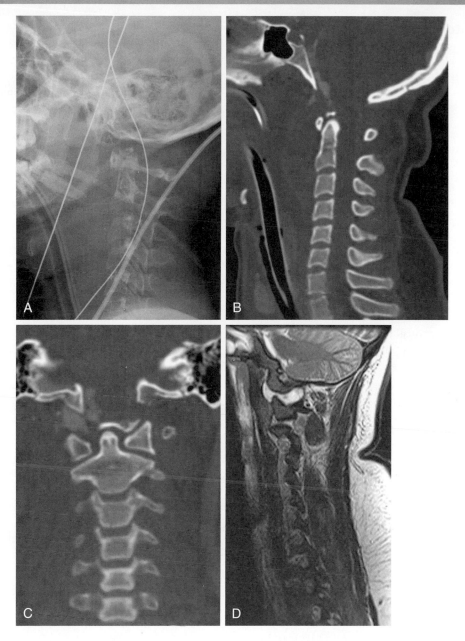

History: A 19-year-old woman (patient 1) who was an unrestrained backseat passenger was ejected in a motor vehicle accident and is unresponsive. A 36-year-old man (patient 2) was involved in a motorcycle accident; he was not wearing a helmet and sustained a head injury.

1. What should be included in the differential diagnosis? (Choose all that apply.)
   a. Rotatory subluxation
   b. Atlantoaxial subluxation
   c. Hangman's fracture
   d. Craniocervical dissociation
   e. Atlantooccipital dissociation

2. The craniocervical junction is composed of the following osseous structures *except:*
   a. Occiput
   b. Atlas
   c. Axis
   d. Clivus

3. Which of the following is the most common spinocerebral injury in fatal cases of atlantooccipital dislocation?
   a. Laceration of the pontomedullary junction
   b. Laceration of the spinal cord
   c. Subdural hemorrhage
   d. Laceration of the midbrain

4. Traumatic craniocervical dissociation is most likely to be associated with injury to which artery?
   a. Common carotid artery
   b. Internal carotid artery
   c. External carotid artery
   d. Vertebral artery

Traumatic Atlantooccipital Dissociation

1. d and e

2. d

3. a

4. d

References

Bellabarba C: Injuries of the craniocervical junction. In Bucholz RW, editor: *Rockwood and Green's fractures in adults*, ed 6, Philadelphia, 2006, Lippincott.

Deliganis A, Baxter AB, Hanson JA: Radiologic spectrum of craniocervical distraction injuries, *Radiographics* 20:S237-S250, 2000.

Vaccaro A: *Spine and spinal cord trauma: Evidence-based management*, New York, 2010, Thieme Medical Publishers.

Cross-Reference

Neuroradiology: The REQUISITES, 3rd ed, pp 578-579.

Comment

Anatomy

Stability of the craniocervical junction depends on the integrity of the osseous components, joint capsules, and ligaments.

Pathophysiology

Disruption of the tectorial membrane (cranial continuation of the posterior longitudinal ligament) and alar ligaments (paired ligaments extending from the odontoid process to the lateral margins of the foramen magnum, limiting lateral rotation of the skull) is required to produce atlantooccipital dislocation. Occipital condyle fractures may be classified as impaction fractures, extensions of occipital skull fractures, or avulsion fractures at the insertions of the alar ligaments. The last are potentially unstable fractures, particularly if displaced.

Imaging

Despite their low sensitivity, plain radiographs are often the first images obtained in patients with cervical spine trauma (Fig. A). Measurements used to help diagnose craniocervical junction injury include the basion-dental interval (<10 mm) and the basion-axial interval (<12 mm). CT scan has greater accuracy for the diagnosis of cervical spine trauma; coronal and sagittal reconstructions allow better depictions of the osseous relationships and of the occipital condyle fractures that may be associated with craniocervical dissociation (Figs. B and C). On CT scan, a space greater than 4 mm between the occipital condyles and C1 is suggestive of atlantooccipital dislocation. Findings that suggest the presence of atlantooccipital injuries include joint subluxation or dislocation, occipital condyle fracture, suboccipital hematoma, injury to the vertebral artery, and fractures through the cranial nerve canals. MRI, particularly short tau inversion recovery (STIR) sequences (Fig. D), is used to assess the spinal cord and ligamentous injury and to detect epidural hematoma.

Management

Nonoperative care is usually implemented until the injury can be surgically reduced and stabilized. Arthrodesis with anatomic realignment is usually indicated for an unstable craniocervical junction or the presence of neurologic injury.

Notes

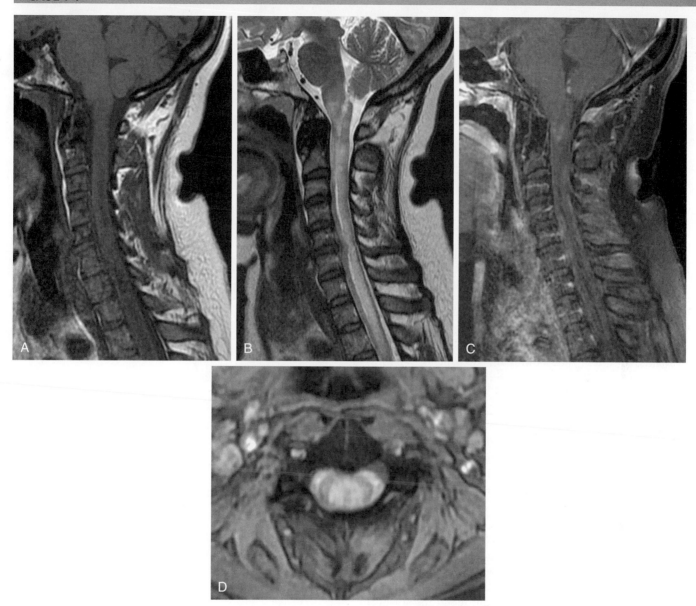

History: A 30-year-old woman presents with a recent onset of upper and lower extremity weakness, sensory deficit, and urinary incontinence.

1. What should be included in the differential diagnosis? (Choose all that apply.)
   a. Acute cord infarction
   b. Neuromyelitis optica (NMO)
   c. Lupus-related longitudinal transverse myelitis (LTM)
   d. Sarcoidosis
   e. Behçet's neuromyelitis

2. What is the most helpful imaging feature in differentiating LTM from other forms of myelitis?
   a. Length of cord involvement
   b. Cross-sectional area of the cord involved
   c. Signal abnormality involving the central gray matter
   d. Pattern of cord enhancement

3. Regarding NMO (Devic's disease) as a cause of LTM, which of the following statements is true?
   a. MRI spinal findings are characteristic of NMO.
   b. Prognosis is better in patients with LTM caused by NMO than in patients with multiple sclerosis–related myelitis.
   c. There are no useful laboratory tests to differentiate NMO-related LTM from other conditions causing LTM.
   d. NMO is one of the most well-recognized causes of LTM.

4. Regarding systemic lupus erythematosus (SLE) as a cause of LTM, which of the following statements is correct?
   a. In patients with LTM affecting the cervical cord, involvement of the brainstem is the rule.
   b. Cord imaging findings are highly variable at presentation in patients with acute SLE-related LTM.
   c. Myelitis is the most common manifestation of central nervous system SLE.
   d. Among the connective tissue disorders, SLE is the one least associated with LTM.

CASE 74

Lupus-Related Longitudinal Transverse Myelitis

1. b, c, d, and e

2. a

3. d

4. b

References

Lehnhardt FG, Impekoven P, Rubbert A, et al: Recurrent longitudinal myelitis as primary manifestation of SLE, *Neurology* 63(10):1976, 2004.

Téllez-Zenteno JF, Remes-Troche JM, Negrete-Pulido RO, et al: Longitudinal myelitis associated with systemic lupus erythematosus: Clinical features and magnetic resonance imaging of six cases, *Lupus* 10(12):851-856, 2001.

Zotos P, Poularas J, Karakitsos D, et al: Lupus related longitudinal myelitis, *J Rheumatol* 37(8):1776, 2010.

Cross-Reference

Neuroradiology: The REQUISITES, 3rd ed, p 549.

Comment

Background

Lupus-related LTM is an infrequent central nervous system complication seen in patients with SLE. In patients with SLE, transverse myelitis is a more frequent myelopathy than LTM.

Imaging

LTM differs from classic transverse myelitis in that it involves a longer segment of the cord—usually more than three contiguous vertebral body segments—and a large cross-sectional area of the cord segments is affected (>50%). On MRI, there is expansion of the cord, with increased signal on T2-weighted images (Figs. A-D). Enhancement is variable and not pathognomonic.

NMO is perhaps the most common entity that causes LTM. NMO has MRI features indistinguishable from other causes of LTM, such as SLE, Behçet's neuromyelitis, and Sjögren's myelitis. The presence of serum NMO-IgG antibodies is characteristic of NMO. In patients with lupus, the serum is negative for this antibody but positive for antiphospholipid antibodies in a significant number of cases.

Management

Treatment for patients with lupus-related LTM includes high doses of corticosteroids and immunosuppressive agents (intravenous cyclophosphamide). Despite aggressive treatment, the prognosis may be poor.

Notes

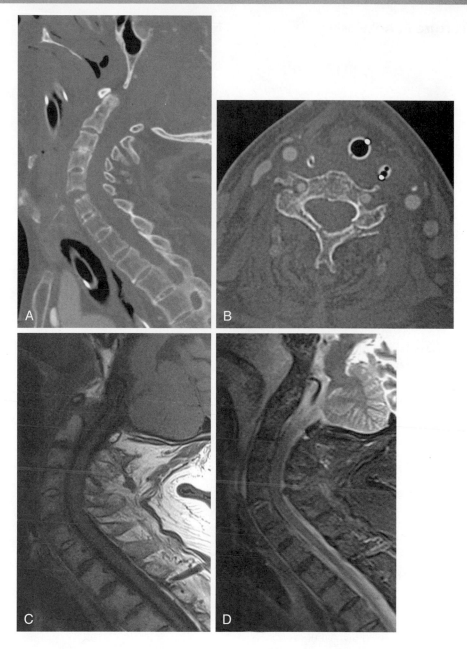

History: An 85-year-old man presents after falling off his bed.

1. What should be included in the differential diagnosis? (Choose all that apply.)
   a. Fracture in a patient with diffuse idiopathic skeletal hyperostosis
   b. Degenerative disk disease
   c. Osteoporotic compression fracture
   d. Fracture in a patient with ankylosing spondylitis
   e. Baastrup's disease

2. Patients with this condition are at significantly increased risk for which type of fracture?
   a. Osteoporotic compression fracture
   b. Odontoid fracture
   c. Three-column fracture
   d. Teardrop fracture

3. Which spine segment is most likely to be involved with fracture in patients with ankylosing spondylitis?
   a. Cervical spine
   b. Thoracic spine
   c. Lumbar spine
   d. Sacrum

4. What is the most common mechanism of cervical spine fractures in patients with ankylosing spondylitis?
   a. Rotation type
   b. Compression
   c. Flexion
   d. Hyperextension

Cervical Spine Fracture in Ankylosing Spondylitis

1. d

2. c

3. a

4. d

References

Caron T, Bransford R, Nguyen Q, et al: Spine fractures in patients with ankylosing spinal disorders, *Spine (Phila Pa 1976)* 35(11):E458-E464, 2010.

Chaudhary SB, Hullinger H, Vives MJ: Management of acute spinal fractures in ankylosing spondylitis, *ISRN Rheumatol* 2011:150484, 2011.

Wang YF, Teng MM, Chang CY, et al: Imaging manifestations of spinal fractures in ankylosing spondylitis, *AJNR Am J Neuroradiol* 26(8):2067-2076, 2005.

Cross-Reference

Neuroradiology: The REQUISITES, 3rd ed, p 534.

Comment

Background

The most serious complication of ankylosing spondylitis is spinal fracture, which can occur with even minor trauma because of the rigidity and osteoporosis that are often seen, especially in older patients or those with long-standing disease. Spinal fractures are four times more common in patients with ankylosing spondylitis than in the general population, and the overall incidence of spinal cord injury is approximately 11 times greater. Fracture must be excluded in any patient with ankylosing spondylitis who complains of new-onset back pain. Fractures typically involve both the anterior and posterior parts of the vertebral column and may be transvertebral or transdiskal.

Pathophysiology

The cervical spine is particularly susceptible to injury because of its oblique facet joints, proximity to the weight of the head, and location at the junction of a fused thoracic area with a more mobile head and neck. Fractures are usually unstable three-column hyperextension fractures (Figs. A-D).

Imaging

Fractures can be difficult to identify on plain radiographs because of spinal ossification, osteoporosis, minor fracture displacement, and poor visibility of the disk space, especially in the cervicothoracic region. CT scan with three-dimensional multiplanar reconstruction can detect occult fractures. MRI is useful to evaluate cord compression and cord signal changes.

Management

Indications for surgical treatment are vertebral instability and the presence of neurologic complications.

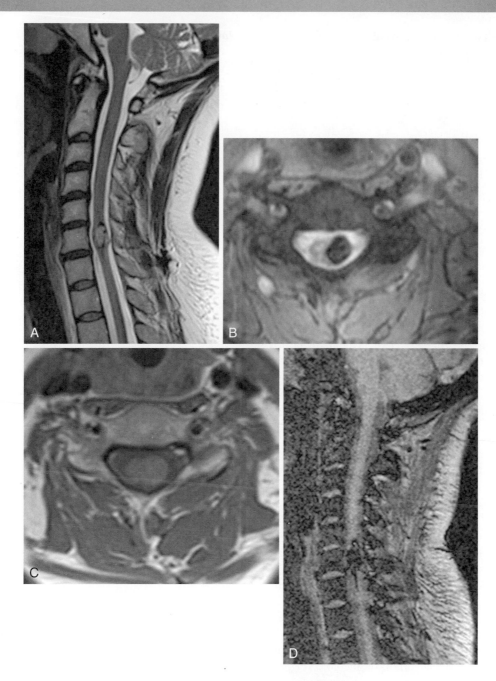

History: A 42-year-old woman with a history of sinonasal cancer is found to have a cord lesion on MRI of the cervical spine.

1. What should be included in the differential diagnosis? (Choose all that apply.)
   a. Intramedullary arteriovenous malformation
   b. Cavernous malformation
   c. Ependymoma
   d. Schwannoma
   e. Meningioma

2. Which of the following intramedullary lesions is least likely to be associated with hematomyelia?
   a. Ependymoma
   b. Hemangioblastoma

   c. Intramedullary arteriovenous malformation
   d. Lymphoma

3. What is the most likely cause of the hypointense rim?
   a. Calcification
   b. Extracellular methemoglobin
   c. Hemosiderin
   d. Chemical shift artifact

4. What additional imaging study would you recommend?
   a. MRI of the brain
   b. Ultrasound of the abdomen
   c. Spinal angiogram
   d. CT scan of the cervical spine

Cavernous Malformation of the Spinal Cord

Notes

1. b

2. d

3. c

4. a

References

Cohen-Gadol AA, Jacob JT, Edwards DA, et al: Coexistence of intracranial and spinal cavernous malformations: A study of prevalence and natural history, *J Neurosurg* 104(3):376-381, 2006.

Zevgaridis D, Medele RJ, Hamburger C, et al: Cavernous haemangiomas of the spinal cord: A review of 117 cases, *Acta Neurochir* 141(3):237-245, 1999.

Cross-Reference

Neuroradiology: The REQUISITES, 3rd ed, p 575.

Comment

Background

Intramedullary cavernous malformations are most often found in women in the third to fifth decades of life and are located predominantly in the thoracic and cervical cord. Spinal cord lesions have an increased frequency of bleeding compared with intracranial lesions. When an intramedullary cavernoma is found, brain imaging is recommended because of the increased risk of additional central nervous system cavernomas. Typically, only one lesion is found because the solitary sporadic form of the disease occurs much more commonly than the multiple sporadic and familial forms. De novo development of intramedullary cavernoma after radiotherapy to the spinal cord has also been described.

Clinical Findings

Patients with intramedullary cavernomas may present with acute neurologic compromise secondary to intramedullary hemorrhage or with chronic progressive myelopathy resulting from microhemorrhages with an associated gliottic reaction.

Imaging

Intramedullary cavernous malformations may have an exophytic component and bulge from the surface of the cord (Fig. A). MRI typically shows a mixed-signal central core surrounded by a hypointense rim of hemosiderin, giving the typical popcorn-like appearance. Central hyperintensity on gradient-echo (Fig. B) and T2-weighted (Fig. A) images and isointensity to hyperintensity on T1-weighted (Fig. C) images usually indicate additional blood breakdown products, such as extracellular methemoglobin. Hypointense areas are accentuated on images that are heavily susceptibility weighted (Fig. D).

Management

For most symptomatic lesions, treatment is total surgical removal to prevent rebleeding and further neurologic compromise.

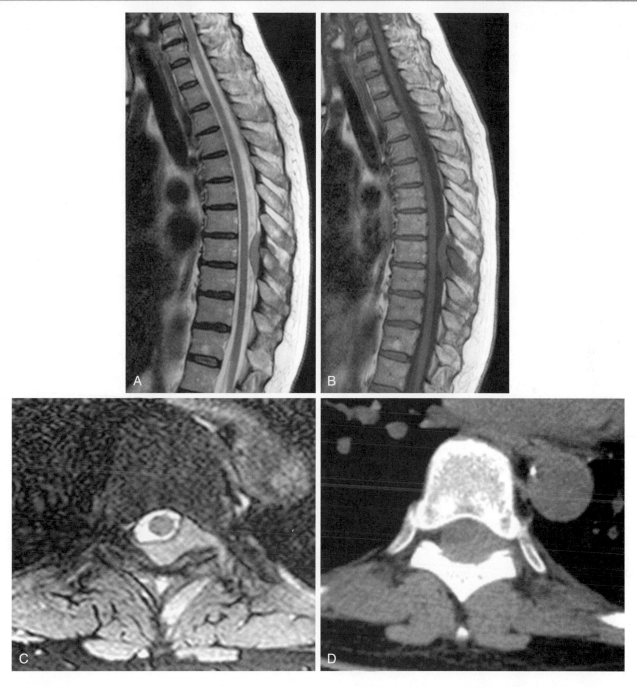

History: A 65-year-old woman presents with midback pain.

1. What should be included in the differential diagnosis? (Choose all that apply.)
   a. Epidural hematoma
   b. Primary epidural lymphoma
   c. Meningioma
   d. Astrocytoma
   e. Metastatic disease

2. What is the predominant location of this lesion?
   a. Intramedullary
   b. Intradural extramedullary
   c. Epidural
   d. Paraspinal

3. What is the most common region of spinal involvement?
   a. Cervical spine
   b. Thoracic spine
   c. Lumbar spine
   d. Sacrum

4. Which of the following imaging features would *not* favor lymphoma over metastatic disease?
   a. Isointense signal relative to cord on T2-weighted images
   b. Involvement of the posterior elements
   c. Increased density on non–contrast-enhanced CT scan
   d. Location within the thoracic spine

Primary Epidural Lymphoma

1. a, b, and e

2. c

3. b

4. d

References

Alameda F, Pedro C, Besses C, et al: Primary epidural lymphoma: Case report, *J Neurosurg* 98(2 Suppl):215-217, 2003.

Boukobza M, Mazel C, Touboul E: Primary vertebral and spinal epidural non-Hodgkin's lymphoma with spinal cord compression, *Neuroradiology* 38(4):333-337, 1996.

Cross-Reference

Neuroradiology: The REQUISITES, 3rd ed, p 565.

Comment

Background

Primary epidural lymphoma is a subset of lymphoma in which there are no other recognizable sites of lymphoma at the time of diagnosis. It occurs in 1% to 6% of patients with non-Hodgkin's lymphoma. The most common region of involvement is the thoracic spine, followed by the lumbar and cervical spine. Patients usually present with backache, followed by symptoms and signs of spinal cord and radicular compression.

Histopathology

Primary epidural lymphoma is often classified as a low-grade or intermediate-grade lesion histologically. In most cases of primary epidural lymphoma, the tumor is located posterior to the spinal cord and has a tendency to spread longitudinally, involving three to four vertebral levels.

Imaging

On MRI, the lesion has homogeneous signal intensity on all pulse sequences (Figs. A-C) and homogeneous enhancement. Relative to cord signal intensity, the tumor is usually isointense on T1-weighted images (see Fig. B) and isointense to hyperintense on T2-weighted images (see Fig. A). Infiltrative growth through the foramen into the paravertebral space is frequent (Fig. D). Adjacent vertebral infiltration occurs in 50% of clinically diagnosed cases, appearing hypointense on T1-weighted images (see Fig. B).

Management

Patients have a potentially favorable outcome if they are diagnosed and treated early because the lesions are very sensitive to radiation and chemotherapy.

Notes

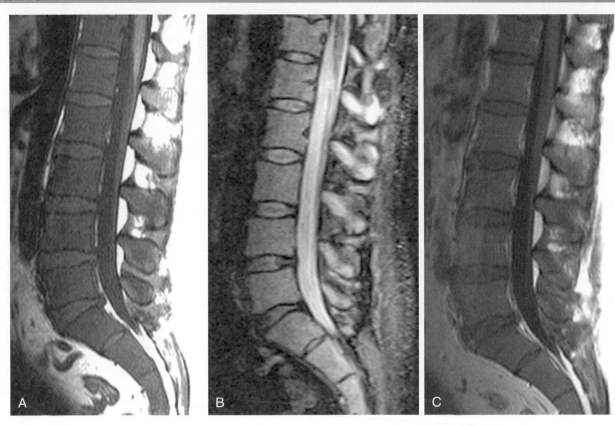

History: A 45-year-old man presents with lower back pain and fever.

1. What should be included in the differential diagnosis? (Choose all that apply.)
   a. Leukemia
   b. Multiple myeloma
   c. Osteomyelitis
   d. HIV
   e. Lymphoma

2. Which of the following conditions results in diffusely hyperintense T1 marrow signal?
   a. Chronic anemia
   b. Postradiation changes
   c. Leukemia
   d. HIV

3. Which of the following findings is *not* found in patients with leukemia?
   a. Diffuse leptomeningeal enhancement
   b. Granulocytic sarcoma
   c. Diffusely decreased T1 marrow signal
   d. Ivory vertebra

4. Which of the following vertebral body signal changes would *not* be expected after bone marrow transplantation?
   a. Central hyperintense band on T1-weighted images
   b. Peripheral isointense region on T1-weighted images
   c. Peripheral hypointense signal on short tau inversion recovery (STIR) images
   d. Central hypointense signal on STIR images

Leukemia

1. a, b, d, and e

2. b

3. d

4. c

References

Ginsberg LE, Leeds NE: Neuroradiology of leukemia, *AJR Am J Roentgenol* 165(3):525-534, 1995.

Moore SG, Gooding CA, Brasch RC, et al: Bone marrow in children with acute lymphocytic leukemia: MR relaxation times, *Radiology* 160(1):237-240, 1986.

Cross-Reference

Neuroradiology: The REQUISITES, 3rd ed, pp 565-566.

Comment

Background

Acute lymphoblastic leukemia is a malignant disease of the bone marrow in which early lymphoid precursors proliferate and replace the normal hematopoietic cells of the marrow. In adults, acute lymphoblastic leukemia is less common than acute myelogenous leukemia.

Imaging

The typical imaging finding in patients with acute leukemia is a diffuse decrease in the signal intensity of the marrow on T1-weighted images (Fig. A). The intervertebral disks appear brighter than or isointense to the diseased marrow. In young adults, it may be difficult to differentiate leukemic infiltration from pure hematopoietic marrow. On STIR images (Fig. B), a variable increase in the signal intensity of the abnormal marrow is observed. After the administration of intravenous contrast medium, the abnormal marrow enhances, and the intervertebral disks appear darker than the enhanced spine (Fig. C). The vertebral signal becomes normal as the disease goes into remission. Involvement of the spine by leukemia can also manifest as abnormal leptomeningeal enhancement or as an intradural, extradural, or paraspinal enhancing mass (chloroma). Leptomeningeal disease can be focal or diffuse. Secondary causes of leptomeningeal enhancement in leukemic patients include infection and meningeal irritation secondary to intrathecal chemotherapy or bleeding.

Management

Treatment is with chemotherapy. Bone marrow transplantation is frequently performed in patients with leukemia.

Notes

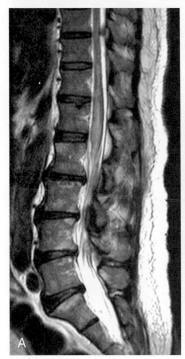

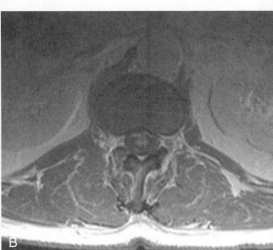

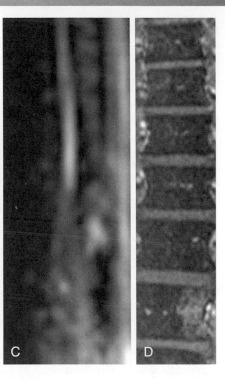

A   B   C   D

History: A 67-year-old man with vascular risk factors suddenly develops low back pain, followed by immediate weakness and sensory disturbance in the bilateral lower extremities.

1. What should be included in the differential diagnosis? (Choose all that apply.)
   a. Multiple sclerosis
   b. Guillain-Barré syndrome
   c. Conus infarction
   d. Meningitis
   e. Sarcoid

2. The findings are most likely due to involvement of which of the following arteries?
   a. Artery of Adamkiewicz
   b. Posterior spinal artery
   c. Radicular artery
   d. Posterior medullary artery

3. Which of the following imaging findings is the most reliable indicator of ischemia of the spinal cord in the acute phase?
   a. Spinal cord enlargement on T1-weighted images
   b. "Pencil" sign on sagittal T2-weighted images
   c. Hyperintense signal on diffusion-weighted imaging, with corresponding low apparent diffusion coefficient
   d. "Snake eyes" configuration on axial T2-weighted images

4. Infarction of which of the following structures may be associated with cord infarction?
   a. Brain
   b. Vertebral body
   c. Bowel
   d. Lower extremity

Conus Infarction

1. c and e

2. a

3. c

4. b

References

Amano Y, Machida T, Kumazaki T: Spinal cord infarcts with contrast enhancement of the cauda equina: Two cases, *Neuroradiology* 40(10):669-672, 1998.

Masson C, Pruvo JP, Meder JF, et al: Study Group on Spinal Cord Infarction of the French Neurovascular Society: Spinal cord infarction: Clinical and magnetic resonance imaging findings and short term outcome, *J Neurol Neurosurg Psychiatry* 75(10):1431-1435, 2004.

Shinoyama M, Takahashi T, Shimizu H, et al: Spinal cord infarction demonstrated by diffusion-weighted magnetic resonance imaging, *J Clin Neurosci* 12(4):466-468, 2005.

Cross-Reference

Neuroradiology: The REQUISITES, 3rd ed, p 571.

Comment

Background

Spinal cord infarction is uncommon and accounts for approximately 1% of all strokes.

Histopathology

Blood is supplied to the cord by the sulcal branches of the anterior spinal artery, which itself is supplied primarily by the artery of Adamkiewicz in the conus region and by radial perforating branches of the pial arterial plexus on the cord surface. The anterior spinal artery supplies approximately the anterior two thirds of the cord and most of the central gray matter. Hypoperfusion in this vascular distribution—owing to pathologic changes in the descending aorta (aneurysm, thrombosis, dissection) or various other causes (small vessel vasculitides, hypotension, pregnancy, sickle cell disease, caisson disease, diabetes, degenerative disease of the spine)—can result in conus infarction.

Imaging

Spin-echo MRI findings include cord enlargement and hyperintense signal on T2-weighted images (Fig. A) in the first few days, with or without gadolinium enhancement (Fig. B). Diffusion-weighted imaging is particularly sensitive to ischemic changes (Fig. C). Abnormal signal and enhancement may demonstrate a double-dot ("owl's eyes" or "snake eyes") pattern in the region of the anterior horns, an H-shaped pattern involving the central gray matter, or a more diffuse pattern involving both gray matter and white matter. Amano and colleagues reported enhancement of the ventral part of the cauda equina, which is composed of motor fiber bundles, in association with conus enhancement (see Fig. B). When infarction results from compromise of a segmental artery, branches supplying the ipsilateral half of the vertebral body may also be affected (Fig. D). Cord atrophy and lack of contrast enhancement are found later (months) in the course of cord infarction.

Management

Treatment includes aspirin and management of the complications of acute paraplegia.

Notes

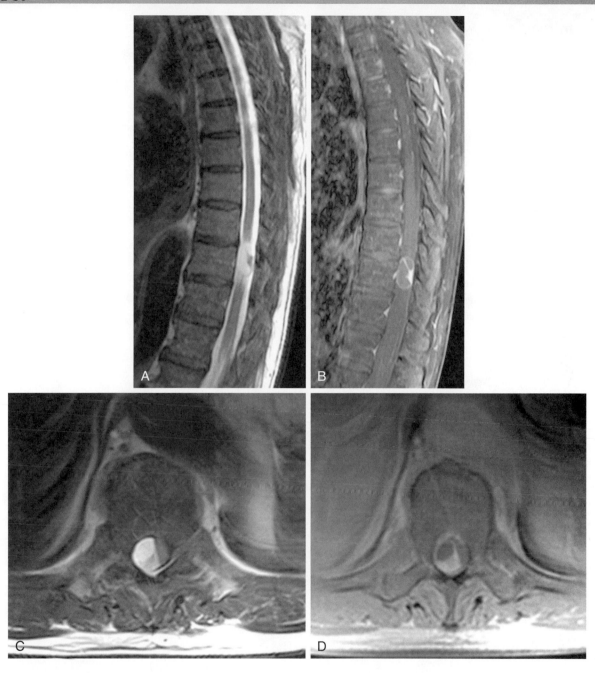

History: A 67-year-old man has a 1-year history of intractable back and right flank pain and right leg tingling.

1. What should be included in the differential diagnosis? (Choose all that apply.)
   a. Meningioma
   b. Astrocytoma
   c. Hemangioblastoma
   d. Schwannoma
   e. Epidural abscess

2. What is the location of this lesion?
   a. Intramedullary
   b. Intradural extramedullary
   c. Epidural
   d. Extraspinal

3. Which of the following statements regarding intradural schwannomas is true?
   a. Schwannomas may be intramedullary in location.
   b. Schwannomas are the second most frequent intradural extramedullary tumor after meningiomas.
   c. Schwannomas usually arise from motor roots.
   d. Cystic changes are more frequent in neurofibromas than in schwannomas.

4. Which of the following lesions is most likely to undergo malignant transformation?
   a. Meningioma
   b. Schwannoma
   c. Neurofibroma
   d. Lipoma

Thoracic Intradural Schwannoma

1. a, c, and d

2. b

3. a

4. c

Reference
Van Goethem JW, van den Hauwe L, Ozsarlak O, et al: Spinal tumors, *Eur J Radiol* 50(2):159-176, 2004.

Cross-Reference
Neuroradiology: The REQUISITES, 3rd ed, pp 561-563.

Comment
Background
Intraspinal schwannomas are usually solitary intradural, extra-medullary lesions, occurring most often in the cervical and thoracic spine. The peak incidence is around the fourth and fifth decades.

Histopathology
Intraspinal schwannomas are well encapsulated and composed of Antoni type A and type B tissue; the latter becomes prominent in larger lesions and is responsible for cyst formation. Larger lesions may appear lobulated and have areas of intrinsic hemorrhage.

Imaging
Schwannomas are mostly solid or heterogeneous solid tumors with cystic changes (Figs. A-D). They are typically isointense to hypointense on T1-weighted images and hyperintense on T2-weighted images (see Figs. A and C). Enhancement is variable; it may be intense and homogeneous, or there may be only peripheral enhancement (see Figs. B and D). More than half of intraspinal schwannomas are purely intradural, and the remaining are purely extradural (25%) or both intradural and extradural (15%).

Management
The treatment of cystic schwannomas involves total excision of the lesion.

Notes

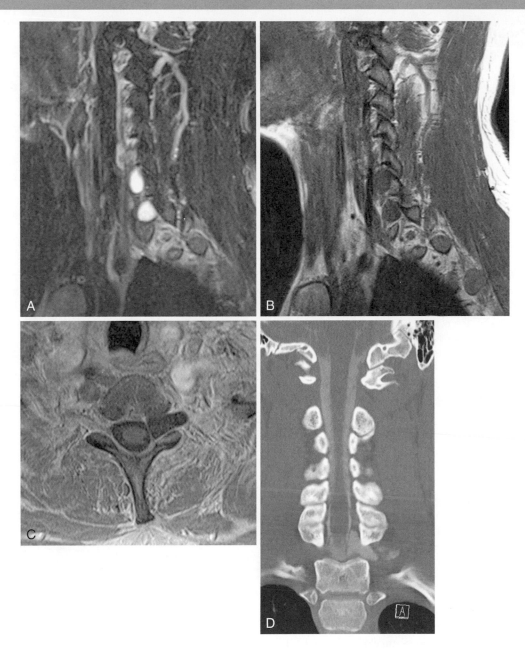

History: A 25-year-old man is injured in a motorcycle collision.

1. What should be included in the differential diagnosis? (Choose all that apply.)
   a. Cystic schwannoma
   b. Pseudomeningocele
   c. Perineural cyst
   d. Synovial sarcoma
   e. Synovial cyst

2. Which of the following cervical roots are most commonly involved in posttraumatic avulsion injury in an adult?
   a. C1 and C2
   b. C3 and C4
   c. C5 and C6
   d. C7 and C8

3. Which of the following imaging modalities is preferred for injury distal to the neural foramen?
   a. Myelography
   b. CT myelography
   c. MRI of the brachial plexus
   d. Ultrasound

4. Which of the following statements regarding traumatic pseudomeningocele is true?
   a. Traumatic pseudomeningoceles are always associated with nerve root avulsion.
   b. About 80% of cases of complete nerve root avulsion are associated with pseudomeningocele.
   c. About 50% of cervical spine levels that demonstrate pseudomeningocele have intact nerve roots.
   d. Clinical and electromyography findings allow the reliable differentiation of a preganglionic and postganglionic nerve lesion in most cases.

Traumatic Pseudomeningocele

1. b and c

2. d

3. c

4. b

References

Bowen BC: Brachial plexus. In Stark DD, Bradley WG Jr, editors: ed 3, *Magnetic resonance imaging*, vol 3, Philadelphia, 1998, Mosby Year Book, pp 1821-1832.

Doi K, Otsuka K, Okamoto Y, et al: Cervical nerve root avulsion in brachial plexus injuries: Magnetic resonance imaging classification and comparison with myelography and computerized tomography myelography, *J Neurosurg* 96(3 Suppl):277-284, 2002.

Cross-Reference

Neuroradiology: The REQUISITES, 3rd ed, p 577.

Comment

Background

Brachial plexus avulsion injury is most commonly caused by a motorcycle accident when the arm and shoulder are severely stretched. Generally, the most common sites of avulsion are C7 and C8.

Pathophysiology

Traumatic pseudomeningocele results from severe traction injury that tears the dura mater and arachnoid walls of the root sleeve, with leakage of cerebrospinal fluid (CSF) into the neural foramen. The enclosed nerve root may or may not be avulsed. After injury, the neural foraminal CSF collection is contiguous with subarachnoid space CSF; however, after healing, some pseudomeningoceles may not communicate with the subarachnoid space and appear as epidural masses.

Imaging

Clinical and electromyography findings may be helpful in differentiating intradural (preganglionic) from peripheral (postganglionic) nerve injury, but they are unreliable in most cases. A combination of conventional myelography and CT myelography is the standard imaging technique for injury to the brachial plexus; however, detection of partial or complete cervical root damage is not fully reliable with either technique. MRI has similar accuracy in detecting cervical root avulsion; however, it provides better information about injury to the brachial plexus distal to the intervertebral foramen (Figs. A-D).

Management

Treatment should be conservative for patients who recover spontaneously within the first few weeks after trauma. Operative treatment is indicated for patients who have nerve root avulsion. Surgery consists of nerve repair and nerve grafting for extraforaminal injury and neurotization or nerve transfer for nerve root avulsion.

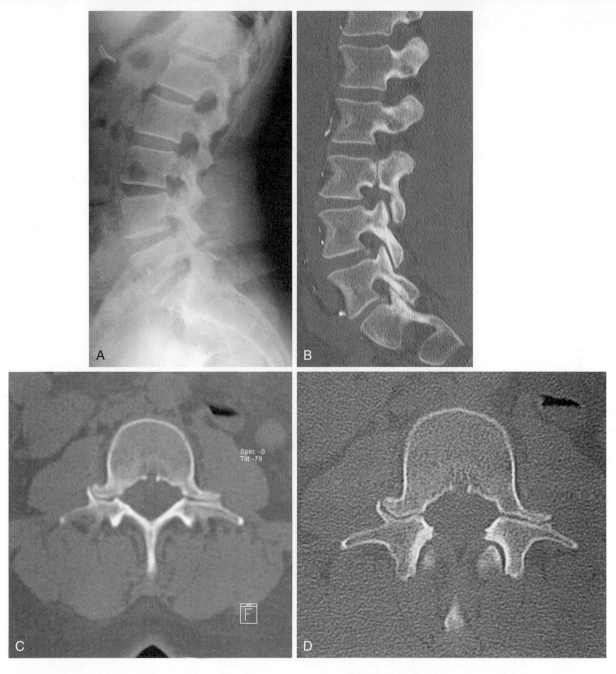

History: A 50-year-old woman presents with persistent low back pain for 6 years, with worsening over the past few months.

1. What should be included in the differential diagnosis? (Choose all that apply.)
   a. Pars interarticularis defects
   b. Retrosomatic clefts
   c. Pedicular fractures
   d. Retroisthmic clefts
   e. Spina bifida

2. Where are retrosomatic clefts most frequently found?
   a. Cervical spine
   b. Thoracic spine
   c. Lumbar spine
   d. Sacrum

3. Which of the following statements regarding retrosomatic clefts is true?
   a. They are more common in men.
   b. They are more frequently unilateral.
   c. Pedicular clefts cannot be differentiated from pars interarticularis defects.
   d. They most frequently occur at a single vertebral level.

4. Which of the following clefts is a result of failure of fusion of the primary ossification centers?
   a. Spina bifida
   b. Retrosomatic clefts
   c. Retroisthmic clefts
   d. Pars interarticularis defects

Pedicular (Retrosomatic) Clefts

1. b and c

2. c

3. d

4. a

References

Chen JJ, Branstetter BF 4th, Welch WC: Multiple posterior vertebral fusion abnormalities: A case report and review of the literature, *AJR Am J Roentgenol* 186(5):1256-1259, 2006.

Kalideen JM, Satyapal KS, Bayat F: Case report: Pedicular cleft associated with bilateral pars interarticularis defects and transverse process hypoplasia of a fifth lumbar vertebra, *Br J Radiol* 67(803):1136-1138, 1994.

Soleimanpour M, Gregg ML, Paraliticci R: Bilateral retrosomatic clefts at multiple lumbar levels, *AJNR Am J Neuroradiol* 16(8):1616-1617, 1995.

Cross-Reference

Neuroradiology: The REQUISITES, 3rd ed, pp 533-534.

Comment

Background

Retrosomatic clefts are defects in the pedicles of the vertebral arch. Recognition of retrosomatic clefts is important because they may be mistaken for traumatic pedicle fractures. Clefts occurring at a single vertebral level without associated disk disease probably have no clinical significance; however, involvement at multiple levels may result in spinal instability.

Pathophysiology

There are six types of posterior neural arch defects. Their origins are congenital or acquired, and there may be a predisposition to defects based on a congenital weakness. Neurocentral synchondroses, paraspinous clefts, and spinous clefts result from failure of fusion of the primary ossification centers. The other three defects—spondylolysis, retrosomatic clefts, and retroisthmic clefts—either have an unknown cause or are presumed to be caused by overuse (e.g., spondylolysis). Retrosomatic cleft represents a hypoplasia or aplasia of the vertebral pedicle. The origin of this defect has not been elucidated. The coexistence of other vertebral anomalies favors a congenital cause, and it is believed to be due to incomplete fusion of anomalous ossification centers. In contrast to pars interarticularis defects, retrosomatic clefts are typically not associated with sclerosis around the defect. Retroisthmic cleft has been described as "laminolysis" because the defect is through the lamina. In contrast to spondylolysis, the defect is dorsal to the inferior articular facet. Retroisthmic cleft is the rarest of the six posterior fusion defects. Although most of these defects occur in the lumbar spine, they may occur anywhere along the spinal column.

Imaging

Imaging of retrosomatic clefts is best done with CT scan (Figs. A-D). Affected pedicles may be elongated, shortened, or thickened, with coexisting contralateral spondylolysis in the same vertebra.

Management

Clefts occurring at a single vertebral level without associated disk disease probably have no clinical significance; however, involvement at multiple levels may result in spinal instability.

Notes

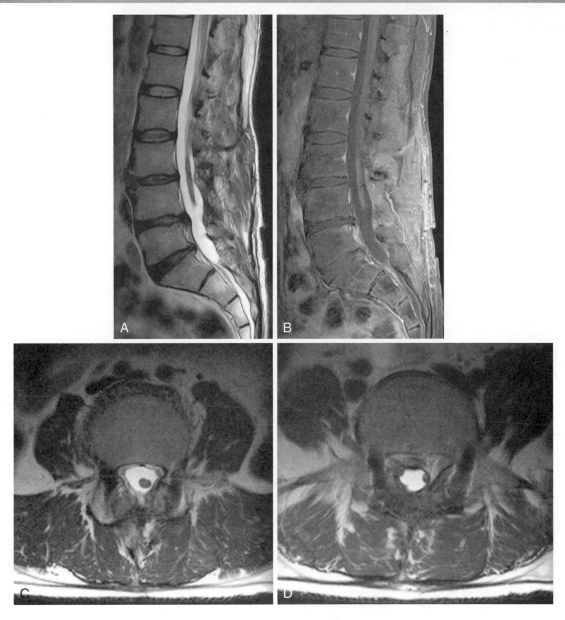

History: A 40-year-old man presents with constant back pain following a laminectomy performed 1 year ago.

1. What should be included in the differential diagnosis? (Choose all that apply.)
   a. Filum lipoma
   b. Chronic arachnoiditis
   c. Meningioma
   d. Diskitis osteomyelitis
   e. Cord tethering

2. Which of the following statements regarding arachnoiditis is true?
   a. Findings should extend over at least five lumbar vertebrae.
   b. When imaging findings are present, the patient is always symptomatic.
   c. There is a direct correlation between the degree of enhancement and the severity of symptoms.
   d. In most cases, arachnoiditis shows little enhancement on MRI.

3. Which of the following findings is not typically seen in the earliest stage of chronic adhesive arachnoiditis?
   a. Arachnoid adhesions in the nerve root sleeves
   b. Arachnoid adhesions between the roots and the walls of the thecal sac
   c. Distortion of the dural sac ending
   d. Arachnoid adhesions between nerve roots

4. Which imaging modality is the least helpful in the diagnosis of chronic arachnoiditis?
   a. Myelography
   b. CT
   c. CT myelography
   d. MRI

Chronic Adhesive Arachnoiditis

1. b and e

2. d

3. c

4. b

References

Etchepare F, Roche B, Rozenberg S, et al: Post–lumbar puncture arachnoiditis: The need for directed questioning, *Joint Bone Spine* 72(2):180-182, 2005.

Georgy BA, Snow RD, Hesselink JR: MR imaging of spinal nerve roots: Techniques, enhancement patterns and imaging findings, *AJR Am J Roentgenol* 166(1):173-179, 1996.

Cross-Reference

Neuroradiology: The REQUISITES, 3rd ed, pp 540-541.

Comment

Background

Arachnoiditis is an inflammation of the arachnoid and subarachnoid space. Symptoms include pain and a burning sensation and are generally stable over time. Increased pain can be observed during trauma or physical effort.

Pathophysiology

Causes of arachnoiditis include infection, subarachnoid hemorrhage, and inflammatory disease such as sarcoidosis. When attributed to local procedures, the mechanism is probably local bleeding or neurotoxicity of a drug. Inflammation produces a fibrinous exudate, causing adhesions between the subarachnoid membrane and contained nerve roots or between the roots themselves. Fibrosis and scarring may also occur, resulting in distortion of anatomic structures. Adhesions may also result in syringomyelia, which can aggravate the neurologic signs.

Imaging

MRI is the imaging study of choice for the diagnosis of arachnoiditis (Figs. A-D). In the lower lumbar spine, the nerve roots of the cauda equina normally have a thin, feathery appearance on myelography, CT myelography, and MRI. On MRI, this appearance is best detected and evaluated with T2-weighted axial images (see Figs. C and D). In patients with arachnoiditis or arachnoidal adhesions, the nerve roots may adhere to the wall of the thecal sac, adhere to one another, or form a conglomerate mass (see Fig. D), which occasionally may be misinterpreted as a tethered cord or thickened filum terminale (see Fig. A). Contrast enhancement is seen in some cases, and the most common pattern of enhancement is a smooth, linear layer outlining the surface of the cord and nerve roots (see Fig. B).

Management

No treatment has been proved to cure arachnoiditis. Treatment is limited to the alleviation of pain and other symptoms. Surgical intervention generally has a poor outcome and provides only temporary relief. Steroid injections are generally discouraged and may worsen the condition.

Notes

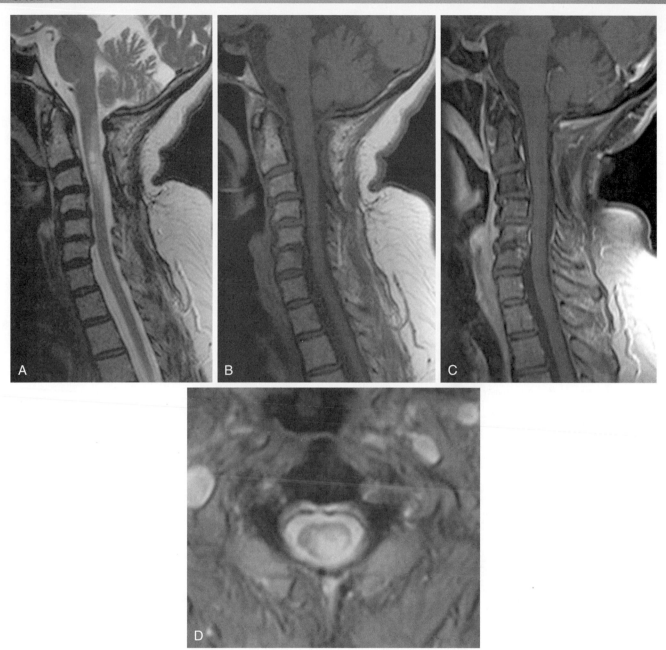

History: A 53-year-old woman presents with left-sided numbness, left arm and hand weakness, and imbalance.

1. What should be included in the differential diagnosis? (Choose all that apply.)
   a. Ependymoma
   b. Acute disseminated encephalomyelitis
   c. Sarcoid
   d. Lymphoma
   e. Astrocytoma

2. Which of the following is *not* an imaging feature of cord astrocytoma?
   a. Lack of contrast enhancement
   b. Lack of cord expansion
   c. Hyperintense T2 signal
   d. Isointense T1 signal

3. What is the most common primary intramedullary neoplasm in an adult?
   a. Ganglioglioma
   b. Lymphoma
   c. Astrocytoma
   d. Ependymoma

4. What is the most common location of spinal cord astrocytomas?
   a. Cervical
   b. Upper thoracic
   c. Lower thoracic
   d. Conus region

Astrocytoma of the Cervical Cord

Notes

1. e

2. b

3. d

4. a

Reference

Seo HS, Kim JH, Lee DH, et al: Nonenhancing intramedullary astrocytomas and other MR imaging features: A retrospective study and systematic review, *AJNR Am J Neuroradiol* 31(3):498-503, 2010.

Cross-Reference

Neuroradiology: The REQUISITES, 3rd ed, pp 556-557.

Comment

Background

Astrocytomas of the spinal cord are unusual and account for approximately 30% of spinal cord tumors. They are the most common childhood intramedullary neoplasm of the spinal cord and are second only to ependymomas in adults. Clinical presentation varies from nonspecific back pain to sensory and motor deficits, depending on the tumor's size and location. The infiltrative nature of astrocytomas leads to a worse prognosis than that associated with ependymomas.

Histopathology

Astrocytomas arise from astrocytes in the spinal cord. Most astrocytomas (75%) are low-grade (World Health Organization grade II) fibrillary astrocytomas. They are most commonly found in the cervical spine.

Imaging

The classic MRI appearance of intramedullary astrocytoma includes cord enlargement and poorly defined margins (Figs. A-D). Intramedullary astrocytoma is typically isointense to hypointense on T1-weighted images (see Fig. B) and hyperintense on T2-weighted images (see Figs. A and D). Peritumoral and tumoral cysts are frequently associated with astrocytomas (see Fig. A). Most intramedullary astrocytomas exhibit at least some enhancement, regardless of cell type or tumor grade. About 20% to 30% of intramedullary astrocytomas show no enhancement (see Fig. C).

Management

The optimal treatment of spinal astrocytomas is controversial. The goal of surgery is to remove the bulk of the tumor when possible, especially in patients with low-grade astrocytomas. Radiation should be considered for high-grade tumors, inoperable tumors, tumors remaining after surgery, and recurring tumors.

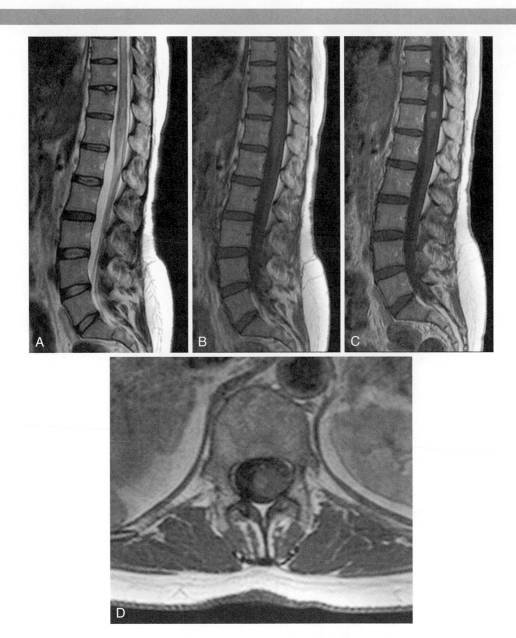

History: A 60-year-old woman presents with paraplegia and sphincter dysfunction.

1. What should be included in the differential diagnosis? (Choose all that apply.)
   a. Hemangioblastoma
   b. Meningioma
   c. Schwannoma
   d. Sarcoid
   e. Metastasis

2. Which of the following tumors is the most common tumor outside the central nervous system (CNS) associated with intramedullary metastases?
   a. Breast cancer
   b. Lung cancer
   c. Melanoma
   d. Lymphoma

3. What is the most likely route for the spread of intramedullary metastases?
   a. Cerebrospinal fluid (CSF) dissemination
   b. Lymphatic spread
   c. Hematogenous spread
   d. Direct spread

4. Which of the following statements regarding spinal cord metastasis is true?
   a. Based on autopsy results of patients with disseminated cancers, the number of patients with brain metastases is approximately 50 times more than the number of patients with spinal cord metastases.
   b. Because of its rich vascularization, the cervical cord is a more common site of intramedullary metastasis than the thoracic spine.
   c. Intramedullary metastases with leptomeningeal disease most likely represent hematogenous spread of disease.
   d. Extra-CNS tumors can extend to the cord by direct invasion from nerve roots or CSF.

Intramedullary Spinal Cord Metastases (Breast Cancer)

1. a, d, and e

2. b

3. c

4. d

References

Crasto S, Duca S, Davini O, et al: MRI diagnosis of intramedullary metastases from extra-CNS tumors, *Eur Radiol* 7(5):732-736, 1997.

Lee SS, Kim MK, Sym SJ, et al: Intramedullary spinal cord metastases: A single-institution experience, *J Neurooncol* 84(1):85-89, 2007.

Villegas AE, Guthrie TH: Intramedullary spinal cord metastasis in breast cancer: Clinical features, diagnosis, and therapeutic consideration, *Breast J* 10(6):532-535, 2004.

Cross-Reference

Neuroradiology: The REQUISITES, 3rd ed, pp 559-560.

Comment

Background

Intramedullary metastases are rare, being found in only 1% to 2% of cancer patients. Myelopathy is the first manifestation in most patients. Urinary and bowel dysfunction predominates in patients with conus medullaris metastasis.

Pathophysiology

Most studies suggest that intramedullary metastases from extra-CNS tumors reach the spinal cord mainly by two routes: (1) arterial circulation to the cord and (2) vertebral venous plexus (Batson's plexus). Extra-CNS tumors can also extend to the cord by direct invasion from nerve roots or CSF.

Imaging

On MRI, intramedullary metastases are most frequently single, oval-shaped, and small, with little or no cord enlargement (Figs. A-D). They are typically isointense to cord on T1-weighted images before contrast agent administration, and they demonstrate homogeneous, nodular enhancement after contrast agent administration (see Figs. B and C). T2-weighted images show surrounding pencil-shaped hyperintensity, representing edema. Larger lesions are more likely to demonstrate central hypointensity on T1-weighted images, peripheral enhancement after contrast agent administration, extensive edema on T2-weighted images (see Fig. A), and cord enlargement. MRI of the brain should be recommended because of potential cerebral metastases and because mimickers of intramedullary metastasis, such as multiple sclerosis or sarcoid, may be favored based on the intracranial findings.

Management

Radiotherapy is the treatment of choice. Other treatment options include chemotherapy and surgery, especially for tumors that are highly radioresistant.

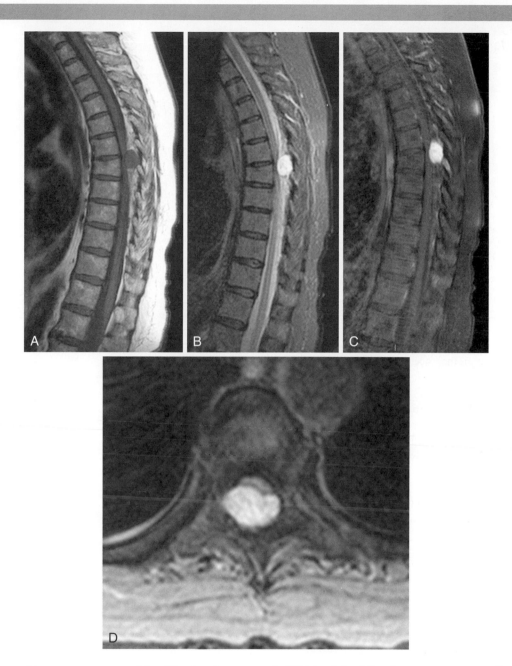

History: A 64-year-old woman presents with midback pain without neurologic deficit.

1. What should be included in the differential diagnosis? (Choose all that apply.)
   a. Lymphoma
   b. Metastasis
   c. Meningioma
   d. Hemangioma
   e. Nerve sheath tumor

2. Which of the following is the most reliable sign to determine the epidural location of a lesion?
   a. Displacement of the cord
   b. Bony involvement
   c. Effacement of epidural fat
   d. Expansion of cerebrospinal fluid spaces

3. Which of the following statements regarding spinal epidural cavernous hemangiomas is true?
   a. The cervical spine epidural space is the most common location.
   b. A purely extradural benign vascular spinal mass lesion is common.
   c. Spinal epidural hemangiomas can be solitary or multiple, with bright signal on T2-weighted images, enhancement, and occasionally a dark rim of T2 signal.
   d. Bone scalloping and foraminal widening are usually present in spinal epidural cavernous hemangiomas.

4. Which of the following lesions should *not* be considered in the differential diagnosis of epidural cavernous hemangioma?
   a. Spinal angiolipoma
   b. Epidural hematoma
   c. Nerve sheath tumor
   d. Meningioma

Thoracic Spine Dorsal Epidural Hemangioma

1. b and d

2. c

3. c

4. d

References

Lee JW, Cho EY, Hong SH, et al: Spinal epidural hemangiomas: Various types of MR imaging features with histopathologic correlation, *AJNR Am J Neuroradiol* 28(7):1242-1248, 2007.

Saghvi D, Munshi M, Kulkami B, et al: Dorsal spinal epidural cavernous hemangioma, *J Craniovertebr Junction Spine* 1(2):122-125, 2010.

Satpathy DK, Das S, Das BS: Spinal epidural cavernous hemangioma with myelopathy: A rare lesion, *Neurol India* 57(1):88-90, 2009.

Cross-Reference

Neuroradiology: The REQUISITES, 3rd ed, p 567.

Comment

Background

Spinal epidural hemangiomas account for about 4% of all epidural tumors and 12% of all spinal hemangiomas. The preoperative differential diagnosis of epidural hemangioma includes schwannoma, angiolipoma, extramedullary hemato-poiesis, hematoma, and less likely tumors such as meningioma or lymphoma. Synovial cysts and disk herniation (on precontrast images) may be included in the differential diagnosis.

Histopathology

Hemangiomas are not vascular neoplasms; rather, they are vascular malformations that, depending on the vascular channels they involve, are classified as capillary, cavernous, arteriovenous, or venous. Spinal epidural hemangiomas are usually of the cavernous type.

Imaging

Cavernous epidural hemangiomas are usually lobulated masses with high T2 signal intensity and intense, homogeneous contrast enhancement on MRI (Figs. A-D).

Management

Preoperative diagnosis of epidural hemangioma is important because of the lesion's high vascularity. Adequate surgical planning is required to control intraoperative bleeding and to avoid incomplete resection of a lesion with the potential to recur. For surgically inaccessible lesions, radiation therapy is the treatment of choice.

Notes

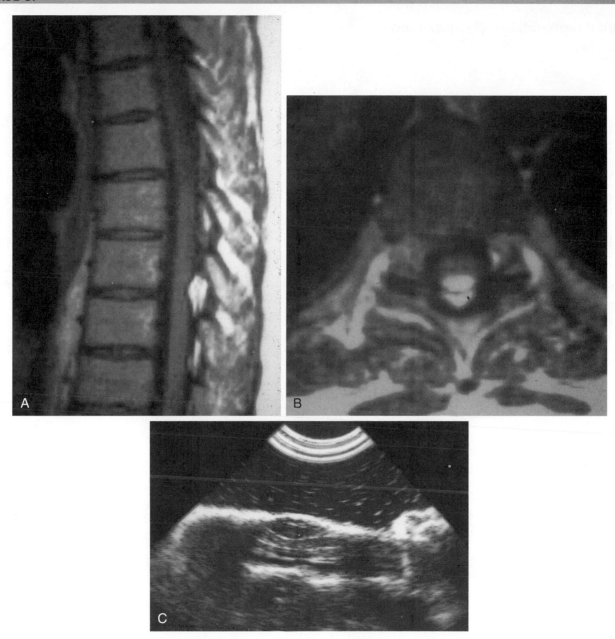

History: A 70-year-old man presents with back pain.

1. What should be included in the differential diagnosis? (Choose all that apply.)
   a. Dermoid
   b. Meningioma
   c. Melanotic melanoma
   d. Iophendylate (Pantopaque) collection
   e. Lipoma

2. Which of the following materials would *not* manifest with hyperintense signal on T1-weighted images?
   a. Hemosiderin
   b. Melanin
   c. Calcifications
   d. Proteinaceous fluid

3. Which of the following is the most common complication associated with residual Pantopaque?
   a. Hydrocephalus
   b. Increased incidence of cord tumors
   c. Syringohydromyelia
   d. Arachnoiditis

4. Which imaging study would be helpful in differentiating retained Pantopaque from lipoma?
   a. MRI
   b. Plain radiographs
   c. Ultrasound
   d. Bone scintigraphy

Retained Iophendylate (Pantopaque)

1. a, c, d, and e

2. a

3. d

4. b

References

Mamourian AC, Briggs RW: Appearance of Pantopaque on MR images, *Radiology* 158(2):457-460, 1986.

Tabor EN, Batzdorf U: Thoracic spinal Pantopaque cyst and associated syrinx resulting in progressive spastic paraparesis: Case report, *Neurosurgery* 39(5): 1040-1042, 1996.

Cross-Reference

Neuroradiology: The REQUISITES, 3rd ed, pp 540-541.

Comment

Background

Iophendylate (Pantopaque) is an oil-based (lipophilic, hydrophobic) iodinated contrast material. Before the introduction of water-soluble (hydrophilic) contrast material, Pantopaque was used for myelography and ventriculography. Although Pantopaque has not been used for decades, it may be retained in the spinal canal for years or decades and is occasionally detected in the intracranial or intraspinal subarachnoid space of older patients.

Pathophysiology

Because of its hydrophobicity, Pantopaque had an extremely slow reabsorption rate. Residual Pantopaque was typically removed from the thecal sac by aspiration after a procedure; however, complete aspiration was infrequent. The most common complication associated with Pantopaque is clinical or subclinical lumbar arachnoiditis. Some investigators have hypothesized that arachnoiditis is more likely to occur when subarachnoid blood (and possibly other factors such as trauma or disk herniation) is present with Pantopaque, resulting in a synergistic effect.

Imaging

The easiest way to diagnose intrathecal Pantopaque is to take a careful history and obtain plain radiographs. If there is a question as to whether the Pantopaque is loculated or mobile, fluoroscopy with the patient in an upright position can be performed. On MRI, Pantopaque is either retained in the subarachnoid space or trapped in the subdural space. Imaging findings are similar and may closely resemble fat (Figs. A-C).

Management

Surgical removal of retained Pantopaque may produce a symptomatic benefit in some cases.

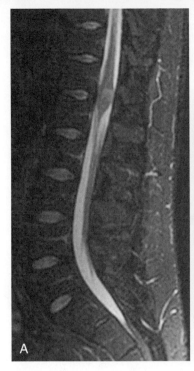
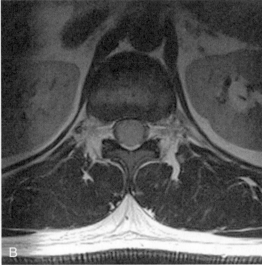
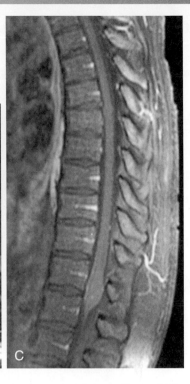

History: A 29-year-old man presents with a 4-week history of numbness in the buttock, perineal area, and lower extremities, as well as difficulty urinating and sexual dysfunction.

1. Which of the following would be included in the differential diagnosis for the imaging findings presented? (Choose all that apply.)
   a. Ganglioglioma
   b. Acute disseminated encephalomyelitis (ADEM)
   c. Astrocytoma
   d. Lymphoma
   e. Cord infarct

2. What is the most common location of spinal cord astrocytomas?
   a. Cervical
   b. Upper thoracic
   c. Lower thoracic
   d. Conus region

3. Which of the following statements regarding spinal cord astrocytomas is true?
   a. Astrocytomas occur more frequently in the region of the conus medullaris compared with ependymomas.
   b. Astrocytomas have a slight female predominance.
   c. Histopathologic grading does not correlate well with clinical behavior.
   d. Most intramedullary astrocytomas exhibit enhancement.

4. What is the most common histologic subtype of spinal cord astroctyoma?
   a. Pilocytic astrocytoma—grade I
   b. Diffuse (fibrillary) astrocytoma (low grade)—grade II
   c. Anaplastic astrocytoma—grade III
   d. Glioblastoma—grade IV

Astrocytoma of the Conus Medullaris

1. a and c

2. a

3. d

4. b

References

Henson JW, Thornton AF, Louis DN: Spinal cord astrocytoma: Response to PCV chemotherapy, *Neurology* 54:518-520, 2000.

Seo HS, Kim JH, Lee DH, et al: Nonenhancing intramedullary astrocytomas and other MR imaging features: A retrospective study and systematic review, *AJNR Am J Neuroradiol* 31:498-503, 2010.

Cross-Reference

Neuroradiology: The REQUISITES, 3rd ed, pp 556-557.

Comment

Background

Astrocytomas are rare tumors that tend to occur in the third to fifth decades of life. Isolated conus astrocytomas may cause symptoms of a lower motor neuron lesion, with or without spinal cord symptoms. Patients may present with various symptoms, ranging from flaccid paralysis or paresis of the lower extremities to spasticity. Patients may also present with urinary and fecal incontinence or constipation.

Histopathology

Astrocytomas arise from astrocytes in the spinal cord. Most cord astrocytomas (75%) are low-grade (World Health Organization grade II) fibrillary astrocytomas. Histopathologic grading correlates well with clinical behavior and, along with the location in the spinal cord, is helpful in determining prognosis.

Imaging

The classic MRI appearance of intramedullary astrocytoma is cord enlargement and poorly defined margins. It is typically isointense to hypointense on T1-weighted images and hyperintense on T2-weighted images (Figs. A and B). Most astrocytomas are central and involve the entire cord. Peritumoral and tumoral cysts are frequently associated with astrocytomas. The frequency of peritumoral edema is less than 50% and is typically small in quantity. Most intramedullary astrocytomas exhibit at least some enhancement, regardless of cell type or tumor grade. About 20% to 30% of intramedullary astrocytomas show minimal or no enhancement (Fig. C).

Management

Surgery and radiation therapy are first-line treatments. Response to chemotherapy has also been described.

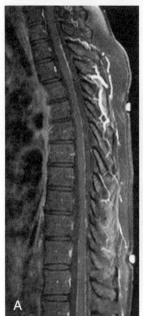 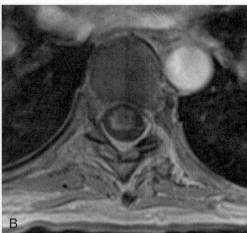 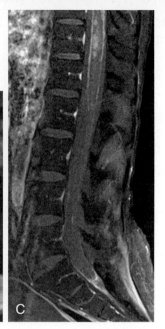

History: A 50-year-old woman presents with leg weakness and numbness.

1. Which of the following should be included in the differential diagnosis for the imaging findings presented? (Choose all that apply.)
   a. Drop metastases
   b. Lymphoma
   c. Meningitis
   d. Sarcoidosis
   e. Intracranial hypotension

2. Which of the following primary central nervous system neoplasms is *least* likely to seed the spinal subarachnoid space?
   a. Oligodendroglioma
   b. Lymphoma
   c. Ependymoma
   d. Dysembryoplastic neuroepithelial tumor (DNET)

3. What percentage of patients with glioblastoma multiforme develop macroscopically evident spinal drop metastases?
   a. 1%
   b. 10%
   c. 25%
   d. 50%

4. Which procedure is best to confirm the diagnosis?
   a. 18F-FDG PET
   b. CT myelography
   c. Lumbar puncture
   d. Serum genetic markers

Glioblastoma Multiforme with Spinal Leptomeningeal Seeding

1. a, b, c, and d

2. d

3. a

4. c

References
Gomori JM, Heching N, Siegal T: Leptomeningeal metastases: Evaluation by gadolinium enhanced spinal magnetic resonance imaging, *J Neurooncol* 36:55-60, 1998.

Karaca M, Andrieu MN, Hicsonmez A, et al: Cases of glioblastoma multiforme metastasizing to spinal cord, *Neurol India* 54:428-430, 2006.

Stark AM, Nabavi A, Mehdorn HM, et al: Glioblastoma multiforme—report of 267 cases treated at a single institution, *Surg Neurol* 63:162-169, 2005.

Cross-Reference
Neuroradiology: The REQUISITES, 3rd ed, pp 559-560.

Comment
Background
Glioblastoma multiforme (GBM) is the most common primary malignancy of the central nervous system. The most common sites for spinal GBM metastases are the lower thoracic and lumbosacral regions.

Pathophysiology
Spread is thought to be due to tumor cells exfoliating into the cerebrospinal fluid (CSF) when the tumor reaches the subarachnoid space. Surgery may enhance the risk of drop metastases, although they have also been reported in people who never had surgery.

Imaging
Postcontrast T1-weighted MRI, without or with fat suppression, is the examination of choice for the detection of spinal leptomeningeal metastases (Figs. A-C). In the study by Gomori and colleagues, leptomeningeal metastases were detected on postcontrast images in approximately 50% of high-risk patients with negative initial CSF cytology or no spinal symptoms. Of the adult gliomas, the one that most commonly spreads via the CSF is GBM. Subarachnoid seeding by intraaxial tumors is hypothesized to occur when the tumor breaks through the ependyma into the ventricular system.

Management
Because cure is not feasible, treatment is solely palliative. Radiation therapy is the most common treatment modality. The advantage of intravenous or intrathecal chemotherapy has not been proved.

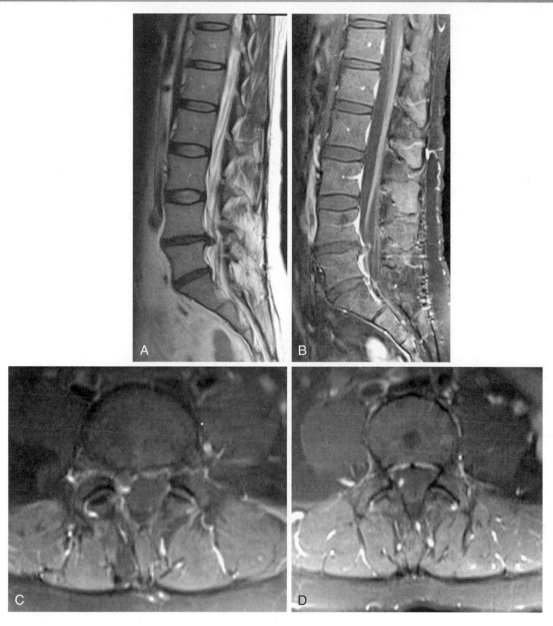

History: A 43-year-old woman presents with back pain radiating to the right leg. The patient has a history of keyhole laminectomy performed 10 years ago.

1. What should be included in the differential diagnosis? (Choose all that apply.)
   a. Dural arteriovenous fistula
   b. Arachnoiditis
   c. Nerve root enhancement secondary to disk herniation
   d. Cytomegalovirus
   e. Guillain-Barré syndrome

2. What is the frequency of lumbar nerve root enhancement on contrast-enhanced MRI after surgery for lumbar disk herniation?
   a. Less than 5%
   b. 25%
   c. 50%
   d. More than 50%

3. What additional intradural structure may produce the findings seen in this case?
   a. Artery of Adamkiewicz
   b. Medullary vein
   c. Radicular vein
   d. Radiculomedullary artery

4. Which of the following statements is true?
   a. The sacral sensory ganglia (dorsal root ganglia) normally enhance.
   b. Nerve root enhancement less than 6 months after surgery is considered abnormal.
   c. Nerve root enhancement has no statistically significant correlation with postoperative sciatica.
   d. The medullary veins are indistinguishable from enhancing nerve roots.

Enhancing Nerve Root with Lumbar Disk Herniation

1. b and c

2. d

3. b

4. a

References

Itoh R, Murata K, Kamata M, et al: Lumbosacral nerve root enhancement with disk herniation on contrast-enhanced MR, *AJNR Am J Neuroradiol* 17(9):1619-1625, 1996.

Lee YS, Choi ES, Song CJ: Symptomatic nerve root changes on contrast-enhanced MR imaging after surgery for lumbar disk herniation, *AJNR Am J Neuroradiol* 30(5):1062-1067, 2009.

Cross-Reference

Neuroradiology: The REQUISITES, 3rd ed, pp 525-526.

Comment

Background

Nerve root enhancement has been observed after lumbosacral surgery in patients with disk herniation. In some patients, enhancement is observed from the site of compression to the conus medullaris. A clinical association between nerve root enhancement and symptoms is highest when recurrent disk herniation is found together with nerve root thickening and displacement.

Pathophysiology

Pathologic enhancement of the sacral and lumbar roots in the cauda equina has been attributed to breakdown of the blood-nerve barrier of these roots from various nonspecific insults, including compression, ischemia, inflammation, active demyelination, and axonal degeneration. For sacral nerves, the sensory ganglia (which lack a blood-nerve barrier) are located within the sacral canal along the course of the dorsal root. Normal enhancement of these ganglia may mimic pathologic enhancement in the sacral region.

Imaging

The enhancing nerve root can be identified by tracking the punctate enhancement on contiguous axial images (Figs. A and B) and the linear enhancement on the sagittal image (Fig. C) to a level of disk herniation (Fig. D). In theory, the large medullary veins, which drain from the midline anterior or posterior median veins on the conus, should be distinguishable from enhancing nerve roots, which originate more laterally from the cord surface.

Management

Spontaneous regression of the herniated disk may result in decompression of the nerve root and resolution of the enhancement. However, prolonged nerve root compression and enhancement may result in intraneural scarring, local demyelination, and wallerian degeneration and should be considered an important indication for surgical treatment.

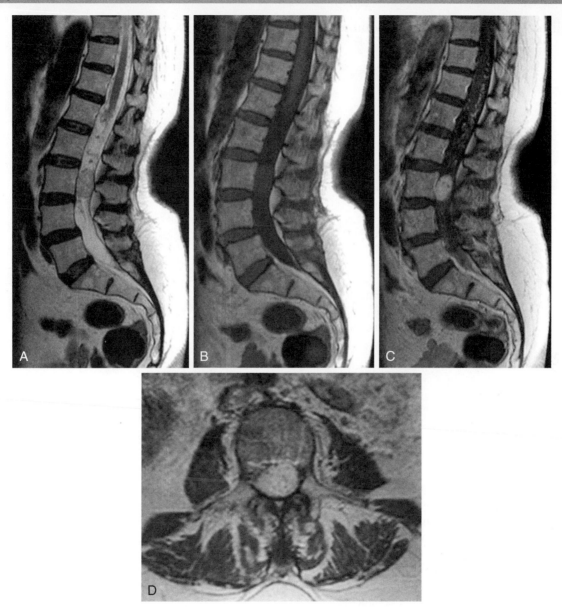

History: A 69-year-old woman presents with a history of worsening back pain for the past 2 years and lower extremity weakness.

1. What should be included in the differential diagnosis? (Choose all that apply.)
   a. Dural arteriovenous fistula
   b. Schwannoma
   c. Meningioma
   d. Hemangioblastoma
   e. Paraganglioma

2. Where in the spinal axis are hemangioblastomas most frequently found?
   a. Cervical spine
   b. Thoracic spine
   c. Lumbar spine
   d. Sacrum

3. Which of the following statements regarding sporadic hemangioblastoma and hemangioblastomas in patients with von Hippel-Lindau (VHL) disease is true?
   a. Patients with VHL disease tend to present with neurologic symptoms at an older age than patients with sporadic disease.
   b. Patients with VHL disease typically have larger tumors than patients with sporadic hemangioblastoma.
   c. Hemangioblastomas in the spine are more often related to VHL disease than are posterior fossa hemangioblastomas.
   d. Hemangioblastomas in patients with VHL disease have a higher frequency of associated cysts compared with sporadic cases.

4. What is the World Health Organization (WHO) classification for hemangioblastomas?
   a. WHO grade I
   b. WHO grade II
   c. WHO grade III
   d. WHO grade IV

Hemangioblastoma of the Cauda Equina

1. d and e

2. b

3. c

4. a

Reference

Biondi A, Ricciardi GK, Faillot T, et al: Hemangioblastomas of the lower spinal region: Report of four cases with preoperative embolization and review of the literature, *AJNR Am J Neuroradiol* 26(4):936-945, 2005.

Cross-Reference

Neuroradiology: The REQUISITES, 3rd ed, pp 558-559.

Comment

Background

Hemangioblastomas are rare tumors accounting for 1% to 5% of all spinal cord tumors. Two thirds are sporadic, and one third of hemangioblastomas are associated with VHL disease. The male-to-female ratio is approximately 2:1. Of spinal hemangioblastomas, 75% are intramedullary.

Histopathology

Hemangioblastomas are composed of abnormal, densely vascular parenchyma consisting of thin-walled, closely packed blood vessels interspersed with large stromal cells.

Imaging

MRI features of spinal hemangioblastoma depend on the size of the tumor. Small (≤10 mm) hemangioblastomas are mostly isointense on T1-weighted images and hyperintense on T2-weighted images. Enhancement after contrast agent administration is homogeneous. Larger tumors tend to be hypointense or have mixed intensity (hypointense/isointense) on T1-weighted images and mixed intensity on T2-weighted images (Figs. A and B). Enhancement after contrast agent administration is heterogeneous (Figs. C and D). Vascular flow voids are commonly seen within or adjacent to medium-sized and large tumors on MRI (see Fig. A). The flow voids represent distended feeding arteries or draining veins. Magnetic resonance angiography (MRA) is a good supplementary technique for tumor characterization and to identify whether the arterial feeders of the tumor give branches to the spinal cord.

Management

Treatment for hemangioblastoma is surgical resection. Embolization of these lesions is possible and can reduce the tumor's vascular supply, facilitating surgery.

Notes

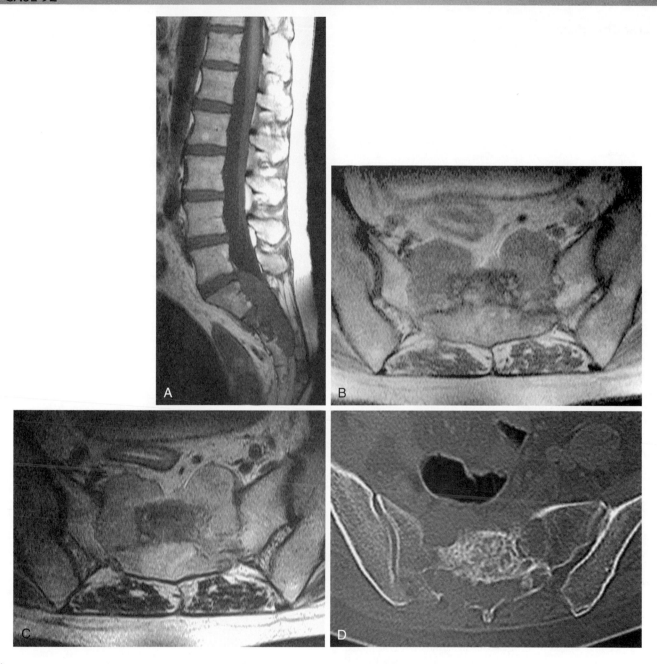

History: A 51-year-old woman with low back pain for the past 2 years presents with cauda equina syndrome.

1. What should be included in the differential diagnosis? (Choose all that apply.)
   a. Metastasis
   b. Meningioma
   c. Chondrosarcoma
   d. Lymphoma
   e. Chordoma

2. What percentage of chordomas originate in the sacrococcygeal region?
   a. 90%
   b. 50%
   c. 35%
   d. 15%

3. Which of the following statements regarding sacral chordomas is true?
   a. Sacral chordomas are typically midline in location.
   b. Sacral chordomas usually extend posteriorly.
   c. Most sacral chordomas invade the rectum.
   d. Sacral chordomas are more common in women than in men.

4. Which joint is most commonly invaded by sacral chordoma?
   a. Facet joint
   b. Femoral joint
   c. Sacroiliac joint
   d. Discovertebral joint

Sacral Chordoma

1. a, c, d, and e

2. b

3. a

4. c

References

Sung MS, Lee GK, Kang HS, et al: Sacrococcygeal chordoma: MR imaging in 30 patients, *Skeletal Radiol* 34(2):87-94, 2005.

York JE, Kaczaraj A, Abi-Said D, et al: Sacral chordoma: 40-year experience at a major cancer center, *Neurosurgery* 44(1):74-79, 1999.

Cross-Reference

Neuroradiology: The REQUISITES, 3rd ed, p 567.

Comment

Background

Chordomas can occur at any age, but they are uncommon in patients younger than 40 years. Chordomas are typically slow growing but locally aggressive. Metastasis is usually a late event and occurs in about one fourth of patients. The presenting symptom in most patients is local pain. Approximately one third of patients also have radiculopathy as a result of irritation of the sciatic nerve. Gluteal muscle infiltration secondary to lateral extension of the tumor is common in sacral chordomas.

Histopathology

Because they originate from notochord remnants, chordomas can involve any segment of the craniospinal axis from the sphenoid to the coccyx. Two types are distinguished histopathologically: typical chordomas, which have a watery, gelatinous matrix, and chondroid chordomas, in which this matrix is replaced by cartilaginous foci.

Imaging

MRI and CT have complementary roles in evaluating chordomas. On MRI, chordomas are lobulated masses (Figs. A-C) that are typically low to intermediate in signal on T1-weighted images (see Fig. A) and heterogeneous in signal on T2-weighted images (see Fig. C). Enhancement is heterogeneous (see Fig. B). CT is helpful in assessing the degree of bone involvement and destruction (Fig. D) and in detecting a pattern of calcification within the lesion.

Management

Sacral chordomas are resistant to radiation and chemotherapy. Radical resection is associated with a significantly longer disease-free interval compared with subtotal removal of the tumor. The addition of radiation after subtotal resection improves the disease-free interval.

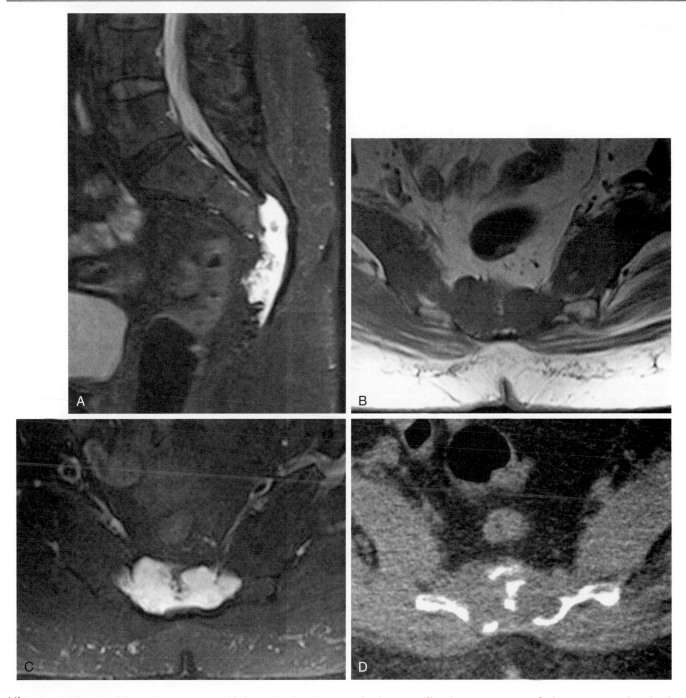

History: A 63-year-old woman presents with lower back pain.

1. What should be included in the differential diagnosis for the imaging findings presented? (Choose all that apply.)
   a. Chordoma
   b. Metastasis
   c. Plasmacytoma
   d. Schwannoma
   e. Ependymoma

2. What is the most common location of chordomas?
   a. Clivus
   b. Cervical spine
   c. Lumbar spine
   d. Sacrococcygeal region

3. Among all primary tumors of the sacrum, what is the frequency of chordoma?
   a. 20%
   b. 40%
   c. 60%
   d. 80%

4. All of the following imaging features are suggestive of chordoma *except:*
   a. Calcification on CT
   b. Origin at the sacrococcygeal junction
   c. Posterior extension
   d. Presence of internal septations

Sacrococcygeal Chordoma

1. a, b, and c

2. d

3. b

4. c

References

Soo MYS, Wong L: Sacrococcygeal chordoma, *J HK Coll Radiol* 5:117-125, 2002.

Sung MS, Lee GK, Kang HS, et al: Sacrococcygeal chordoma: MR imaging in 30 patients, *Skeletal Radiol* 34(2):87-94, 2005.

Cross-Reference

Neuroradiology: The REQUISITES, 3rd ed, p 567.

Comment

Background

Sacrococcygeal chordomas are found predominantly in adults 50 to 65 years old. Chordomas are typically slow growing but locally aggressive, and gluteal muscle infiltration secondary to lateral extension of the tumor is common.

Histopathology

Chordomas arise from remnants of the notochord and can involve any segment of the craniospinal axis from the sphenoid to the coccyx. Typical chordomas consist of mucin-containing physaliphorous cells, purely cystic mucinous pools, or sometimes both.

Imaging

Chordomas typically arise from the lower three segments of the sacrum and coccyx, whereas metastases and other tumors typically arise from the first and second sacral segments. The classic features of sacrococcygeal chordoma include a soft tissue mass with aggressive destruction of bone and invasion of adjacent soft tissues (Figs. A-D). On MRI, the lesion is of intermediate to low signal intensity on T1-weighted images (see Fig. B) and high intensity on T2-weighted images (see Figs. A and C). The presence of mucinous pools accounts for the hyperintense lobulations of the mass seen on T2-weighted images. Hypointense septations represent fibrous strands between the lobular components of the tumor (see Fig. C).

Management

The treatment of choice in sacral chordoma is wide surgical resection. Obtaining tumor-free margins at the initial surgery reduces the risk of local recurrence and is the primary factor in improved survival.

Notes

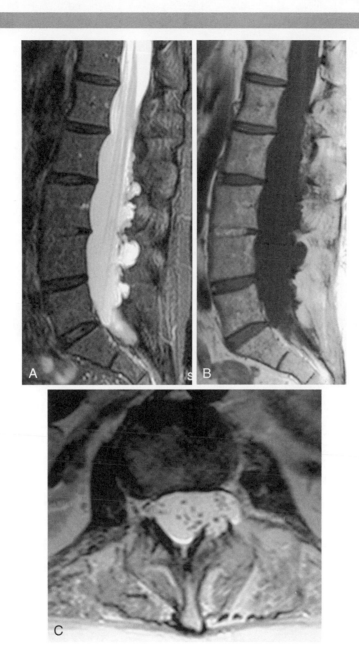

History: A 55-year-old man presents with cauda equina syndrome.

1. What should be included in the differential diagnosis? (Choose all that apply.)
   a. Neurofibromatosis type 1
   b. Neurofibromatosis type 2
   c. Systemic lupus erythematosus
   d. Marfan syndrome
   e. Ankylosing spondylitis

2. What imaging feature is helpful in suggesting ankylosing spondylitis as the underlying diagnosis rather than other causes of dural ectasia?
   a. Location within the cervical spine
   b. Involvement of more than three consecutive vertebral body segments
   c. Predominant involvement of the posterior elements
   d. Posterior vertebral body scalloping

3. What is the most likely mechanism of dural ectasia in patients with ankylosing spondylitis?
   a. Small vessel angiitis involving the vasa vasorum of the nerve roots
   b. Previous spinal irradiation for treatment of ankylosing spondylitis
   c. Nerve root damage from increased pulsatile forces transmitted through the cerebrospinal fluid
   d. Chronic inflammatory process

4. Which of the following conditions is most specifically associated with ankylosing spondylitis?
   a. Biapical pulmonary fibrosis
   b. Urethritis
   c. Dactylitis
   d. Malar rash

Dural Ectasia in Ankylosing Spondylitis

1. a, d, and e

2. c

3. d

4. a

Reference
Liu CC, Lin YC, Lo CP, et al: Cauda equina syndrome and dural ectasia: Rare manifestations in chronic ankylosing spondylitis, *Br J Radiol* 84(1002):e123-e125, 2011.

Cross-Reference
Neuroradiology: The REQUISITES, 3rd ed, pp 534, 535, 537.

Comment
Background
Ankylosing spondylitis is a seronegative spondyloarthropathy affecting primarily the spine and sacroiliac joints. Cauda equina syndrome is a rare neurologic manifestation in patients with long-standing ankylosing spondylitis. Dural ectasia is a condition in which the spinal dural sac is enlarged; this usually involves the lumbosacral region, where the cerebrospinal fluid pressure is greatest. It is occasionally seen in patients with Marfan syndrome, neurofibromatosis type 1, Ehlers-Danlos syndrome, and long-standing ankylosing spondylitis; however, the bony erosion in ankylosing spondylitis involves predominantly the posterior elements rather than the posterior aspect of the vertebral bodies, as seen in the other conditions.

Pathophysiology
The mechanism of dural ectasia formation in patients with ankylosing spondylitis is unclear. One possible explanation is that the inflammatory process in ankylosing spondylitis results in adhesions of the dura mater that reduce the compliance and elasticity of the lower dural sac and its ability to dampen the fluctuations in cerebrospinal fluid pressure, which results in dural ectasia and bony erosion.

Imaging
CT shows expansion of the spinal canal, with remodeling and erosion of the posterior elements of the vertebrae, including the pedicles. MRI reveals characteristic expansion of the lumbar spinal canal, with scalloping of the laminae and spinous processes (Figs. A-C).

Management
There is no effective medical or surgical treatment for dural ectasia; it is presumably an end result of the chronic inflammatory process.

Notes

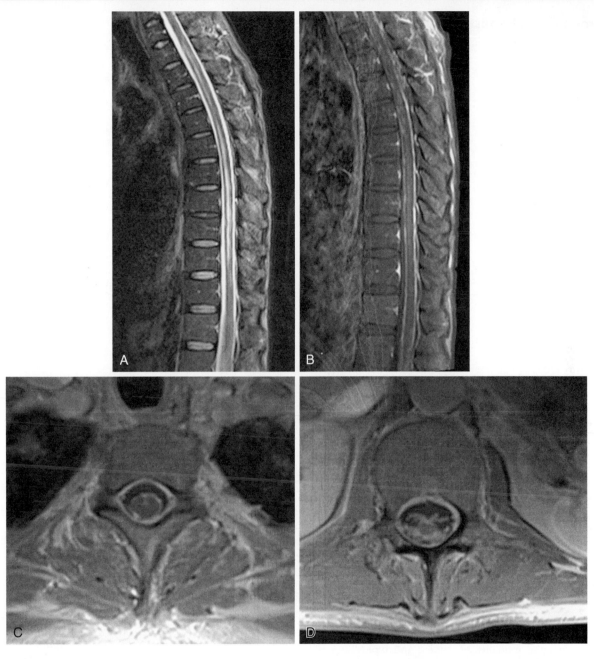

History: A 44-year-old man with a history of a left heel skin lesion removed 5 years ago presents with back pain.

1. What should be included in the differential diagnosis? (Choose all that apply.)
   a. Sarcoid
   b. Tuberculous meningitis
   c. Multiple sclerosis
   d. Lymphoma
   e. Leptomeningeal carcinomatosis

2. Which of the following lesions is *least* likely to manifest with leptomeningeal carcinomatosis?
   a. Lung cancer
   b. Breast cancer
   c. Melanoma
   d. Bladder cancer

3. Where along the spinal axis is leptomeningeal metastasis *most* likely to be found?
   a. Cervical cord
   b. Thoracic cord
   c. Cauda equina
   d. Thecal sac terminus

4. Which of the following primary leptomeningeal tumors containing melanin is unlikely to manifest with isolated diffuse involvement of the subarachnoid space?
   a. Pigmented meningioma
   b. Primary leptomeningeal melanomatosis
   c. Diffuse melanosis
   d. Meningeal melanocytoma

CASE 95

Leptomeningeal Metastases (Malignant Melanoma)

1. a, b, d, and e

2. d

3. c

4. a

References

Chamberlain MC: Leptomeningeal metastasis, *Curr Opin Neurol* 22(6):665-674, 2009.

Gomori JM, Heching N, Siegal T: Leptomeningeal metastases: Evaluation by gadolinium enhanced spinal magnetic resonance imaging, *J Neurooncol* 36(1):55-60, 1998.

Holtz AJ: The sugarcoating sign, *Radiology* 208(1):143-144, 1998.

Cross-Reference

Neuroradiology: The REQUISITES, 3rd ed, pp 559-560.

Comment

Background

Diffuse leptomeningeal metastatic disease, or carcinomatosis, has become more common as the longevity of patients with cancer has increased and as techniques for identifying malignant cells in the cerebrospinal fluid have improved.

Histopathology

Leptomeningeal carcinomatosis occurs with the invasion and subsequent proliferation of neoplastic cells in the subarachnoid space; this may cause multifocal or diffuse infiltration of the leptomeninges in a sheetlike fashion along the surface of the spinal cord. This multifocal seeding of the leptomeninges by malignant cells is called leptomeningeal carcinomatosis if the primary malignancy is a solid tumor and lymphomatous meningitis or leukemic meningitis if it is not a solid tumor. Leptomeningeal metastases may result from hematogenous spread or intrathecal cerebrospinal fluid spread (drop metastases) of malignant cells.

Imaging

MRI is the imaging modality of choice and typically demonstrates peripheral linear or nodular enhancement of the cord surface and conus (Figs. A-D). Linear enhancement has been called the "sugarcoating" or "frosting" sign. In addition, thickening and linear or nodular enhancement of the cauda equina roots are often seen (see Fig. D).

Management

The therapeutic management of leptomeningeal carcinomatosis includes intrathecal administration of chemotherapy and radiotherapy. Treatment is controversial, and no straightforward guidelines exist in the literature.

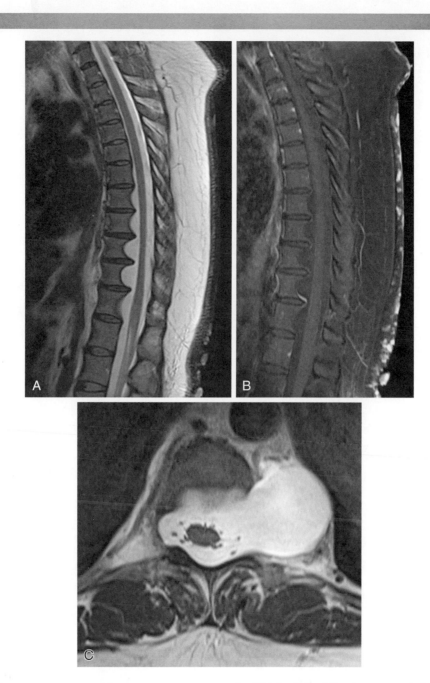

History: A 46-year-old woman presents with cutaneous lesions.

1. What should be included in the differential diagnosis? (Choose all that apply.)
   a. Neurofibromatosis type 1
   b. Marfan syndrome
   c. Arachnoid cyst
   d. Spinal cord tumor
   e. Acromegaly

2. All of the following conditions may cause posterior scalloping *except:*
   a. Achondroplasia
   b. Communicating hydrocephalus
   c. Morquio syndrome
   d. Down syndrome

3. Which of the following tumors is *least* likely to cause localized posterior vertebral scalloping?
   a. Schwannoma
   b. Lymphoma
   c. Lipoma
   d. Ependymoma

4. Which of the following statements is *false?*
   a. Posterior scalloping can be diagnosed with plain radiographs.
   b. Dural ectasia is a highly characteristic indicator of Marfan syndrome.
   c. Dural ectasia is typically more marked in the cervical spine.
   d. Minor posterior vertebral body scalloping can be seen in normal individuals.

Posterior Vertebral Body Scalloping in Neurofibromatosis Type 1

1. a, b, and e

2. d

3. b

4. c

References
Wakely SL: The posterior vertebral scalloping sign, *Radiology* 239(2):607-609, 2006.
Woon CY: Dural ectasia: A manifestation of type 1 neurofibromatosis, *CMAJ* 182(13):1448, 2010.

Cross-Reference
Neuroradiology: The REQUISITES, 3rd ed, pp 534, 535, 537.

Comment
Background
Posterior vertebral scalloping appears on imaging as an exaggeration of the normal concavity of the posterior surface of one or more vertebral bodies. It is often seen in patients with neurofibromatosis type 1 secondary to dural ectasia. The complications of progressive vertebral body erosion include angular deformities and vertebral fractures and dislocations. Neurologic deficit rarely occurs because the spinal canal is widened.

Pathophysiology
Dural ectasia is thought to cause posterior vertebral scalloping owing to loss of the normal protection provided to the vertebral body by a strong, intact dura.

Imaging
Classic radiologic findings include erosion of the central posterior vertebral body, wedging and posterior scalloping of the vertebral body, pedicle erosion, foraminal enlargement, and kyphosis (Figs. A to C).

Management
Dural ectasia leads to tremendous erosion and deformation of the anterior column and may progress, compromising support function. Early surgical stabilization may be necessary to prevent severe deformity and late complications.

Notes

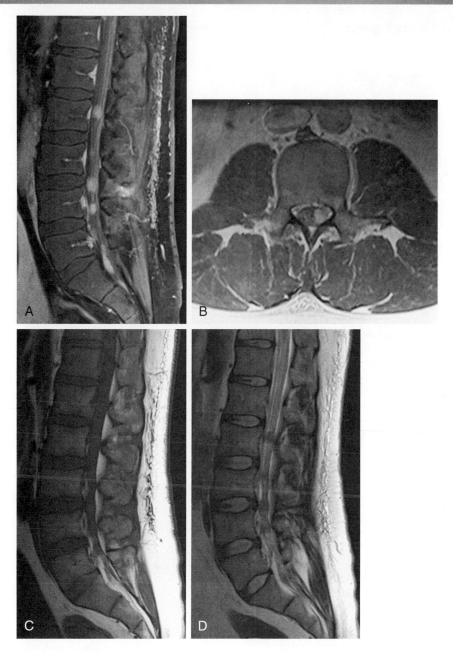

History: A 38-year-old African American man presents with bilateral lower extremity pain, weakness, and sensory loss.

1. What should be included in the differential diagnosis? (Choose all that apply.)
   a. Nerve sheath tumor
   b. Metastasis
   c. Sarcoidosis
   d. Guillain-Barré syndrome
   e. Infectious leptomeningitis

2. Which of the following cerebrospinal fluid abnormalities is not supportive of neurosarcoidosis?
   a. Elevated angiotensin-converting enzyme levels
   b. Low total protein
   c. Elevated white blood cell count
   d. Presence of oligoclonal bands

3. Which of the following manifestations of neurosarcoidosis is the most common?
   a. Parenchymal brain lesions
   b. Peripheral neuropathy
   c. Myopathy
   d. Cranial neuropathy

4. Which imaging study would you recommend next for this patient?
   a. CT myelography
   b. 18F-FDG PET/CT
   c. MRI of the brain and spine
   d. CT scan of the brain

Sarcoidosis of the Cauda Equina

1. a, b, c, and e

2. b

3. d

4. c

References
Kaiboriboon K, Olsen TJ, Hayat GR: Cauda equina and conus medullaris syndrome in sarcoidosis, *Neurologist* 11(3):179-183, 2005.

Spencer TS, Campellone JV, Maldonado I, et al: Clinical and magnetic resonance imaging manifestations of neurosarcoidosis, *Semin Arthritis Rheum* 34(4):649-661, 2005.

Cross-Reference
Neuroradiology: The REQUISITES, 3rd ed, pp 546, 547.

Comment
Background
Sarcoidosis is a multisystem granulomatous disease of unknown etiology. Sarcoidosis can affect patients of all ages and races, but it is most common in the third and fourth decades of life, and African Americans and whites of northern European descent have the highest disease incidence. Women are more frequently affected than men. Approximately 5% of patients have involvement of the nervous system. Central nervous system involvement is the initial presentation in about half of these patients, making the diagnosis difficult.

Histopathology
Definitive diagnosis of neurosarcoidosis requires the exclusion of other causes of neuropathy and the identification of noncaseating sarcoid granulomas by histologic analysis.

Imaging
Spinal neurosarcoidosis can manifest with a spinal cord mass, leptomeningitis, and lumbosacral nerve root masses. The MRI enhancement pattern in patients with sarcoidosis is nonspecific. In cases involving the cauda equina, enhancement is leptomeningeal, with linear enhancement or small nodules that are often dura-based and demonstrate intense enhancement (Figs. A and B). The lesions are hypointense or isointense in signal on T1-weighted images (Fig. C) and isointense or hyperintense on T2-weighted images (Fig. D).

Management
Diagnosis and early treatment of neurosarcoidosis with corticosteroids can minimize neurologic complications and decrease disease morbidity rates; however, with delayed diagnosis and treatment, the disease typically resolves only partially and may recur.

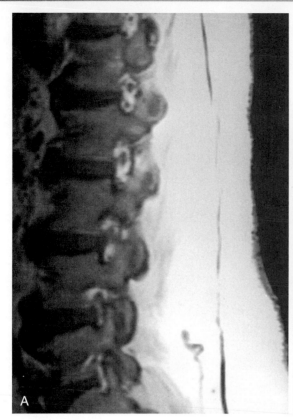

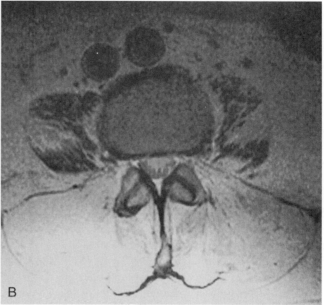

History: A 52-year-old man presents with progressive lower extremity weakness.

1. What should be included in the differential diagnosis? (Choose all that apply.)
   a. Muscular dystrophy
   b. Lipoma
   c. Dermatomyositis
   d. Spinal muscular atrophy
   e. Lumbar plexopathy

2. What is the inheritance pattern of Duchenne's muscular dystrophy?
   a. Autosomal recessive
   b. Autosomal dominant
   c. X-linked
   d. Mitochondrial

3. What anatomic structure does the low-signal-intensity stripe located between the spine and the skin on the parasagittal image represent?
   a. Interspinous ligament
   b. Posterior thoracolumbar fascia
   c. Middle thoracolumbar fascia
   d. Anterior thoracolumbar fascia

4. What is "pseudohypertrophy" in the context of Duchenne's muscular dystrophy?
   a. Hypertrophy of the urinary bladder wall secondary to incontinence
   b. Hypertrophy of the subcutaneous fat
   c. Hypertrophy of one limb
   d. Enlargement of certain muscle groups

Duchenne's Muscular Dystrophy

1. a, c, and d

2. c

3. b

4. d

References

Mercuri E, Pichiecchio A, Allsop J, et al: Muscle MRI in inherited neuromuscular disorders: Past, present, and future, *J Magn Reson Imaging* 25(2):433-440, 2007.

Ozsarlak O, Schepens E, Parizel PM, et al: Hereditary neuromuscular diseases, *Eur J Radiol* 40(3):184-197, 2001.

Cross-Reference

Neuroradiology: The REQUISITES, 3rd ed, p 528.

Comment

Background

Muscular dystrophy refers to a collection of genetically determined myopathies characterized by progressive atrophy or degeneration of individual muscle cells. Traditionally, muscular dystrophies are subdivided according to the pattern of initial muscle involvement. Duchenne's muscular dystrophy is the most severe form of muscular dystrophy and is inherited as an X-linked recessive disorder, predominantly in boys. It is initially characterized by symmetric and selective involvement of the proximal pelvic girdle muscles in the early stage of the disease process; the calf and proximal shoulder girdle muscles become involved in the late stage. In patients with Duchenne-type muscular dystrophy, complete paralysis and death usually ensue within the first 2 decades of life. The patient in this case has a benign variant of the Duchenne type that may not begin until the fourth decade and has a minimal effect on life span.

Histopathology

Duchenne's muscular dystrophy is caused by a defective gene for dystrophin (a protein in the muscles). The lack of dystrophin makes muscle fibers susceptible to mechanical damage, leading to their replacement by fat. Dystrophin is found not only in skeletal muscle but also in smooth muscle and in the brain.

Imaging

MRI of muscle is increasingly being used as a diagnostic tool because various inherited neuromuscular disorders show a specific pattern of muscle involvement. MRI is also helpful in determining the severity of fatty infiltration. On T1-weighted images, hyperintense fatty infiltration interspersed between the diseased muscles is typically seen (Figs. A and B). The posterior layer of the thoracolumbar fascia is prominent on MRI (see Fig. A) because it is outlined by the fatty replaced muscle and the subcutaneous fat.

Management

There is no known cure for Duchenne's muscular dystrophy. Treatment is aimed at controlling symptoms to improve quality of life.

Notes

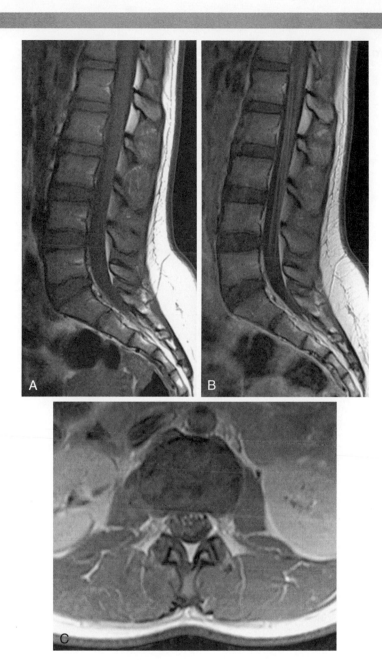

History: A 16-year-old girl presents with lower extremity weakness and a history of fever, headache, and sore throat 3 weeks prior.

1. What should be included in the differential diagnosis? (Choose all that apply.)
   a. Cytomegalovirus infection
   b. Chronic inflammatory demyelinating polyneuropathy
   c. Sarcoidosis
   d. Guillain-Barré syndrome (GBS)
   e. Vitamin B$_{12}$ deficiency

2. Which of the following findings on physical examination is atypical of GBS?
   a. Symmetric ascending motor weakness
   b. Pronounced sensory involvement
   c. Hyporeflexia
   d. Areflexia

3. Which of the following is *not* a risk factor for GBS?
   a. *Campylobacter jejuni* infection
   b. Recent vaccination
   c. Previous trauma
   d. Recent viral illness

4. What enhancement pattern of the cauda equina roots is strongly suggestive of GBS?
   a. Isolated enhancement of the ventral roots
   b. Isolated enhancement of the dorsal roots
   c. Diffuse enhancement of the nerve roots
   d. Nodular enhancement of the roots

Guillain-Barré Syndrome

1. a, b, c, and d

2. b

3. c

4. a

References

Byun WM, Park WK, Park BH, et al: Guillain-Barré syndrome: MR imaging findings in eight patients, *Radiology* 208(1):137-141, 1998.

Zuccoli G, Panigrahy A, Bailey A, et al: Redefining the Guillain-Barré spectrum in children: Neuroimaging findings of cranial nerve involvement, *AJNR Am J Neuroradiol* 32(4):639-642, 2011.

Cross-Reference

Neuroradiology: The REQUISITES, 3rd ed, pp 540-541, 548.

Comment

Background

GBS is an acute, rapidly progressing inflammatory polyradiculopathy that causes acute neuromuscular failure. Cranial nerve involvement is frequently seen in GBS, with the facial nerve being affected most often. Patients with GBS initially present with progressive and ascending weakness of the extremities and areflexia. Symptoms progress rapidly and may include facial nerve palsies, autonomic dysfunction, pain, numbness, paresthesia, and respiratory failure. Diagnosis is usually established on the basis of the clinical presentation. Cerebrospinal fluid analysis shows an elevated protein level without pleocytosis.

Pathophysiology

GBS is a postinfectious, immune-mediated disease. A mild respiratory or gastrointestinal tract infection precedes the onset of symptoms in 75% of patients with GBS. Many of the infectious agents are thought to induce the production of antibodies that cross-react with specific gangliosides and glycolipids found in myelin of the peripheral nervous system.

Imaging

MRI is frequently ordered to exclude other causes of motor weakness, such as cord compression and transverse myelitis. MRI in patients with GBS shows thickening and marked enhancement of the nerve roots in the conus medullaris and cauda equina (Figs. A-C). Byun and colleagues suggested that enhancement solely of the anterior roots (Fig. C) is strongly suggestive of GBS.

Management

GBS does not respond to corticosteroids. Treatment consists of supportive therapy, plasmapheresis, and infusion of immunoglobulin.

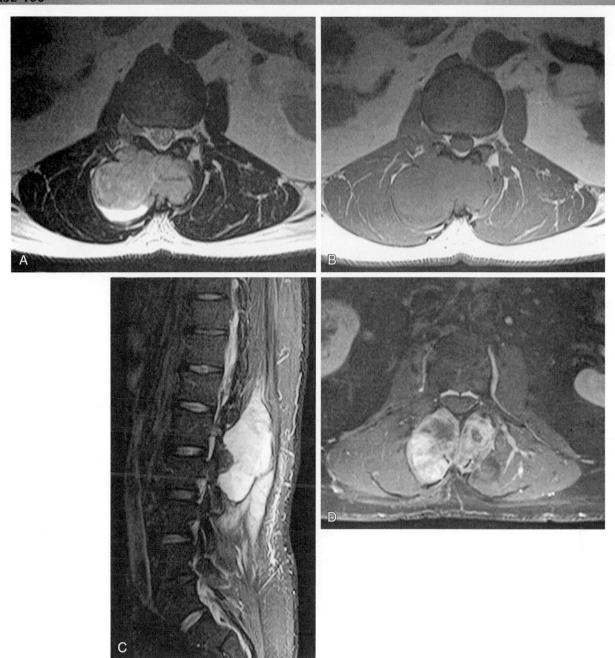

History: A 54-year-old man presents with midback swelling.

1. What should be included in the differential diagnosis? (Choose all that apply.)
   a. Fibromatosis
   b. Abscess
   c. Organized hematoma
   d. Sarcoma
   e. Metastasis

2. What is the most common type of soft tissue sarcoma in adults?
   a. Pleomorphic undifferentiated sarcoma
   b. Liposarcoma
   c. Synovial cell sarcoma
   d. Fibrosarcoma

3. Which of the following is the *least* common location of soft tissue sarcomas?
   a. Around the knee
   b. Thigh
   c. Proximal arm
   d. Paraspinal soft tissues

4. Which of the following statements regarding fibrosarcoma is true?
   a. Secondary fibrosarcoma is less aggressive than primary fibrosarcoma.
   b. Infantile fibrosarcoma has a better prognosis compared with fibrosarcoma in adults.
   c. Fibrosarcoma has been noted to arise from hemangioma.
   d. Soft tissue fibrosarcomas often manifest as painful masses.

Paraspinal Fibrosarcoma

1. a, d, and e

2. a

3. d

4. b

Reference
Ilaslan H, Schils J, Nageotte W, et al: Clinical presentation and imaging of bone and soft-tissue sarcomas, *Cleve Clin J Med* 77(Suppl 2):S2-S7, 2010.

Cross-Reference
Neuroradiology: The REQUISITES, 3rd ed, pp 565-566.

Comment

Background
Soft tissue sarcomas originating in the paraspinal muscles are rare tumors that are often diagnosed late because of a low clinical index of suspicion. Fibrosarcoma represents about 10% of musculoskeletal sarcomas. Fibrosarcoma of the soft tissues usually affects individuals 35 to 55 years old and most often manifests as a painless mass. Because these tumors frequently arise deep to the muscular fascia, they may become extremely large before diagnosis.

Histopathology
Fibrosarcomas are tumors of mesenchymal cell origin, composed of malignant fibroblasts in a collagen background. They can occur as a soft tissue mass or as a primary or secondary (arising from a preexisting lesion or after radiotherapy) bone tumor. Similar to other soft tissue sarcomas, no definite cause can be identified; however, genetic mutations may play a role in their development.

Imaging
MRI findings are nonspecific. Soft tissue sarcoma is generally a large mass deep to fascia. A pseudocapsule or capsule is commonly seen, which may produce well-defined margins (Figs. A and B). On T2-weighted images, soft tissue sarcomas are heterogeneous in signal (see Fig. A); high signal changes surrounding the lesion (Fig. C) are thought to represent peritumoral edema. Heterogeneous enhancement is typically seen (Fig. D).

Management
Patients with paraspinal soft tissue tumors should undergo complete staging before biopsy. Wide en bloc resection should be performed. If the tumor involves the lamina, bone should be resected en bloc. Adjuvant radiotherapy is recommended if wide margins cannot be achieved.

Notes

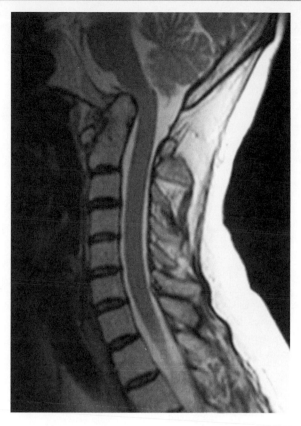

History: A 41-year-old woman presents with neck pain.

1. What should be included in the differential diagnosis? (Choose all that apply.)
   a. Achondroplasia
   b. Rheumatoid arthritis
   c. Psoriatic arthritis
   d. Os odontoideum
   e. Atlantoaxial subluxation

2. What term best describes the imaging findings in this case?
   a. Platybasia
   b. Basilar invagination
   c. Basilar impression
   d. Cranial settling

3. Chamberlain's line is drawn between which anatomic landmarks?
   a. Posterior edge of the hard palate and the opisthion
   b. Posterior edge of the hard palate and the undersurface of the occipital squamosal surface
   c. Basion and opisthion
   d. Tuberculum sella and basion

4. What is the frequency of cranial settling in patients with rheumatoid arthritis?
   a. Less than 1%
   b. 5% to 8%
   c. 22% to 25%
   d. 42% to 45%

Cranial Settling in Rheumatoid Arthritis

1. b and c

2. d

3. a

4. b

References

Kim DH, Hilibrand AS: Rheumatoid arthritis in the cervical spine, *J Am Acad Orthop Surg* 13(7):463-474, 2005.

Smoker WR: MR imaging of the craniovertebral junction, *Magn Reson Imaging Clin N Am* 8(3):635-650, 2000.

Cross-Reference

Neuroradiology: The REQUISITES, 3rd ed, pp 300, 301.

Comment

Background

The term *cranial settling* is applied to upward migration (vertical subluxation) of the odontoid process caused by loss of the supporting ligamentous structures. It is typically associated with rheumatoid arthritis but also occurs in nonrheumatoid conditions, such as psoriatic arthritis.

Histopathology

Synovitis with pannus formation in patients with rheumatoid arthritis affects the diarthrodial joints, including the anterior atlantodental, transverse dental, and lateral atlantoaxial joints. The inflammation ultimately leads to laxity of the joint capsules and ligaments, with resultant abnormal joint mobility. As the disease progresses, the inflammation produces erosion of the lateral C1 masses, the occipital condyles, and the articular facets of C2. The skull and C1 settle onto the cervical spine, causing the odontoid process to be located at an abnormally high position, often severely impinging on the brainstem or cervicomedullary junction.

Imaging

On MRI, the cervicomedullary angle is an effective indicator of cord distortion from cranial settling and superior migration of the odontoid (see the figure). This angle incorporates lines drawn along the anterior aspects of the cervical cord and along the medulla. The normal range is 135 to 175 degrees. Angles less than 135 degrees indicate basilar invagination and have been associated with myelopathy.

Management

Occipitocervical fusion is the procedure of choice in patients with cranial settling. Preoperatively, cervical traction can be used to attempt a gradual reduction.

Notes

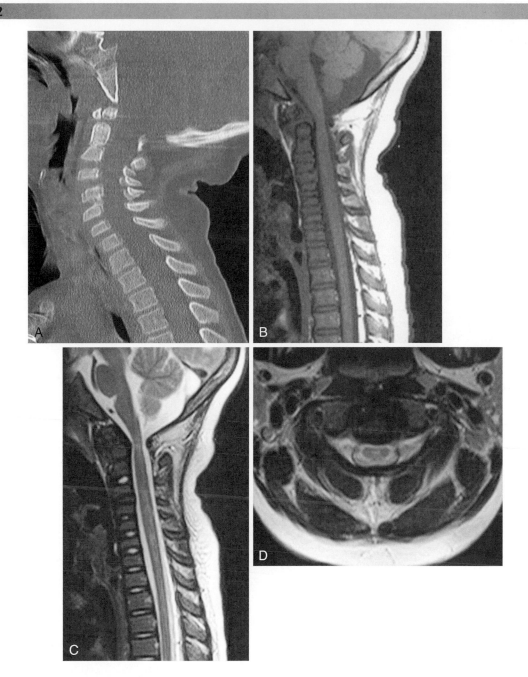

History: The patient is a 6-year-old child with Down syndrome.

1. What should be included in the differential diagnosis? (Choose all that apply.)
   a. Odontoid fracture nonunion
   b. Klippel-Feil syndrome
   c. Atlantoaxial subluxation
   d. Os odontoideum
   e. Persistent ossiculum terminale

2. All of the following are odontoid anomalies occurring in childhood and adolescence *except:*
   a. Aplasia
   b. Hypoplasia
   c. Os odontoideum
   d. Subdental synchondrosis

3. What does the horizontal dark line within C2 on sagittal MRI represent?
   a. Hahn cleft
   b. Fracture line
   c. Normal synchondrosis
   d. Inferior cortical margins of C2, which is fused with C3

4. Which of the following features does not favor congenital os odontoideum over an old odontoid fracture with nonunion?
   a. Hypoplasia of the dens
   b. Smooth sclerotic margins of the dens and ossicle
   c. Wide gap between the dens and ossicle
   d. Hypertrophy of the anterior arch of C1

Os Odontoideum

1. a and d

2. d

3. c

4. b

References

Barnes PD, Kim FM, Crawley C: Developmental anomalies of the craniocervical junction and cervical spine, *Magn Reson Imaging Clin N Am* 8(3):651-674, 2000.

Smoker WR: MR imaging of the craniovertebral junction, *Magn Reson Imaging Clin N Am* 8:635-650, 2000.

Cross-Reference

Neuroradiology: The REQUISITES, 3rd ed, pp 580-581.

Comment

Background

Os odontoideum is an uncommon craniovertebral junction abnormality characterized by a separate ossicle superior to the dens. Many cases are found incidentally, and others are diagnosed when patients become symptomatic. An increased incidence of os odontoideum has been reported in congenital conditions such as Down syndrome, Morquio syndrome, the Klippel-Feil spectrum of anomalies, and spondyloepiphyseal dysplasia.

Pathophysiology

Proposed etiologies for os odontoideum include congenital (proatlas remnant or hypertrophied ossiculum terminale) and acquired (odontoid fracture) mechanisms. The ossicle may be located near the dens tip (expected location; orthotopic os) or near the basion (anterior lip of the foramen magnum; dystopic os). Odontoid anomalies can produce craniocervical instability. Determining the nature and degree of instability is more important than establishing the origin of the anomaly. Anterior displacement of the os-atlas complex relative to the body of the axis in the neutral lateral position and increased range of motion (instability) during flexion and extension can result in cord compression.

Imaging

Radiologic evaluation is used to confirm the diagnosis and estimate the degree of spinal instability. Initial evaluation includes plain radiographs with flexion and extension views. On CT, os odontoideum appears as a round or oval ossicle with a smooth, uniform cortex separated from the base of the axis by a wide gap (Fig. A). The ossicle border does not directly match up with the axis body. The os fragment often moves with the atlas, and the atlantodental interval does not reflect the abnormal motion of the segment. Direct measurement of the motion of C1 on the body of C2 is more useful. MRI (Figs. B-D) is used to assess cord compression and cord signal changes.

Management

Treatment of odontoid anomalies often requires immobilization and traction to achieve reduction, followed by surgical stabilization.

Notes

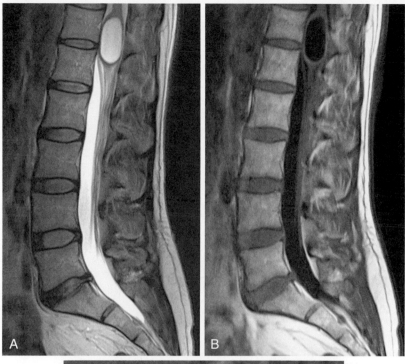

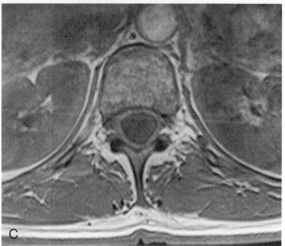

History: A 48-year-old woman presents with back pain and bilateral lower extremity weakness.

1. What should be included in the differential diagnosis? (Choose all that apply.)
   a. Dermoid cyst
   b. Syringomyelia
   c. Ependymoma
   d. Astrocytoma
   e. Ventriculus terminalis cyst

2. Which of the following statements regarding cystic ventriculus terminalis is true?
   a. It is typically found in the midthoracic cord.
   b. Pulsatile cerebrospinal fluid (CSF) flow is typically seen on cine images.
   c. No ependymal lining is found on pathologic examination.
   d. The cyst is typically larger in diameter in adults than in children.

3. Cystic dilatation of the ventriculus terminalis in children may be associated with all of the following congenital anomalies *except:*
   a. Tethered cord syndrome
   b. Diastematomyelia
   c. Chiari I malformation
   d. Lumbosacral lipoma

4. Which of the following imaging features is *not* characteristic of a ventriculus terminalis cyst?
   a. Location within the distal spinal cord
   b. Well-defined margins
   c. Rim enhancement
   d. Hypointense signal on T1-weighted images

Ventriculus Terminalis Cyst

1. b and e

2. d

3. b

4. c

References
Ciappetta P, D'urso PI, Luzzi S, et al: Cystic dilation of the ventriculus terminalis in adults, *J Neurosurg Spine* 8(1):92-99, 2008.
Ganau M, Talacchi A, Cecchi PC, et al: Cystic dilation of the ventriculus terminalis, *J Neurosurg Spine* 17(1):86-92, 2012.
Liccardo G, Ruggeri F, De Cerchio L, et al: Fifth ventricle: An unusual cystic lesion of the conus medullaris, *Spinal Cord* 43(6):381-384, 2005.

Cross-Reference
Neuroradiology: The REQUISITES, 3rd ed, pp 318-319.

Comment
Background
Persistent terminal ventricle, also known as ventriculus terminalis or fifth ventricle, is an ependyma-lined cavity within the conus medullaris. Ventriculus terminalis can be seen at any age. Studies have shown that it is smallest in middle age and largest in early childhood.

Embryology and Histopathology
The mechanism of isolated dilatation of the ventriculus terminalis with cyst formation is unclear, and various theories have been proposed; however, it is thought to result from abnormal closure of the communication with the upper part of the central canal by ependyma.

Imaging
Ventricular dilatation cyst appears on MRI as a rounded cavity with well-defined borders that is filled with fluid of the same intensity as CSF on both T1 and T2 sequences; there is no enhancement after injection of contrast agent (Figs. A-C). A contrast study should always be performed to exclude the possibility of a cystic intramedullary neoplasm.

Management
Asymptomatic patients and those with mild symptoms can be managed conservatively. In patients with neurologic disturbances, surgical treatment should be considered. Fenestration of the cyst and excision of a window from the cyst wall to prevent recurrence is an effective surgical technique.

Notes

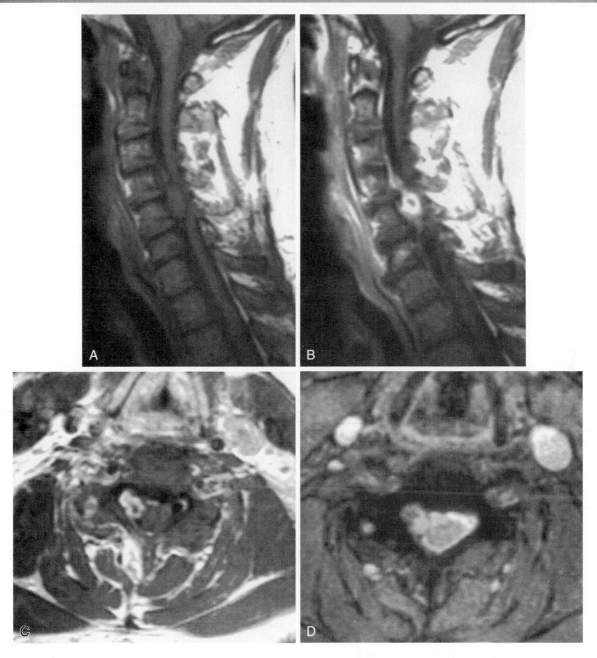

History: A 66-year-old man presents with neck pain and right arm pain and weakness.

1. What should be included in the differential diagnosis? (Choose all that apply.)
   a. Schwannoma
   b. Synovial cyst
   c. Sequestered disk fragment
   d. Meningioma
   e. Epidural abscess

2. At what level along the spinal axis is a sequestered disk most commonly seen?
   a. Cervical spine
   b. Thoracic spine
   c. Lumbar spine
   d. Sacral spine

3. Which of the following is *least* likely to show a "dural tail"?
   a. Neurosarcoid
   b. Meningioma
   c. Epidural metastasis
   d. Schwannoma

4. Which of the following statements regarding a sequestered disk is true?
   a. The sequestered fragment is in continuity with the parent disk.
   b. Sequestered disk is the same as migrated disk.
   c. The enhancement surrounding the sequestered fragment is due to infection.
   d. Peridiskal scar tissue in patients who have not undergone surgery is histologically identical to the epidural scar tissue seen in patients who have undergone surgery.

Sequestered Cervical Disk Herniation

1. a, b, c, and d

2. c

3. a

4. d

References

Ross JS, Modic MT, Masaryk TJ, et al: Assessment of extradural degenerative disease with Gd-DTPA-enhanced MR imaging: Correlation with surgical and pathologic findings, *AJR Am J Roentgenol* 154(1):151-157, 1990.

Tofuku K, Koga H, Kawabata N, et al: Dorsally sequestered cervical disc herniation, *Spine (Phila Pa 1976)* 32(26):E837-E840, 2007.

Cross-Reference

Neuroradiology: The REQUISITES, 3rd ed, pp 524-526.

Comment

Background

Although more common in the lumbar spine, sequestered disk fragments may also be observed in the cervical spine. A sequestered cervical disk fragment has the potential to migrate not only superiorly and inferiorly in the ventral epidural space but also around the dural sac and nerve root. The path of migration of a disk fragment is determined by the anatomy of the anterior epidural space.

Histopathology

The patient in the present case underwent surgery for a preliminary diagnosis of spinal tumor. Pathologically, the resected mass was composed of dense connective tissue, fibrocartilage, cartilage, bone fragments, and a mesenchymal reaction. No tumor was detected.

Imaging

The nonenhancing center of the mass at C5 (Figs. A-C) is the sequestered or "free" fragment. By definition, this fragment is not in continuity with the parent herniated disk at C4-5 (see Fig. B). MRI is useful for differentiating sequestered disk herniation from other epidural mass lesions, such as extradural tumors. Peripheral enhancement around the extradural disk fragment is commonly found (see Figs. A-C). The enhancement is due to the vascular fibrous (scar) tissue that surrounds the fragment and to the accumulation of contrast material in the adjacent epidural venous plexus. In this case, the sequestered disk fragment has migrated (i.e., has been displaced) caudad. Sequestered disk fragments often appear heterogeneous, whereas tumors usually appear homogeneous on T2-weighted images (Fig. D).

Management

Early resection of a herniated disk with sufficient surgical decompression of the spinal cord is required to prevent a poor postoperative course, especially in patients with an acute onset and rapid progression of paralysis.

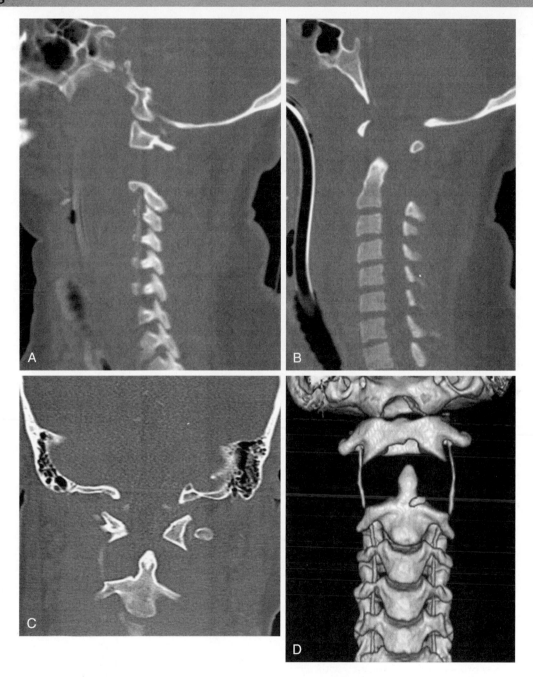

History: A 16-year-old pedestrian was hit by a car.

1. What should be included in the differential diagnosis? (Choose all that apply.)
   a. Vertebral artery laceration
   b. C1-C2 vertical distraction
   c. Occipital condyle fracture
   d. Craniocervical dissociation
   e. Atlantooccipital dislocation

2. Which of the following best defines the craniocervical junction?
   a. Functional unit between C1 and C3
   b. Functional unit including the occiput to C2
   c. Functional unit including the foramen magnum and C1
   d. Functional unit between the occiput and C3

3. Which mechanism of injury is the most common in craniocervical dissociation?
   a. Distraction injury
   b. Rotational injury
   c. Compression injury
   d. Translational injury

4. Which of the following statements regarding traumatic craniocervical dissociation is true?
   a. Children have a greater risk of craniocervical dissociation after deceleration injury than do adults.
   b. Plain radiographs are highly sensitive in diagnosing traumatic craniocervical dissociation.
   c. The normal atlantooccipital interval is less than 10 mm.
   d. Traumatic craniocervical dissociation is common and rarely results in death or neurologic compromise.

Traumatic Craniocervical Dissociation

1. b, d, and e

2. b

3. a

4. a

References

Cooper Z, Gross JA, Lacey JM, et al: Identifying survivors with traumatic craniocervical dissociation: A retrospective study, *J Surg Res* 160(1):3-8, 2010.

Deliganis A, Baxter AB, Hanson JA: Radiologic spectrum of craniocervical distraction injuries, *Radiographics* 20:S237-S250, 2000.

Junewick JJ: Pediatric craniocervical junction injuries, *AJR Am J Roentgenol* 196(5):1003-1010, 2011.

Cross-Reference

Neuroradiology: The REQUISITES, 3rd ed, pp 578-579.

Comment

Anatomy

The craniocervical junction is a functional unit composed of the occiput, atlas, and axis. Stability depends on the integrity of these osseous components, joint capsules, and ligaments. Ligaments provide most of the stabilization and include the tectorial membrane (cranial continuation of the posterior longitudinal ligament), alar ligaments (which extend from the odontoid process to the lateral margins of the foramen magnum), and cruciform ligament (vertically oriented bands of the transverse ligament that extend to the anterior foramen magnum and posterior body of the axis). Stabilization is provided to a lesser extent by the anterior longitudinal ligament, which extends cranially as the anterior atlantooccipital and atlantoaxial ligaments.

Pathophysiology

Traumatic craniocervical dissociation refers to disruption of the single functional joint between the occiput and C2. The most important of these injuries are atlantooccipital dissociation and atlantoaxial vertical distraction. Craniocervical dissociation injury is rare and usually results in immediate death or high morbidity, particularly with neurologic injuries and respiratory problems. It is associated with cervicomedullary dysfunction, lower cranial nerve palsies (cranial nerves IX through XII), and vertebrobasilar arterial injury. These injuries are usually associated with hyperextension or hyperflexion distraction mechanisms, often encountered in motor vehicle accidents.

Imaging

Plain radiographs are readily available and are often the first imaging modality used to evaluate the craniocervical junction, although radiography offers relatively poor sensitivity and specificity in the detection of injury. CT scan has greater accuracy for the diagnosis of cervical spine trauma, with sagittal (Figs. A and B), coronal (Fig. C), and three-dimensional (Fig. D) reconstructions allowing better depictions of the osseous relationships. On CT scan, the normal basion-dental interval should remain less than 12 mm, and the normal C1-C2 lateral mass interval should be less than 2.6 mm. MRI complements CT scan in the evaluation of cervical spine injury and has an important role in the assessment of spinal cord and ligamentous injuries and epidural hematomas.

Management

Nonoperative care is usually implemented until the injury can be surgically reduced and stabilized. Arthrodesis with anatomic realignment is usually indicated for an unstable craniocervical junction or the presence of neurologic injury.

Notes

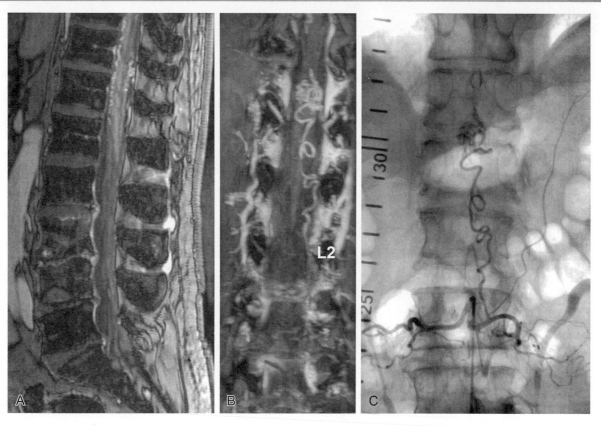

History: A 60-year-old man presents with progressive numbness in the lower extremities for the past year and recent urinary incontinence.

1. What should be included in the differential diagnosis? (Choose all that apply.)
   a. Hemangioblastoma
   b. Cavernous malformation
   c. Leriche syndrome
   d. Dural arteriovenous fistula (DAVF)
   e. Glomus arteriovenous malformation (AVM)

2. Which of the four commonly accepted types of spinal vascular malformations is most likely in this patient?
   a. Type I
   b. Type II
   c. Type III.
   d. Type IV

3. Which of the following patients best fits the demographic for the lesion in this case?
   a. 50-year-old woman
   b. 20-year-old woman
   c. 12-year-old boy
   d. 60-year-old man

4. What is the most common location of spinal DAVF along the spinal axis?
   a. High cervical spine (at the level of the foramen magnum)
   b. Lower cervical spine (below C2 and above T1)
   c. Thoracolumbar region
   d. Sacral spine

Dural Arteriovenous Fistula (L2)

1. d

2. a

3. d

4. c

References

Bowen BC, Fraser K, Kochan JP, et al: Spinal dural arteriovenous fistulas: Evaluation with magnetic resonance angiography, *AJNR Am J Neuroradiol* 16(10):2029-2043, 1995.

Krings T, Geibprasert S: Spinal dural arteriovenous fistulas, *AJNR Am J Neuroradiol* 30(4):639-648, 2009.

Saraf-Lavi E, Bowen BC, Quencer RM, et al: Detection of spinal dural arteriovenous fistulae with MRI and contrast-enhanced MR angiography: Sensitivity, specificity, and prediction of vertebral level, *AJNR Am J Neuroradiol* 23(5):858-867, 2002.

Cross-Reference

Neuroradiology: The REQUISITES, 3rd ed, pp 572-574.

Comment

Background

Spinal DAVF is the most commonly encountered spinal vascular malformation; however, it is still an underdiagnosed entity. Because the presenting clinical symptoms are nonspecific, the neuroradiologist is often the first to raise the possibility of this diagnosis. Patients typically present with progressive myelopathy.

Pathophysiology and Classification

Spinal DAVF is presumed to be an acquired disease, although the exact etiology is unknown. A commonly accepted classification scheme for spinal vascular malformations is that of Anson and Spetzler, in which four types of spinal AVM are described. Type I is DAVF, which is subclassified into type IA (single feeding artery) and type IB (multiple feeding arteries). The nidus is located within or on the dura mater of the proximal nerve root sleeve in the neural foramen.

Imaging

Spinal DAVF can occur anywhere from the level of the foramen magnum to the sacrum; identifying the arteriovenous shunt location may be challenging, especially in cases in which cord edema is extensive. Noninvasive evaluation of the shunt location is extremely helpful to guide invasive conventional angiography. Contrast-enhanced spinal magnetic resonance angiography (MRA; Figs. A and B) has contributed greatly to diagnosing and demonstrating the level of the fistula, and it helps avoid unnecessary superselective injections of all possible arterial feeders. Two methods can be used: the standard three-dimensional (3D) time-of-flight (TOF) technique, and dynamic bolus-injected contrast-enhanced MRA. Although the 3D TOF technique offers good spatial resolution, only normal (large) veins are depicted, whereas dynamic contrast-enhanced MRA allows the differentiation of normal spinal cord arteries and veins. MRA shows increased tortuosity, length, and size of the intradural vessels (see Fig. A). The fistula level is diagnosed by following the dominant and often tortuous draining medullary vein to the foraminal level (see Fig. B). Selective spinal angiography (Fig. C) is necessary to confirm the diagnosis and the fistula level.

Management

Treatment consists of interruption of the draining medullary vein, either surgically or by superselective endovascular embolization with a liquid embolic agent. Careful angiographic evaluation is required before treatment of this lesion to identify the artery of Adamkiewicz and confirm that it is not supplied by the same segmental artery as the fistula to prevent cord infarction.

Notes

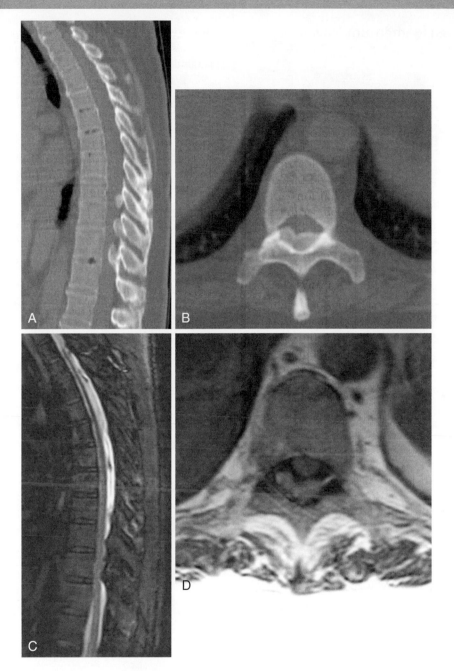

History: A 61-year-old woman presents with myelopathy.

1. What should be included in the differential diagnosis? (Choose all that apply.)
   a. Calcified epidural hematoma
   b. Ossification of the ligamentum flavum (OLF)
   c. Ossification of the posterior longitudinal ligament (OPLL)
   d. Synovial cyst
   e. Meningioma

2. What is the most common region of involvement along the spinal axis?
   a. Cervical spine
   b. Thoracic spine
   c. Lumbar spine
   d. Sacrum

3. What acquired spinal abnormality is associated with OLF?
   a. Spondylolysis
   b. Spondylolisthesis
   c. OPLL
   d. Schmorl's nodes

4. What metabolic disorder can cause the findings shown in this case?
   a. Rickets
   b. Gout
   c. Fluorosis
   d. Hyperlipidemia

Ossification of the Ligamentum Flavum

1. a and b

2. b

3. c

4. c

References
Kang KC, Lee CS, Shin SK, et al: Ossification of the ligamentum flavum of the thoracic spine in the Korean population, *J Neurosurg Spine* 14(4):513-519, 2011.

Shiokawa K, Hanakita J, Suwa H, et al: Clinical analysis and prognostic study of ossified ligamentum flavum of the thoracic spine, *J Neurosurg* 94(2 Suppl): 221-226, 2001.

Sugimura H, Kakitsubata Y, Suzuki Y, et al: MRI of ossification of ligamentum flavum, *J Comput Assist Tomogr* 16(1):73-76, 1992.

Cross-Reference
Neuroradiology: The REQUISITES, 3rd ed, p 531.

Comment

Background

OLF is an acquired degenerative disease seen mainly in Asian adults and affecting approximately 20% of individuals older than 65 years. The disease has also been described in non-Asian adults. It is most common in the thoracic spine and can be unilateral, bilateral, or bridging. Thoracic OLF is usually asymptomatic but may result in myelopathy, radiculopathy, or a combination of the two. The most common symptoms are motor dysfunction and sensory deficit in the lower extremities. The disease usually has an insidious onset and a very slow progression.

Pathophysiology

The development and pathogenesis of OLF are poorly understood. Thoracic OLF most commonly involves the T9-T12 levels, where greater mobility may result in frequent mechanical injury.

Imaging

CT with reformatted images is an excellent tool for evaluating OLF (Fig. A). OLF can be classified as unilateral, bilateral, or bridged according to the location on axial CT images. CT typically demonstrates dense sclerosis (usually V-shaped) along the anterior margin of the lamina and facets on axial images (Fig. B). A potential advantage of CT over MRI is the better detection of neural foraminal extension of OLF by CT. MRI can differentiate areas of ossification containing fatty marrow from areas of bone with dense sclerosis (Fig. C). When fatty marrow is absent, OLF demonstrates hypointensity on both T1-weighted and T2-weighted images. MRI can also provide information about the presence of associated disease, such as OPLL or disk herniation, and evidence of cord compression with edema or myelomalacia (Fig. D).

Management

The best treatment in symptomatic patients with myelopathy is surgical decompression.

Notes

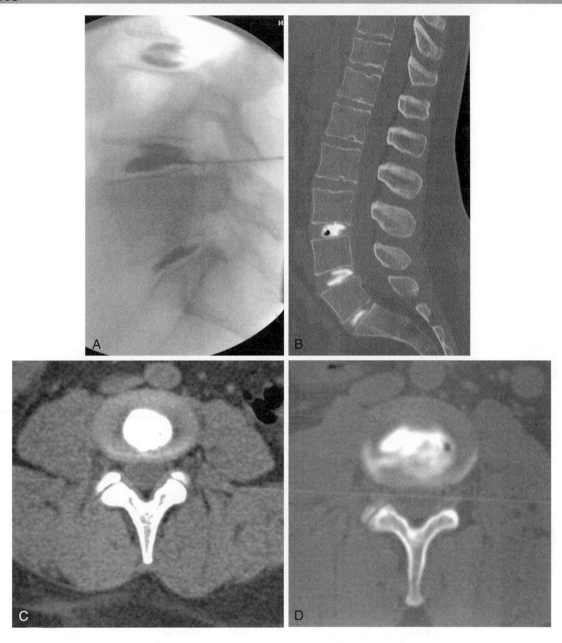

History: A 35-year-old man presents with severe back pain and right posterior thigh and buttock pain.

1. Which of the following should be included in the differential diagnosis for the imaging findings presented? (Choose all that apply.)
   a. Diskitis osteomyelitis
   b. Extruded disk
   c. Annular fissure
   d. Leak of contrast material into the epidural space
   e. Vertebral body compression fracture

2. What is the main use for diskography?
   a. To repair annular fissure
   b. To evaluate for cord compression
   c. To better delineate disk morphology
   d. To determine which disk level, if any, is responsible for a patient's neurologic symptoms

3. Which of the following is the most common serious complication of lumbar diskography?
   a. Exacerbation of pain
   b. Diskitis
   c. Disk herniation
   d. Epidural abscess

4. According to the Modified Dallas Discogram classification system, extension of contrast material to the outer third of the annulus, as seen on an axial CT image, constitutes what grade?
   a. Grade II
   b. Grade III
   c. Grade IV
   d. Grade V

Diskography

1. c

2. d

3. b

4. b

References

Schellhas KP: Discography, *Neuroimaging Clin N Am* 10(3):579-596, 2000.

Walker J 3rd, El Abd O, Isaac Z, et al: Discography in practice: A clinical and historical review, *Curr Rev Musculoskelet Med* 1(2):69-83, 2008.

Cross-Reference

Neuroradiology: The REQUISITES, 3rd ed, p 521.

Comment

Background

Diskography was first developed to determine intervertebral disk morphology and pathology. The advent of CT and MRI led to diminished interest in this procedure, but the use of diskography has recently increased because of its capacity to demonstrate which disk level is responsible for a patient's clinical symptoms. The key to determining the responsible disk level or levels is to obtain a detailed description of the patient's symptoms and evaluate whether it is concordant with the pain elicited during diskography. Another important step is to access the disk on the side contralateral to the pain. If the patient describes right lower extremity pain, the suspected disk should be entered on the left side. This avoids confusion between pain secondary to the disk pathology and pain caused by the procedure.

Imaging and Classification

Diskograms are typically performed in the lumbar spine under fluoroscopic guidance (Fig. A). When performing diskography, it is imperative to follow sterile technique to avoid complications such as diskitis osteomyelitis. Immediately after diskography, CT is performed (Figs. B-D). A CT scan is needed to confirm contrast agent injection into the nucleus pulposus; it can also assess degeneration of the annulus and annular disruption.

The Modified Dallas Discogram system is the "gold standard" for the CT classification of annulus disruption. Six grades are described. Grade 0 is a normal disk (Fig. A); no contrast material has leaked from the confines of the nucleus pulposus. Grade I is leak of contrast material into the inner third of the annulus, grade II is leak of contrast material into the outer two thirds of the annulus, and grade III is leak of contrast material through all layers of the annulus. Grade III tears are believed to be painful because the outer third of the disk has nerve fibers. Grade IV is a grade III tear in which contrast material has spread circumferentially (>30 degrees) around the disk; this often resembles a ship anchor (Fig. D). Grade IV represents the merging of a full-thickness radial tear with a concentric annular tear. Most severe is a grade V tear, which is a grade III or IV tear that has completely ruptured the outer layers of the disk, with contrast material leaking into the epidural space. This type of tear can induce a severe inflammatory reaction, causing chemical radiculopathic pain.

Management

Diskography is recommended for patients with persistent pain in whom disk abnormalities are suspected and to help in surgical planning when fusion is being considered. Diskography of suspected disks before surgery may improve surgical outcomes.

Notes

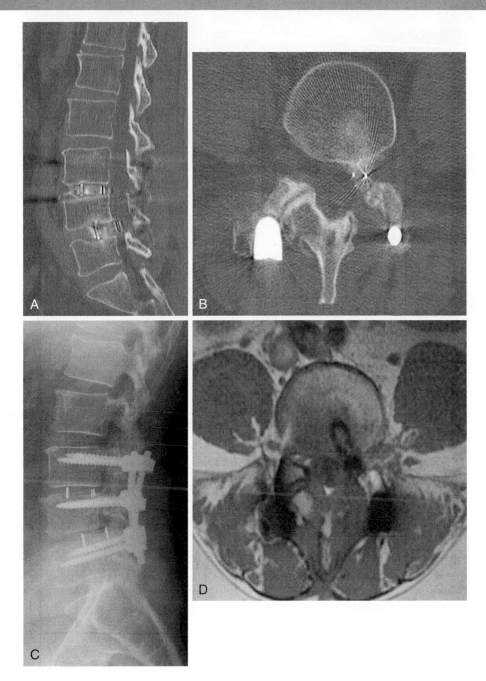

History: A 58-year-old man who underwent back surgery 1 year ago presents with low back pain and radiculopathy.

1. What should be included in the differential diagnosis? (Choose all that apply.)
   a. Disk herniation
   b. Diskitis osteomyelitis
   c. Posterior disk cage migration
   d. Meningioma
   e. Retropulsed bone fragment

2. What is the reported rate of cage migration?
   a. Less than 0.5%
   b. Less than 2%
   c. 5%
   d. More than 10%

3. All of the following imaging findings support the diagnosis of a migrated cage rather than disk herniation *except:*
   a. Presence of bilateral transpedicular screws
   b. Rectangular-shaped appearance of the abnormality on axial images
   c. Abnormality marginated by a dark rim on T1-weighted and T2-weighted images
   d. Modic type I end-plate changes

4. Which structure does the extruded disk cage likely affect in this case?
   a. Descending left L4 nerve root
   b. Exiting left L4 nerve root
   c. Descending left L5 nerve root
   d. Exiting right L5 nerve root

Posteriorly Migrated Disk Cage

1. c

2. b

3. d

4. c

Reference

Elias WJ, Simmons NE, Kaptain GJ, et al: Complications of posterior lumbar interbody fusion when using a titanium threaded cage device, *J Neurosurg* 93(1 Suppl):45-52, 2000.

Cross-Reference

Neuroradiology: The REQUISITES, 3rd ed, pp 537-540.

Comment

Background

Posterior lumbar interbody fusion (PLIF) was first reported in the 1940s, and since then, numerous variations in the technique have been described. The reported incidence of posterior cage migration is less than 2% in more recent literature. The use of intraoperative fluoroscopy is mandatory to confirm proper placement of the cages. Common indications for PLIF include symptomatic spinal stenosis, low-grade spondylolisthesis, segmental instability, and diskogenic pain. The PLIF procedure may be supplemented with posterior instrumentation—either standard pedicular fixation or translaminar screws. Complications include cage migration (as in this case), pseudarthrosis, implant subsidence, epidural hemorrhage, and laceration of the dura.

Pathophysiology

PLIF allows posterior decompression of the neural elements while stabilizing the affected spinal motion segments. The objectives of this procedure are to restore the weight-bearing capacity to the more physiologic ventral position and maintain disk space height, which indirectly opens and decompresses the neural foramina. Numerous techniques have been reported, including the use of autologous iliac crest bone graft, allograft bone, and bone chips. More recently, titanium and carbon fiber cages have been used to maintain disk height and prevent the complication of late graft collapse. To promote spinal fusion, the fusion cage is packed with cancellous bone and inserted into the disk space after meticulous end-plate decortication.

Imaging

CT is the modality of choice for detecting a posteriorly migrated disk cage. Axial and sagittal images show one or more of the markers posterior to the vertebral body cortex and within the spinal canal (Figs. A and B). Lateral plain films are also sensitive (Fig. C). MRI shows a well-defined extradural defect with a geometric shape. The cage is typically marginated by a dark rim on T1-weighted images, representing the peripheral metallic frame of the cage (Fig. D).

Management

Depending on the extent of posterior migration and the associated symptoms, treatment ranges from conservative management to urgent reoperation and cage removal.

Notes

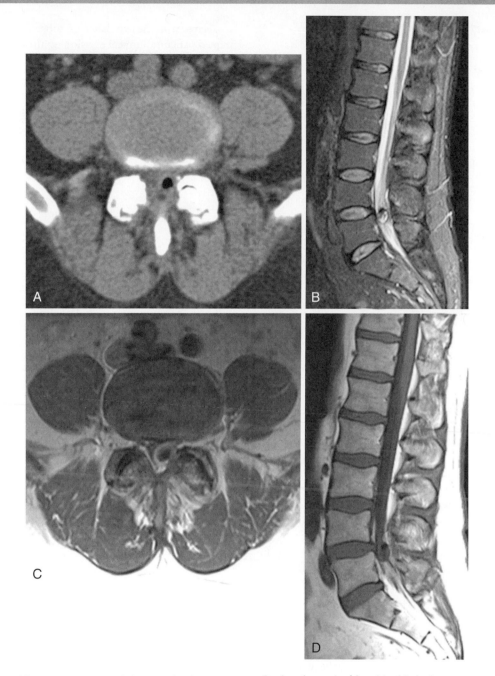

History: A 55-year-old man presents with back and left hip pain and numbness of the left lower extremity.

1. What should be included in the differential diagnosis? (Choose all that apply.)
   a. Tarlov cyst
   b. Cystic schwannoma
   c. Synovial cyst
   d. Migrated sequestered disk fragment
   e. Ganglion cyst

2. What is the likely etiology of this lesion?
   a. Baastrup's disease
   b. Facet joint degenerative changes
   c. Degenerative disk disease
   d. Spondylolysis

3. At what spinal level is this lesion most commonly found?
   a. L2-3
   b. L3-4
   c. L4-5
   d. L5-S1

4. What would be the most likely explanation for sudden exacerbation of chronic back pain in this patient?
   a. Cyst rupture
   b. Infection of the cyst
   c. Malignant degeneration to synovial sarcoma
   d. Hemorrhage within the cyst

Lumbar Juxta-articular (Synovial) Cyst

1. c and e

2. b

3. c

4. d

References

Jackson DE Jr, Atlas SW, Mani JR, et al: Intraspinal synovial cysts: MR imaging, *Radiology* 170(2):527-530, 1989.

Martha JF, Swaim B, Wang DA, et al: Outcome of percutaneous rupture of lumbar synovial cysts: A case series of 101 patients, *Spine J* 9(11):899-904, 2009.

Swartz PG, Murtagh FR: Spontaneous resolution of an intraspinal synovial cyst, *AJNR Am J Neuroradiol* 24(6):1261-1263, 2003.

Cross-Reference

Neuroradiology: The REQUISITES, 3rd ed, pp 531, 532.

Comment

Background

Pain with or without radiculopathy is commonly present with synovial cysts and may be due to mass effect of the cyst on the dorsal roots or to the underlying facet arthritis. Spontaneous resolution of symptoms, which is rare, has been attributed to decompression of the cyst into the adjacent facet joint as inflammation resolves.

Histopathology

Synovial cyst results when the synovial lining protrudes through a defect or rupture of a degenerated facet joint. There is usually communication with the adjacent facet joint.

Imaging

Although the diagnosis of synovial cyst can be made with CT scan (Fig. A), the cysts are more conspicuous on MRI. The findings that help characterize a synovial cyst are its location (epidural, posterolateral); its apparent continuity with a hypointense, hypertrophic (degenerated) left facet joint; and its hypointense rim on T2-weighted image (Fig. B). Cysts may have variable signal intensity, depending on whether they contain synovial or other watery fluid, hemorrhage or proteinaceous material, or gas. The hypointensity of the rim on T2-weighted images has been attributed to the presence of a fibrous capsule with hemosiderin deposits, fine calcifications, or both. On images obtained after the administration of a contrast agent, peripheral enhancement of the cyst is seen (Fig. C). An air-filled cyst (Fig. D) may be indistinguishable from an osteophyte on MRI, but the two are easily distinguished on CT (see Fig. A).

Management

Symptomatic synovial cysts may be treated conservatively. Percutaneous aspiration of a synovial cyst is ineffective in the long term because the cysts tend to refill. Corticosteroid injection into the lumbar facet joint with attempted cyst rupture is correlated with the avoidance of subsequent surgery in half of treated patients. Surgical excision of the cyst is highly effective for pain relief and appears to be the definitive treatment for these lesions.

Notes

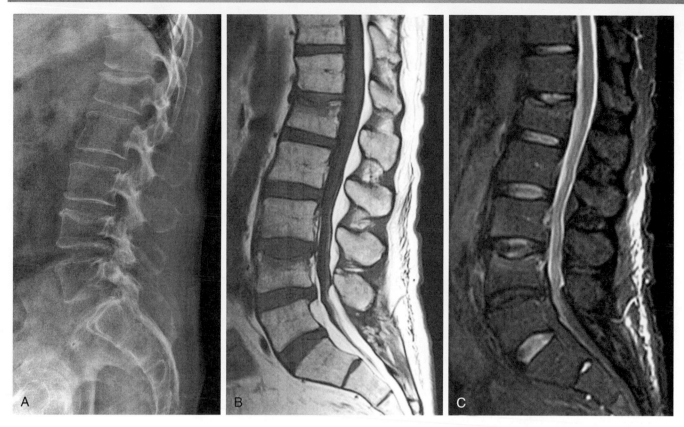

History: A 49-year-old man presents with back pain.

1. What should be included in the differential diagnosis? (Choose all that apply.)
   a. Degenerative type I Modic end-plate changes
   b. Pathologic fractures
   c. Osteoporotic compression fractures
   d. Scheuermann's disease
   e. Diskitis osteomyelitis

2. All of the following are typically associated with degenerative end-plate changes *except:*
   a. Disk space narrowing
   b. Osteophytes
   c. Disk desiccation
   d. End-plate signal abnormality that spares the cortex

3. Which of the following MRI features is suggestive of benign fracture?
   a. Posterior element involvement
   b. Paravertebral extension
   c. Low-signal-intensity band
   d. Epidural mass

4. Which of the following imaging modalities provides the best assessment of osteoporosis?
   a. CT
   b. Ultrasound
   c. MRI
   d. Bone scan

Acute Osteoporotic Compression Fractures

1. b and c

2. d

3. c

4. a

References

Abdel-Wanis ME, Solyman MT, Hasan NM: Sensitivity, specificity and accuracy of magnetic resonance imaging for differentiating vertebral compression fractures caused by malignancy, osteoporosis, and infections, *J Orthop Surg (Hong Kong)* 19(2):145-150, 2011.

Baker LL, Goodman SB, Perkash I, et al: Benign versus pathologic compression fractures of vertebral bodies: Assessment with conventional spin-echo, chemical-shift, and STIR MR imaging, *Radiology* 174(2):495-502, 1990.

Cross-Reference

Neuroradiology: The REQUISITES, 3rd ed, p 566.

Comment

Background

Differentiating benign and malignant vertebral fractures may be difficult, particularly when there is no history of malignancy. This is especially true in elderly patients, who are predisposed to both osteoporosis and malignancies. Symptoms may be nonspecific, and the only complaint may be back pain.

Histopathology

Both malignant and acute benign fractures may manifest with low T1-weighted and high T2-weighted signals on MRI; this is attributed to an increased focal water content resulting from hemorrhage or edema. After the acute stage, hematoma and edema decrease. However, in malignant fractures, the infiltrating abnormal soft tissue and associated reactive response continue to show low T1-weighted and high T2-weighted signal patterns.

Imaging

Radiographs are of limited use in differentiating between benign and malignant fractures; however, they can reveal diffuse osteopenia and loss of vertebral body height (Fig. A). MRI is superior to other diagnostic tools in differentiating benign from malignant compression spinal fractures. In the case shown, the bands of low signal intensity on the T1-weighted image (Fig. B) and high signal intensity on the short tau inversion recovery (STIR) image (Fig. C) could represent an acute benign fracture or a pathologic fracture. Diffusion-weighted and fat-saturated postcontrast T1-weighted MRI may help differentiate between benign and pathologic fractures. Pathologic fractures may show evidence of restricted diffusion (although this remains controversial) and diffuse vertebral body enhancement, in addition to features of cortical destruction, involvement of posterior elements, and signal abnormalities of unfractured vertebrae. Baker and colleagues found that chronic benign fractures usually demonstrate a marrow signal that is isointense relative to normal vertebrae on all pulse sequences. High signal intensity was observed in only about 10% of chronic benign fractures.

Management

Having a vertebral fracture is a strong risk factor for subsequent fractures. Treatment is largely determined by the presence of symptoms, particularly pain. Management includes conservative treatment, vertebroplasty, kyphoplasty, or surgery.

Notes

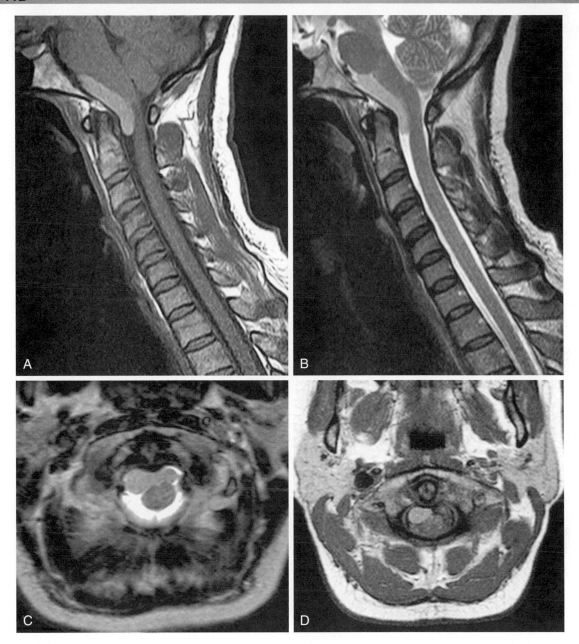

History: A 40-year-old woman has a mass in the craniocervical junction that was found incidentally on a CT scan of the neck obtained for a thyroid mass.

1. What should be included in the differential diagnosis? (Choose all that apply.)
   a. Cystic schwannoma
   b. Arachnoid cyst
   c. Neurenteric cyst
   d. Infectious cyst
   e. Epidermoid

2. All of the following anomalies are associated with neurenteric cyst *except:*
   a. Spina bifida
   b. Fused vertebrae
   c. Hemivertebra
   d. Short pedicle

3. Where along the spinal axis do neurenteric cysts most commonly occur?
   a. Craniocervical junction
   b. Cervicothoracic spine
   c. Lumbar spine
   d. Sacral spine

4. Which of the following statements regarding neurenteric cyst is true?
   a. Females are more commonly affected than males.
   b. Associated bony abnormalities of the spine are found in 10% of cases.
   c. Associated cardiac abnormalities may be present.
   d. Intraspinal cysts are usually dorsal in location.

Neurenteric (Enterogenous) Cyst

1. b, c, d, and e

2. d

3. b

4. c

References

Savage JJ, Casey JN, McNeill IT, et al: Neurenteric cysts of the spine, *J Craniovertebr Junction Spine* 1(1):58-63, 2010.

Wagner HJ, Seidel A, Reusche E, et al: A craniospinal enterogenous cyst: Case report, *Neuropediatrics* 29(4):212-214, 1998.

Cross-Reference

Neuroradiology: The REQUISITES, 3rd ed, p 99.

Comment

Background

Neurenteric (or enterogenous) cysts account for approximately 1% of spinal axis tumors. Most patients are younger than 40 years at the time of diagnosis and have slowly progressive myelopathy. Males are more commonly affected than females. About 50% of patients have other congenital anomalies, such as vertebral defects and fistulous communications with cysts in the mediastinum, thorax, or abdomen.

Histopathology

Neurenteric cysts are heterotopic rests of epithelium, reminiscent of gastrointestinal and respiratory tissue, resulting from inappropriate partitioning of the embryonic notochordal plate during week 3 of gestation. The cyst is identified histopathologically by the presence of mucin-secreting columnar or cuboidal epithelium that is usually lacking cilia, similar to epithelium of the gastrointestinal tract.

Imaging

CT has an essential role in evaluating the osseous malformations associated with these lesions. On MRI, the signal characteristics can vary from cerebrospinal fluid (CSF)–like to hyperintense on T1-weighted and T2-weighted images (Figs. A-D). The variation in signal is due to the fact that neurenteric cysts are lined by mucin-secreting cells. The cyst fluid may be rich in macromolecules, which can shorten T1 without significantly altering T2, resulting in hyperintensity on both T1-weighted and T2-weighted images. The effect is analogous to that described for mucoceles and chronic secretions in the paranasal sinuses. The cyst is generally found in the cervical region anterior to the cord in an intradural extramedullary location.

Management

Total surgical excision is the treatment of choice to avoid cyst recurrence.

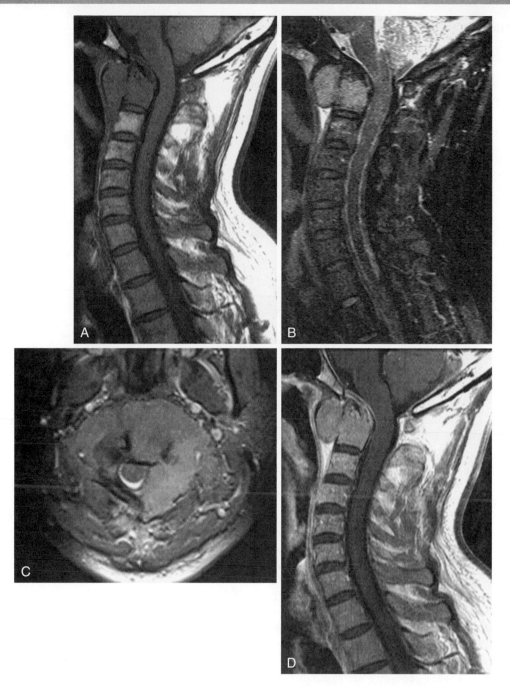

History: A 48-year-old man presents with increasing neck pain.

1. What should be included in the differential diagnosis? (Choose all that apply.)
   a. Atypical hemangioma
   b. Metastasis
   c. Plasmacytoma
   d. Rheumatoid arthritis
   e. Calcium pyrophosphate dihydrate deposition disease

2. This condition can progress to which of the following?
   a. Paget's disease
   b. Leukemia
   c. Osteosarcoma
   d. Multiple myeloma

3. Where along the spinal axial skeleton does solitary plasmacytoma of bone most commonly occur?
   a. Cervical spine
   b. Thoracic spine
   c. Lumbar spine
   d. Sacrum

4. Which of the following MRI patterns is characteristic of solitary vertebral plasmacytoma?
   a. "Mini brain"
   b. "Owl's eye"
   c. "Polka dot"
   d. "Salt and pepper"

Plasmacytoma

1. a, b, and c

2. d

3. b

4. a

References

Afonso PD, Almeida A: Solitary plasmacytoma of the spine: An unusual presentation, *AJNR Am J Neuroradiol* 31(1):E5, 2010.

Major NM, Helms CA, Richardson WJ: The "mini brain": Plasmacytoma in a vertebral body on MR imaging, *AJR Am J Roentgenol* 175(1):261-263, 2000.

Cross-Reference

Neuroradiology: The REQUISITES, 3rd ed, p 570.

Comment

Background

Solitary plasmacytoma of bone is uncommon, occurring in approximately 5% of patients with plasma cell myeloma. These tumors occur more frequently in younger age groups and have a better prognosis than multiple myeloma. They are typically found in male patients with a median age of 55 years.

Histopathology

By strict definition, the diagnosis requires histologic evidence of a monoclonal plasma cell infiltrate in one bone lesion, absence of other bone lesions, and a lack of marrow plasmacytosis elsewhere. Because of the distribution of hematopoietic cells, the spine is one of the most commonly affected sites.

Imaging

Solitary plasmacytoma of the spine is predominantly lytic and typically involves the vertebral body and the posterior elements, with epidural extension and compression of the sac or cord. Occasionally, it may manifest as an expansile lesion with a soft tissue mass, fractures, or, rarely, osteosclerosis. On MRI, vertebral plasmacytoma is typically expansile, hypointense on T1-weighted images (Fig. A), and hyperintense on T2-weighted images (Figs. B and C); it enhances on postcontrast images (Fig. D). The "mini brain" pattern on axial MRI is reportedly characteristic of solitary vertebral plasmacytoma. In this pattern, curvilinear structures with low signal intensity on all imaging sequences extend partially through the vertebral body. These structures, which probably represent thick cortical struts resulting from compensatory hypertrophy of residual trabecular bone, resemble sulci seen in the brain. The pattern has not been described for other primary or metastatic bone lesions and is postulated to result from the less aggressive nature of plasmacytoma.

Management

Although local radiotherapy is effective for the primary tumor, multiple myeloma develops in most patients within a few years.

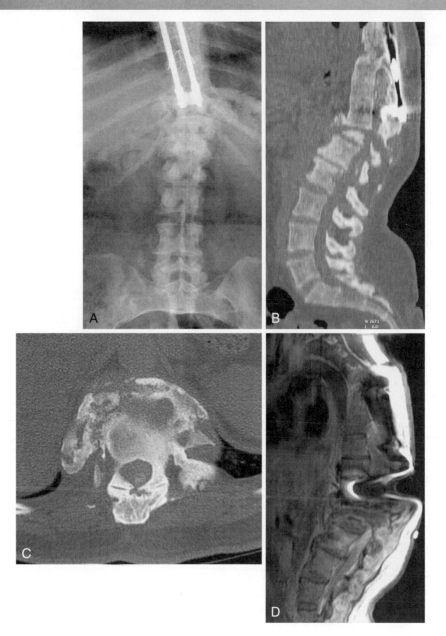

History: A 37-year-old woman who sustained a spinal cord injury 15 years ago in a motor vehicle accident and was stabilized with posterior instrumentation now presents with spasticity in her lower extremities and a change in posture.

1. What should be included in the differential diagnosis for the imaging findings presented? (Choose all that apply.)
   a. Vertebral osteomyelitis
   b. Neuropathic spine arthropathy
   c. Metastatic disease
   d. Degenerative changes
   e. Ankylosing spondylitis

2. What is the most common spinal location for these changes?
   a. Cervical spine
   b. Thoracic spine
   c. Lumbar spine
   d. Sacral spine

3. What is the most common cause of neuropathic spine arthropathy in the United States?
   a. Diabetes mellitus
   b. Spinal cord injury
   c. Tabes dorsalis
   d. Syringomyelia

4. Which of the following imaging findings favors the diagnosis of diskitis osteomyelitis over spinal neuropathic arthropathy?
   a. Vacuum disk
   b. Central enhancement of the disk
   c. Osseous debris
   d. Spondylolisthesis

Neuropathic Spinal Arthropathy (Charcot Spine)

1. a, b, and c

2. c

3. a

4. b

References

Jones EA, Manster BJ, May DA, et al: Neuropathic osteoarthropathy: Diagnostic dilemmas and differential diagnosis, *Radiographics* 20:S279-S293, 2000.

Lacout A, Lebreton C, Mompoint D, et al: CT and MRI of spinal neuroarthropathy, *AJR Am J Roentgenol* 193(6):W505-W514, 2009.

Wagner SC, Schweitzer ME, Morrison WB, et al: Can imaging findings help differentiate spinal neuropathic arthropathy from disk space infection? Initial experience, *Radiology* 214(3):693-699, 2000.

Cross-Reference

Neuroradiology: The REQUISITES, 3rd ed, pp 534-535.

Comment

Background

Neuropathic spinal arthropathy, also known as Charcot spine, is a progressive, destructive process that involves the vertebral bodies, intervertebral disks, and facets. It is more frequently found in female patients (71% of cases).

Pathophysiology

Neuropathic spinal arthropathy occurs when neurologic damage causes loss of the protective proprioceptive reflexes. Underlying mechanisms include excessive loads to the thoracolumbar spine by the transfer activities of paraplegic patients in the presence of impaired pain and proprioceptive sensation. Other possible mechanisms are iatrogenic instability and concentration of loads to the lower adjacent segment fused by a previous operation (as in this case). The diagnosis may be complicated in patients with posttraumatic paralysis because they often have a neurogenic bladder, which predisposes them to bacteremia and an increased risk of diskitis osteomyelitis, mimicking neuropathic arthropathy.

Imaging

When two adjacent vertebral bodies are affected, differentiation between neuropathic arthropathy and diskitis osteomyelitis may be difficult. Findings on plain radiographs (Fig. A) and CT scans (Figs. B and C) that favor neuropathic arthropathy include joint disorganization, debris, a vacuum phenomenon in the disk space, facet involvement, and spondylolisthesis. MRI findings that favor neuropathic arthropathy include diffuse vertebral body hypointensity on T1-weighted images, diffuse hyperintensity on T2-weighted images, and diffuse enhancement on postcontrast T1-weighted images. Patients with diskitis osteomyelitis tend to have more localized vertebral body signal abnormalities and enhancement, involving the adjacent vertebral end-plates. Rim enhancement of the disk on postcontrast T1-weighted images favors neuropathic arthropathy (Fig. D), and central enhancement favors diskitis. CT and MRI findings that are not useful for differentiation include end-plate erosion, end-plate sclerosis, loss of disk height, paraspinal soft tissue mass, and osteophyte formation.

Management

A combined anterior and posterior approach with extensive débridement, autogenous bone grafting, and posterior instrumentation is the main therapeutic modality.

Notes

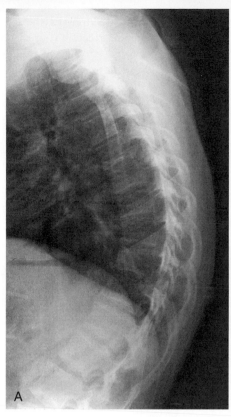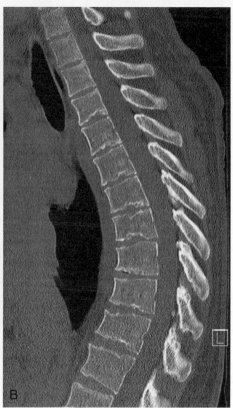

History: A 23-year-old man presents with back pain.

1. What should be included in the differential diagnosis for the imaging findings presented? (Choose all that apply.)
   a. Postural kyphosis
   b. Compression fractures
   c. Ankylosing spondylitis
   d. Scheuermann's kyphosis
   e. Morquio syndrome

2. Which of the following statements regarding Scheuermann's kyphosis is true?
   a. In the classic form, the apex is localized between T4 and T6.
   b. In type II, the apex is localized between T10 and T12.
   c. Type II is the most common form of Scheuermann's kyphosis.
   d. Type II occurs more frequently and in a slightly younger age group than type I.

3. Sorenson's criteria for the diagnosis of Scheuermann's kyphosis include all of the following *except:*
   a. More than 5 degrees of anterior wedging of at least three consecutive vertebrae at the apex of the kyphosis
   b. Vertebral end-plate irregularities
   c. Thoracic kyphosis of more than 45 degrees
   d. More than five Schmorl's nodes involving the thoracic vertebral end-plates

4. Which of the following is the imaging modality of choice for evaluating an adolescent with suspected Scheuermann's kyphosis?
   a. Plain radiograph
   b. CT myelogram
   c. MRI
   d. Bone scan

Scheuermann's Kyphosis

1. b and d

2. b

3. d

4. a

References

Papagelopoulos PJ, Mavrogenis AF, Savvidou OD, et al: Current concepts in Scheuermann's kyphosis, *Orthopedics* 31(1):52-58; quiz 59-60, 2008.
Soo CL, Noble PC, Esses SI: Scheuermann kyphosis: Long-term follow-up, *Spine J* 2(1):49-56, 2002.

Cross-Reference

Neuroradiology: The REQUISITES, 3rd ed, p 528.

Comment

Background

Scheuermann's kyphosis is the most common cause of kyphotic deformity in adolescents and the second most common spinal deformity after idiopathic scoliosis. There are two forms of Scheuermann's kyphosis—the classic thoracic type (type I), and the thoracolumbar or lumbar type (type II). Patients commonly present between 12 and 15 years of age. Type II has a lower apex, which is frequently associated with increased lumbar lordosis. It occurs in a slightly older age group than the classic type and tends to be more painful, but it rarely leads to progressive deformity.

Pathophysiology

The etiology of Scheuermann's kyphosis is controversial. A genetic component appears to be present. Mechanical factors have a significant role, and heavy lifting seems to be a contributing factor in many patients.

Imaging

Common radiographic findings include accentuated thoracic kyphosis (>45 degrees overall for some criteria), vertebral body wedging, Schmorl's nodes, end-plate irregularities, and disk space narrowing (Figs. A and B). Not all of the typical radiographic findings are required for the diagnosis of Scheuermann's kyphosis, and there is no absolute consensus among radiologists concerning the specific imaging features of this condition. According to Sorenson's criteria, a minimum of three contiguous apical vertebrae wedged by at least 5 degrees each is required; Drummond's criterion is two wedged vertebrae. Other investigators argue that the diagnosis depends on the rigidity of the kyphotic curve evaluated on lateral plain radiographs in hyperextension.

Management

Most patients seek medical attention because of the kyphotic deformity. Scheuermann's kyphosis can be either static or progressive. There are no predictors of disease progression at the present time, and the optimal treatment is controversial. Treatment options include physical therapy, bracing, and surgical correction. Surgical correction is usually reserved for patients with severe kyphosis (>75 degrees). These treatment options provide similar functional outcomes at long-term follow-up.

Notes

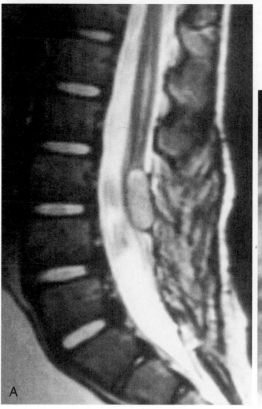

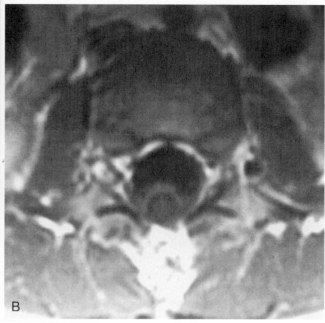

History: A 10-year-old boy presents with back pain.

1. What should be included in the differential diagnosis? (Choose all that apply.)
   a. Teratoma
   b. Meningioma
   c. Epidermoid cyst
   d. Ventriculus terminalis cyst
   e. Dermoid

2. What is the most likely etiology of this lesion?
   a. Congenital
   b. Iatrogenic
   c. Genetic mutation
   d. Posttraumatic

3. Which imaging technique can differentiate this lesion from a ventriculus terminalis cyst?
   a. Functional MRI
   b. Diffusion-weighted imaging
   c. MRI perfusion
   d. Susceptibility-weighted imaging

4. All of the following MRI findings are characteristic of epidermoid cyst *except:*
   a. Hypointense signal on T1-weighted images
   b. Hyperintense signal on T2-weighted images
   c. Thick peripheral enhancement
   d. Restricted diffusion

Epidermoid Cyst

1. c and d

2. a

3. b

4. c

References

Gupta S, Gupta RK, Gujral RB, et al: Signal intensity patterns in intraspinal dermoids and epidermoids on MR imaging, *Clin Radiol* 48(6):405-413, 1993.

Naidich TP, Blaser SI, Delman BN, et al: Congenital anomalies of the spine and spinal cord. In Atlas SW, editor: *Magnetic resonance imaging of the brain and spine*, ed 3, Philadelphia, 2002, Lippincott Williams & Wilkins, pp 1527-1631.

Cross-Reference

Neuroradiology: The REQUISITES, 3rd ed, p 552.

Comment

Background

Spinal epidermoid cysts are slow-growing benign lesions that may be congenital or acquired. Congenital spinal epidermoid cysts result from inclusion of ectodermal tissue during closure of the neural tube between the third and fourth weeks of fetal life. Acquired epidermoid cysts result from implantation of viable skin elements during back surgery, trauma, or lumbar puncture.

Fifteen percent of all central nervous system epidermoid and dermoid tumors are located in the spine. Spinal epidermoid and dermoid tumors occur with approximately equal frequency. Most epidermoids are found in the lumbar region, whereas most dermoids are in the thoracolumbar region. According to various reports, 20% to 25% of cases have an associated dermal sinus.

Histopathology

Spinal dermoid cysts are similar to epidermoids in their squamous epithelial structure; however, dermoid cysts contain dermal appendages, such as sweat glands and hair follicles.

Imaging

Epidermoid cysts are intradural extramedullary in most cases; rarely, they may be intramedullary. The signal characteristics of epidermoid and dermoid tumors are variable and depend on their keratin, collagen, cholesterol, and water composition. In general, dermoid cysts contain mainly fatty tissue and show hyperintense signal areas on T1-weighted images, in contrast to the generally hypointense signal of epidermoids. This variability in signal probably explains why the cystic mass shown is not isointense relative to cerebrospinal fluid on T1-weighted or T2-weighted images (Fig. A). Minimal or no contrast enhancement in the wall of the cyst is typical (Fig. B). It is difficult to determine whether the mass is intramedullary or extramedullary, and sometimes these lesions have both components.

Management

Management is by surgical removal.

Notes

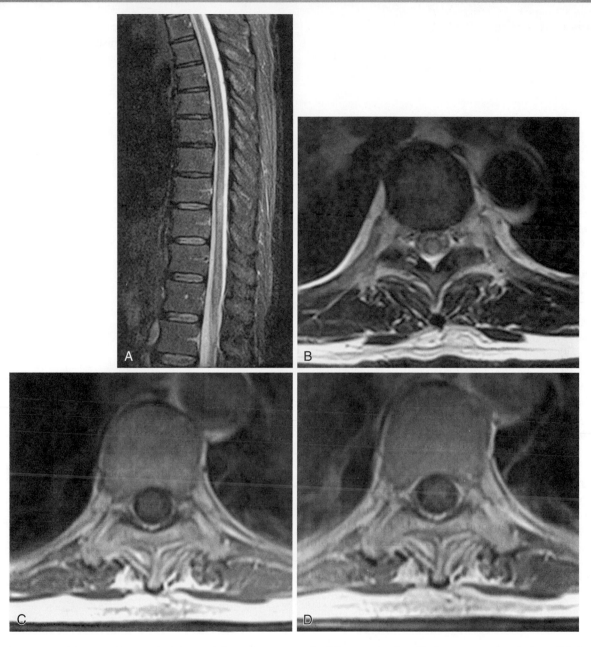

History: A 60-year-old man with HIV is admitted for rash localized to the groin and left buttock area and decreased sensation in the lower extremities.

1. What should be included in the differential diagnosis? (Choose all that apply.)
   a. Lymphoma
   b. Multiple sclerosis
   c. Sarcoid
   d. Viral myelitis
   e. Cord infarct

2. All of the following are common opportunistic viral infections of the spinal cord in adults with AIDS *except:*
   a. JC virus
   b. Cytomegalovirus
   c. Herpes simplex virus
   d. Varicella-zoster virus (VZV)

3. What mechanism likely accounts for viral myelitis in patients with VZV?
   a. Hematogenous spread
   b. Cerebrospinal fluid spread
   c. Direct invasion
   d. Lymphatic spread

4. Which of the following imaging findings is the *least* typical of VZV myelitis?
   a. Diffuse cord hyperintensity on T2-weighted images
   b. Focal enhancing lesion
   c. Multifocal cord lesions
   d. Hematomyelia

Varicella-Zoster Virus Myelitis

1. a, b, c, and d

2. a

3. c

4. d

References

Esposito MB, Arrington JA, Murtaugh FR, et al: MR of the spinal cord in a patient with herpes zoster, *AJNR Am J Neuroradiol* 14(1):203-204, 1993.
Hirai T, Korogi Y, Hamatake S, et al: Case report: Varicella-zoster virus myelitis—serial MR findings, *Br J Radiol* 69(828):1187-1190, 1996.

Cross-Reference

Neuroradiology: The REQUISITES, 3rd ed, pp 548-549.

Comment

Background

Herpes zoster infection (shingles) represents a reactivation of latent VZV infection and usually manifests as peripheral or cranial neuropathy. Myelitis is a relatively rare central nervous system complication of VZV infection, with an acute onset. Shortly after the appearance of the typical cutaneous rash in a dermatomal distribution, a self-limited paraparesis develops, with or without sensory loss and sphincter dysfunction.

Histopathology

The pathogenesis may be direct viral invasion of the cord, vasculitis with ischemic necrosis, or an immunologic-parainfectious mechanism. Direct invasion is often inferred from the eccentric location of the enhancement near the dorsal root entry zone and the correspondence between the level of the cord lesion and the dermatomal distribution of the skin lesions in patients with shingles. VZV has been isolated from the brain and spinal cord, indicating that direct invasion does occur.

Imaging

MRI findings in documented cases of VZV myelitis include diffuse cord hyperintensity on T2-weighted images, extending over several levels and probably representing edema, and less extensive focal (Figs. A-D) or multifocal lesions with enhancement on postcontrast T1-weighted images (see Fig. D). In some cases, the enhancement has been attributed to blood-cord barrier breakdown, in association with inflammatory changes caused by direct viral invasion. Other MRI findings, such as marked enhancement of inflammatory tissue surrounding and involving the dorsal root ganglion and extending to the paravertebral soft tissues, have also been described.

Management

The cerebrospinal fluid shows increased levels of protein and pleocytosis. Cerebrospinal fluid polymerase chain reaction can be used to detect VZV DNA. Treatment includes antiviral therapy (e.g., acyclovir) and steroid therapy. Clinical outcomes range from spontaneous recovery to ascending progression and death. VZV immune globulin has been approved by the U.S. Food and Drug Administration in high-risk groups, such as immunocompromised patients, pregnant women, and infants.

Notes

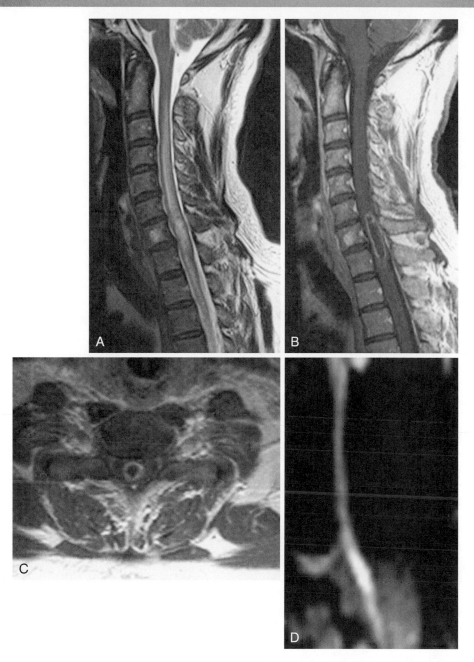

History: A 57-year-old man presents with a history of neck pain and right upper and lower extremity weakness and hypoesthesia.

1. What should be included in the differential diagnosis? (Choose all that apply.)
   a. Ependymoma
   b. Metastasis
   c. Intramedullary abscess
   d. Multiple sclerosis
   e. Cord infarction

2. What is the location of this lesion?
   a. Epidural
   b. Intradural extramedullary
   c. Intramedullary
   d. Extraspinal

3. What is the most commonly identified causative organism?
   a. *Staphylococcus*
   b. *Streptococcus*
   c. *Mycobacterium tuberculosis*
   d. Gram-negative bacterium

4. Which of the following MRI sequences would be most helpful in narrowing the differential diagnosis?
   a. Susceptibility-weighted imaging
   b. Diffusion-weighted imaging (DWI)
   c. T1-weighted images with contrast agent administration
   d. T2-weighted images

Intramedullary Abscess (*Streptococcus*)

1. a, b, c, and d

2. c

3. a

4. b

Reference

Murphy KJ, Brunberg JA, Quint DJ, et al: Spinal cord infection: Myelitis and abscess formation, *AJNR Am J Neuroradiol* 19(2):341-348, 1998.

Cross-Reference

Neuroradiology: The REQUISITES, 3rd ed, pp 546-547.

Comment

Background

Intramedullary abscess is uncommon. Almost half the cases occur in the first 2 decades of life.

Pathophysiology

Staphylococcus and *Streptococcus* are the most common organisms found in intramedullary abscesses. Predisposing factors include prior trauma or surgery, diabetes, immunocompromise, intravenous drug abuse, and congenital abnormalities such as a dermal sinus. Tuberculous and schistosomal abscesses have also been reported. In 25% of patients, a primary source of infection is never found. A rapid onset of symptoms portends a bad outcome.

Imaging

Typical MRI features include enlargement of the spinal cord with hypointensity on T1-weighted images, increased signal on T2-weighted images (Fig. A), and peripheral contrast enhancement (Figs. B and C). Similar to brain abscess, restricted fluid motion on DWI (Fig. D) can be useful in differentiating pyogenic abscess from tumors and other entities. A temporal sequence of MRI findings has been described—analogous to the sequence that occurs with brain cerebritis or abscess—and recognition of this sequence may aid in differentiating cord infection from other intramedullary lesions. Initially, there is diffuse intramedullary hyperintensity on T2-weighted images, with a localized zone of poorly defined marginal enhancement on T1-weighted images. After the initiation of medical therapy (at least 1 week of treatment), the T2 signal abnormalities markedly decrease in size, and the enhancement pattern becomes well defined and ringlike, with central low signal. This progression of findings is similar to that described for the evolution from cerebritis to intracranial abscess with capsule formation.

Management

The only treatment that offers a chance of achieving a favorable outcome is early surgical drainage, followed by appropriate antimicrobial therapy.

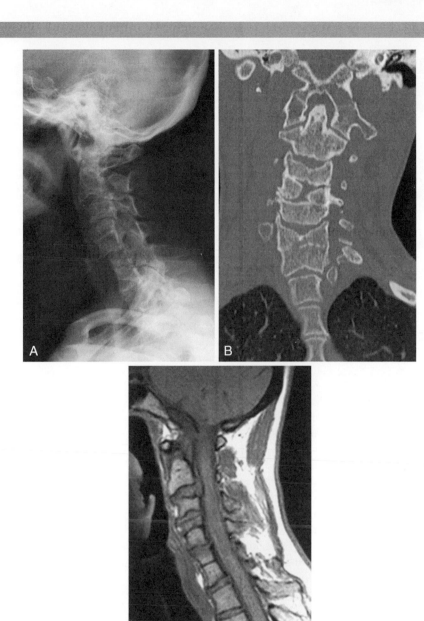

History: A 49-year-old woman presents with headache, neck pain, and cold sensation in the hands.

1. What should be included in the differential diagnosis? (Choose all that apply.)
   a. Congenital fusion
   b. Klippel-Feil syndrome
   c. Rheumatoid arthritis
   d. Ankylosing spondylitis
   e. Iatrogenic fusion

2. All of the following findings on MRI of the cervical spine may be associated with Klippel-Feil syndrome *except:*
   a. Basilar invagination
   b. Congenitally absent cervical pedicle
   c. Degenerative disk disease
   d. Syringomyelia

3. Which of the following is *not* part of the classic clinical triad of Klippel-Feil syndrome?
   a. Macroglossia
   b. Restricted motion
   c. Low posterior hairline
   d. Short neck

4. Which of the following signs helps differentiate congenital fusion from acquired fusion secondary to infection or surgery?
   a. "Trolley track" sign
   b. "Y" sign
   c. "Shiny corner" sign
   d. "Wasp-waist" sign

Klippel-Feil Syndrome

1. a and b

2. b

3. a

4. d

References

Floemer F, Magerkurth O, Jauckus C, et al: Klippel-Feil syndrome and Sprengel deformity combined with an intraspinal course of the left subclavian artery and a bovine aortic arch variant, *AJNR Am J Neuroradiol* 29(2):306-307, 2008.

Tracy MR, Dormans JP, Kusumi K: Klippel-Feil syndrome: Clinical features and current understanding of etiology, *Clin Orthop Relat Res* (424)183-190, 2004.

Ulmer JL, Elster AD, Ginsberg LE, et al: Klippel-Feil syndrome: CT and MR of acquired and congenital abnormalities of cervical spine and cord, *J Comput Assist Tomogr* 17(2):215-224, 1993.

Cross-Reference

Neuroradiology: The REQUISITES, 3rd ed, pp 594-595.

Comment

Background

Klippel-Feil syndrome is a congenital disorder characterized by failure of cervical segmentation. Patients with Klippel-Feil syndrome usually present with the disease during childhood but may present later in life. Scoliosis, spina bifida, and rib anomalies can also occur. The syndrome is associated with numerous abnormalities affecting the renal, nervous, and vascular systems, as well as abnormalities of the inner, middle, and outer ears. One third of patients have Sprengel's deformity, which is caused by tethering of the scapula to the cervical spine by a fibrous band or an anomalous bone (omovertebral bone). As a result, the scapula has an elevated position, and shoulder motion is limited. Klippel-Feil syndrome is also associated with cervical spondylosis and intervertebral disk herniation.

Pathophysiology

The etiology of Klippel-Feil syndrome and its associated conditions is unknown. It is believed to result from faulty segmentation along the embryo's developing axis during the third to eighth weeks of gestation.

Imaging

Plain radiography is the initial diagnostic modality and includes frontal and lateral views of the cervical spine (Fig. A). CT can better evaluate spinal stenosis and associated vertebral body anomalies (Fig. B). MRI (Fig. C) is indicated in patients with neurologic deficits and for the evaluation of additional findings, such as syringomyelia.

Management

Surgery is indicated in cases of progressive deformities, spinal stenosis, and instability of the cervical spine. Neurologic deficit and pain are additional indications for surgery.

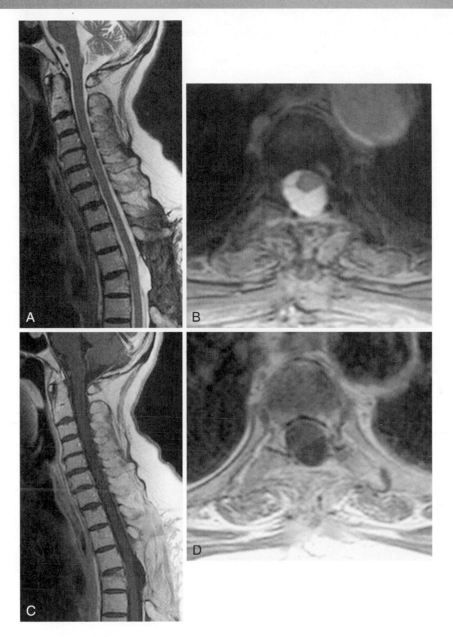

History: A 74-year-old woman who underwent T3-4 laminectomy for resection of an intradural meningioma 3 months earlier now presents with midscapular pain.

1. What should be included in the differential diagnosis? (Choose all that apply.)
   a. Congenital arachnoid cyst
   b. Neurenteric cyst
   c. Cystic schwannoma
   d. Intradural abscess
   e. Acquired arachnoid cyst

2. All of the following imaging findings favor the diagnosis of acquired arachnoid cyst over congenital intradural arachnoid *except:*
   a. Location lateral to the spinal cord
   b. Location in the lumbar spine
   c. Evidence of prior spine surgery
   d. Presence of an intramedullary syrinx

3. Acquired arachnoid cyst may develop secondary to all of the following causes *except:*
   a. Trauma
   b. Prior surgery
   c. Disk herniation
   d. Infection

4. What is the frequency of syringomyelia in patients with congenital intradural arachnoid cysts?
   a. Less than 1%
   b. Less than 10%
   c. 25%
   d. More than 50%

Acquired Arachnoid Cyst (Postsurgical)

1. a and e

2. d

3. c

4. b

Reference

Khosla A, Wippold FJ: CT myelography and MR imaging of extramedullary cysts of the spinal canal in adult and pediatric patients, *AJR Am J Roentgenol* 178(1):201-207, 2002.

Cross-Reference

Neuroradiology: The REQUISITES, 3rd ed, p 551.

Comment

Background

Intradural spinal arachnoid cysts are uncommon and may be congenital, idiopathic, or acquired. Causes of acquired spinal arachnoid cysts include trauma, infection, inflammation, and hemorrhage. Iatrogenic causes include spinal injection, lumbar puncture, and surgery. The most common clinical findings are paraparesis, neuropathic pain, gait disturbances, hypoesthesia or dysesthesia, and, rarely, incontinence. There may be postural accentuation of pain because the cyst enlarges in different positions.

Pathophysiology

Congenital or developmental arachnoid cysts differ from secondary or acquired arachnoid cysts; the latter are loculations of cerebrospinal fluid (CSF) surrounded by arachnoid scarring and probably result from arachnoiditis. They are also associated with an increased frequency of syringohydromyelia.

Imaging

The T3-4 cystic mass mildly deforming the cord has signal characteristics approximating CSF on T2-weighted images (Figs. A and B) and postcontrast T1-weighted images (Figs. C and D). The cyst fluid may appear hyperintense to CSF on T2-weighted images because of the flow-dephasing effects on the bulk of the CSF outside the cyst, which decreases the relatively high signal of the CSF in the subarachnoid space (see Fig. A).

Management

Treatment includes cyst excision, cyst fenestration with laminectomy or hemilaminectomy, or cyst drainage with or without MRI guidance.

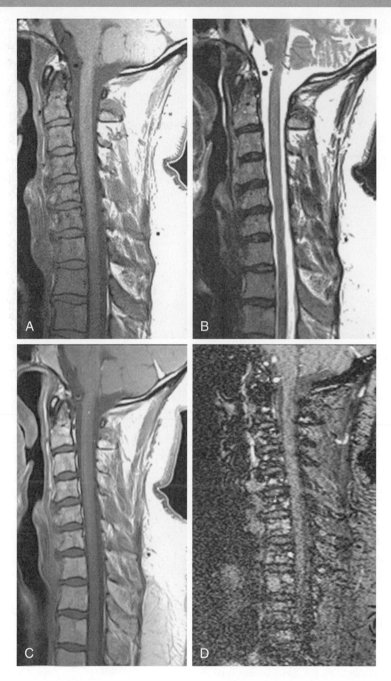

History: A 54-year-old man presents with neck and back pain.

1. What should be included in the differential diagnosis? (Choose all that apply.)
   a. Metastatic disease
   b. Multiple myeloma
   c. Lymphoma
   d. Diskitis osteomyelitis
   e. Chronic anemia

2. Which of the following skeletal sites is most commonly involved on a skeletal survey in patients with multiple myeloma?
   a. Ribs
   b. Skull
   c. Vertebrae
   d. Pelvis

3. What is an advantage of plain radiography over MRI in the evaluation of patients with multiple myeloma?
   a. Lower false-negative rate
   b. Better evaluation of diffuse bone marrow involvement
   c. Easier examination for the patient to tolerate
   d. Better detection of cortical bone lesions

4. Which of the following MRI features is typical of multiple myeloma?
   a. H-shaped vertebra
   b. "Salt-and-pepper" pattern
   c. "Fluid" sign
   d. Geographic pattern

Multiple Myeloma

1. a, b, and c

2. c

3. d

4. b

Reference
Healy CF, Murray JG, Eustace SJ, et al: Multiple myeloma: A review of imaging features and radiological techniques, *Bone Marrow Res* 583439, 2011.

Cross-Reference
Neuroradiology: The REQUISITES, 3rd ed, p 570.

Comment
Background
Multiple myeloma is the most common primary malignant neoplasm of the skeletal system and predominantly affects patients in the seventh decade of life. Presenting symptoms include bone pain, pathologic fractures, weakness, anemia, infection (often pneumococcal), hypercalcemia, spinal cord compression, and renal failure. In 30% of cases, the diagnosis is incidental. Most patients have more than one site of bony involvement, and pathologic fractures are very common.

Histopathology
Multiple myeloma is a neoplastic disorder of plasma B cells characterized by bone marrow infiltration and overproduction of monoclonal immunoglobulins.

Imaging
Skeletal survey is the initial imaging modality in the evaluation of patients with multiple myeloma. Characteristic findings are multiple destructive lytic lesions of the skeleton and severe demineralization. A major disadvantage of plain radiography is its high false-negative rate (30% to 70%), leading to a significant underestimation in the diagnosis and staging of patients with multiple myeloma, especially those with diffuse bone marrow involvement. Diffuse osteopenia as a result of multiple myeloma cannot be distinguished from senile or postmenopausal osteoporosis on plain radiographs. CT has a higher sensitivity than plain radiography in detecting small lytic lesions.

MRI (Figs. A-D) is the most sensitive imaging modality for detecting diffuse and focal multiple myeloma in the spine. Lesions in multiple myeloma typically have low signal intensity on T1-weighted images (see Fig. A), have high signal intensity on T2-weighted and short tau inversion recovery (STIR) images (see Fig. B), and generally show enhancement (see Fig. C). Five different patterns of marrow infiltration have been identified: a normal appearance, despite minor microscopic plasma cell infiltration; focal involvement; homogeneous diffuse infiltration; combined diffuse and focal infiltration; and heterogeneous bone marrow secondary to punctate infiltration with the interposition of fat islands, also known as the "salt-and-pepper" pattern.

Management
Multiple myeloma is incurable, and management focuses on treating the disease process and associated complications. Treatment includes drug therapy, autologous stem cell transplantation, radiation, and surgery in some cases.

Notes

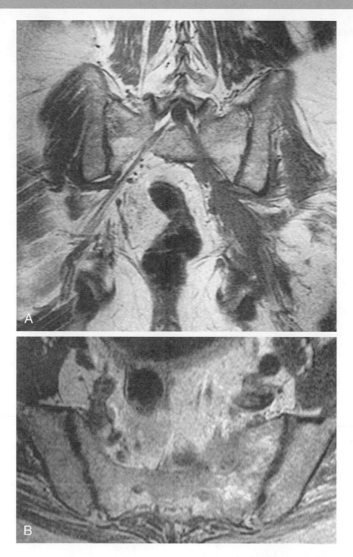

History: A 63-year-old woman presents with left-sided sciatica.

1. What should be included in the differential diagnosis? (Choose all that apply.)
   a. Plexiform neurofibroma
   b. Guillain-Barré syndrome
   c. Osteochondroma
   d. Metastatic infiltration
   e. Charcot-Marie-Tooth disease

2. Which nerve levels contribute to the sacral plexus?
   a. L1-S2
   b. L4-S3
   c. S1-S4
   d. L4-S4

3. A lesion in the sacral plexus would be expected to cause all of the following *except:*
   a. Abnormal patellar reflexes
   b. Atrophy of the gluteus maximus
   c. Atrophy of the erector spinae
   d. Sciatica

4. All of the following may produce sciatica *except:*
   a. Foraminal lesion at L4-5
   b. Lesion in the lateral recess at L4-5
   c. Lesion in the foramen of L5-S1
   d. Lesion in the lateral recess of L5-S1

Metastatic Tumor Infiltration of Sacral Nerves and Plexus

1. a and d

2. d

3. c

4. a

References

Bowen BC: Lumbosacral plexus. In Stark DD, Bradley WG Jr, editors: ed 3, *Magnetic resonance imaging*, vol 3, Philadelphia, 1998, Mosby-Year Book, pp 1907-1916.

Filler AG, Haynes J, Jordan SE, et al: Sciatica of nondisc origin and piriformis syndrome: Diagnosis by magnetic resonance neurography and interventional magnetic resonance imaging with outcome study of resulting treatment, *J Neurosurg Spine* 2(2):99-115, 2005.

Cross-Reference

Neuroradiology: The REQUISITES, 3rd ed, pp 515-516.

Comment

Background

The term *sciatica* describes a syndrome of acute pain radiating into the leg. The pain of sciatica is usually in the distribution of S1 (down the back of the leg to the heel), L5 (down the lateral surface of the leg to the instep), or both because these two roots are most commonly affected by degenerative disk disease. However, the symptoms may be mimicked by lesions in the pelvis involving the sacral plexus or lesions in the gluteal and upper thigh region involving the sciatic nerve.

Imaging

In this case, the coronal T1-weighted image (Fig. A) demonstrates the course of the normal right S1 root exiting the anterior foramen, continuing inferiorly and laterally to join the sacral plexus (at the parasagittal level of the sacroiliac joint), and then continuing into the upper portion of the thigh as the sciatic nerve. The corresponding left neural structures are infiltrated by a mass that tracks along the left S1 root superiorly. The postcontrast axial image (Fig. B) shows enhancement of the mass enveloping the S1 root and eroding the anterior surface of the sacrum. The left S2 root in the neural foramen is also enhanced and enlarged compared with the normal right S2 root. This finding is consistent with retrograde, perineural spread of tumor, which in this case was proved by biopsy to be metastatic from a primary lung carcinoma.

Management

Treatment is surgical resection and radiation therapy.

Figures for this case are from Bowen BC: Lumbosacral plexus. In: Stark DD, Bradley WG Jr, Eds: *Magnetic Resonance Imaging,* third edition, Vol 3. Philadelphia, Mosby–Year Book, 1998, pp 1907–1916.

Challenge

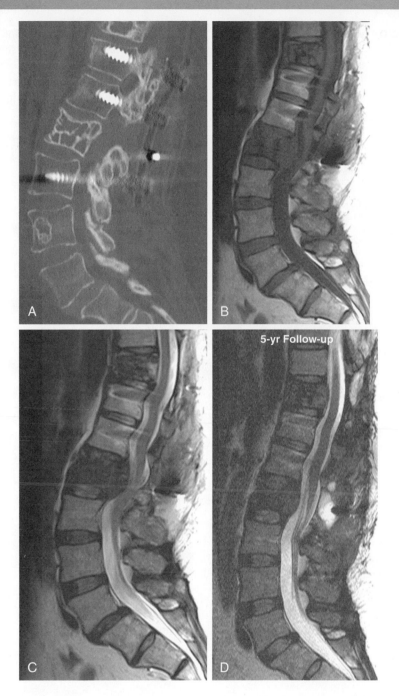

History: A 53-year-old woman presents with a long history of back pain and hysterectomy 10 years ago.

1. What should be included in the differential diagnosis? (Choose all that apply.)
   a. Benign metastasizing leiomyoma (BML)
   b. Vertebral body metastasis
   c. Brown tumor
   d. Chordoma
   e. Lymphoma

2. Where does BML most commonly occur?
   a. Pelvic cavity
   b. Lymph nodes
   c. Vertebra
   d. Lung

3. Which of the following imaging findings provides the best clue to the diagnosis of BML in this case?
   a. T2 hypointensity
   b. Lack of significant interval growth
   c. Enhancement of the lesion on postcontrast images
   d. Presence of a vertebral body collapse

4. Which of the following causes of multiple vertebral body lesions is unlikely to manifest as a hypointense lesion on T2-weighted images?
   a. Brown tumor
   b. Metastatic prostate cancer
   c. Multiple myeloma
   d. Lymphoma

Benign Metastasizing Leiomyoma

1. a, b, c, and e

2. d

3. b

4. c

References

Alessi G, Lemmerling M, Vereecken L, et al: Benign metastasizing leiomyoma to skull base and spine: A report of two cases, *Clin Neurol Neurosurg* 105(3):170-174, 2003.

Awonuga AO, Shavell VI, Imudia AN, et al: Pathogenesis of benign metastasizing leiomyoma: A review, *Obstet Gynecol Surv* 65(3):189-195, 2010.

Kang MW, Kang SK, Yu JH, et al: Benign metastasizing leiomyoma: Metastasis to rib and vertebra, *Ann Thorac Surg* 91(3):924-926, 2011.

Cross-Reference

Neuroradiology: The REQUISITES, 3rd ed, pp 565-566.

Comment

Pathophysiology

BMLs are slow-growing metastatic lesions associated with a current or prior history of uterine leiomyoma. They are characterized by a benign histology with low mitotic indices, lack of nuclear pleomorphism, and no evidence of invasion despite multiple distant lesions. The pathogenesis of BML is poorly understood. Female gonadal steroids likely play a major role; however, occasional reported cases in postmenopausal women who are not receiving hormone replacement therapy suggest that other factors may be involved. In most cases, BML occurs in the pelvic cavity, lung, and lymph node; rarely, it occurs in the vertebra or skull base.

Clinical Findings

It has been suggested that the primary lesions in BML may be low-grade sarcomas with metastatic potential; however, the clinical course of BML is much less aggressive than that of a true leiomyosarcoma. Patients with BML are often asymptomatic and have an indolent course. Nevertheless, patients with histologically benign-appearing BMLs can occasionally present with debilitating symptoms or life-threatening complications and death.

Imaging

On CT, BML appears as a nonexpansive osteolytic lesion (Fig. A). On MRI, the lesions are hypointense on both T1-weighted images (Fig. B) and T2-weighted images (Figs. C and D) and demonstrate enhancement. Larger lesions may cause vertebral body collapse and epidural extension, as seen in this case.

Management

Surgery is the treatment of choice for symptomatic leiomyoma metastases causing secondary neurologic deficit. Nonsymptomatic or small lesions can be treated first with trial hormonal therapy. Postoperatively, hormonal therapy should be considered if, on histologic examination, estrogen and progesterone receptors are found to be positive. Lesions increasing in size even with trial hormonal therapy should be considered for surgery. Bilateral oophorectomy has been advocated as the treatment of choice to stop further growth and to reduce the size of the tumors.

Notes

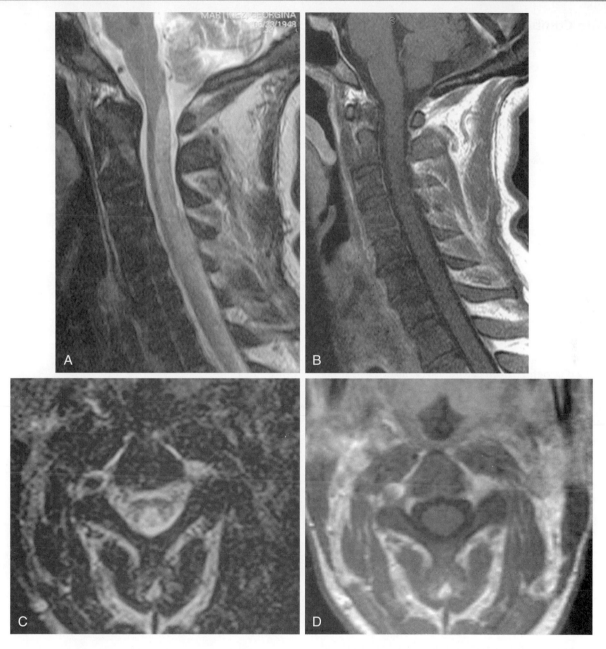

History: A 57-year old woman presents with difficulty walking and bilateral upper extremity weakness for the past several weeks.

1. What should be included in the differential diagnosis? (Choose all that apply.)
   a. Multiple sclerosis
   b. Wallerian degeneration
   c. Spinal dural arteriovenous fistula
   d. Subacute combined degeneration (SCD)
   e. Vacuolar myelopathy

2. Which of the following conditions is *not* associated with vitamin B_{12} deficiency?
   a. AIDS
   b. Alcoholism
   c. Multiple sclerosis
   d. Metformin therapy

3. What commonly used anesthetic agent has been implicated in vitamin B_{12} deficiency?
   a. Propofol
   b. Amobarbital
   c. Nitrous oxide
   d. Ketamine

4. Which imaging finding is *least* likely to be seen with SCD?
   a. High signal intensity on T2-weighted images in the posterior columns
   b. Contrast enhancement
   c. Expansion of the spinal cord
   d. Low signal intensity on T1-weighted images in the posterior columns

CASE 124

Subacute Combined Degeneration

1. b, d, and e

2. c

3. c

4. d

References

Ravina B, Loevner LA, Bank W: MR findings in subacute combined degeneration of the spinal cord: A case of reversible cervical myelopathy, *AJR Am J Roentgenol* 174(3):863-865, 2000.

Renard D, Dutray A, Remy A, et al: Subacute combined degeneration of the spinal cord caused by nitrous oxide anaesthesia, *Neurol Sci* 30(1):75-76, 2009.

Tian C: Hyperintense signal on spinal cord diffusion-weighted imaging in a patient with subacute combined degeneration, *Neurol India* 59(3):429-431, 2011.

Cross-Reference

Neuroradiology: The REQUISITES, 3rd ed, pp 549-550.

Comment

Background

SCD is the manifestation of vitamin B_{12} deficiency in the spinal cord. The causes of vitamin B_{12} (cyanocobalamin) deficiency can be divided into three main categories: (1) inadequate intake (e.g., vegetarianism), (2) malabsorption (e.g., pernicious anemia, gastrectomy, intestinal infections, Crohn's disease, tropical sprue), and (3) other conditions (e.g., nitrous oxide anesthesia, transcobalamin II deficiency). The most common cause of vitamin B_{12} deficiency in the United States is pernicious anemia.

Histopathology

Histopathologic studies demonstrate degeneration of myelin sheaths and axonal loss in the posterior, lateral, and sometimes anterior columns.

Imaging

Sagittal T2-weighted images reveal increased signal intensity of variable length in the posterior columns (Fig. A). On cross-sectional images, the signal abnormality appears as an inverted "V" (Fig. C). This configuration reflects greater involvement of the lateral than the medial portions of the dorsal columns and corresponds to relative sparing of proprioceptive sensation in the lower extremities. Lesions typically occur in the thoracic and cervical cord, most often exceeding several vertebral bodies in length. The hyperintensity may or may not be associated with postcontrast enhancement on T1-weighted images (Figs. B and D). Cord enlargement has been observed in some cases. Restricted diffusion in the posterior columns has also been described. Lateral column hyperintensity is uncommon, even in cases with histologic and clinical evidence of lateral column involvement.

Management

Therapy with vitamin B_{12} results in partial to full recovery, depending on the duration and extent of neurodegeneration. Vitamin B_{12} supplements must be taken throughout life to prevent symptoms from recurring.

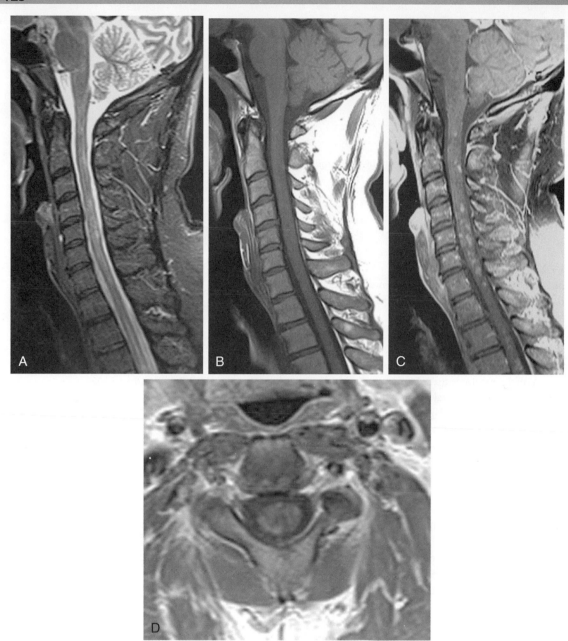

History: A 43-year-old man with a history of recurrent bilateral optic neuritis and increasing lower extremity numbness for the past 3 years presents with mild spastic paraparesis.

1. What should be included in the differential diagnosis? (Choose all that apply.)
   a. Sarcoid
   b. Metastatic disease
   c. Infection
   d. Lymphoma
   e. Vitamin B_{12} deficiency

2. What spinal region is most often involved with this disease?
   a. Cervical region
   b. Thoracic region
   c. Lumbar region
   d. Sacral region

3. In what percentage of sarcoid spinal cord lesions is leptomeningeal infiltration present?
   a. Less than 1%
   b. 25%
   c. 60%
   d. More than 90%

4. All of the following statements regarding sarcoidosis are true *except:*
   a. Spinal cord involvement is the usual initial manifestation of the disease.
   b. Dura-based sarcoid granulomatous masses are rare.
   c. Diagnosis and early treatment of neurosarcoidosis with steroids can minimize neurologic complications.
   d. Elevated serum angiotensin-converting enzyme levels can be found.

Cervical Sarcoidosis

1. a, b, c, and d

2. a

3. c

4. b

Reference

Smith JK, Matheus MG, Castillo M: Imaging manifestations of neurosarcoid-osis, *AJR Am J Roentgenol* 182(2):289-295, 2004.

Cross-Reference

Neuroradiology: The REQUISITES, 3rd ed, pp 546-547.

Comment

Background

Sarcoidosis is a systemic disease most commonly affecting African Americans (females more than males) in the third and fourth decades of life.

Histopathology

Sarcoidosis manifests histopathologically as noncaseating granulomas of unknown etiology. Spinal neurosarcoidosis can manifest as intramedullary, intradural extramedullary, extradural, or vertebral lesions. Intramedullary involvement occurs in less than 1% of sarcoidosis cases and often causes severe neurologic sequelae.

Imaging

The spinal manifestations of sarcoidosis are similar to the intracranial findings, and there can be both intramedullary and extramedullary involvement. Involvement of the cord may be extensive (Figs. A-D) and infiltrative, with cord enlargement and associated hyperintensity on T2-weighted images (see Fig. A) and hypointensity on T1-weighted images. The enhancement pattern may be patchy, circumscribed focal enhancement or broad-based and peripheral enhancement, extending from the spinal cord surface to the center of the cord, suggesting inflammation that extends from the leptomeninges via the perivascular spaces inward. In the chronic stages, cord atrophy without enhancement and gliosis may be present. The diagnosis of neurosarcoidosis requires the exclusion of other diseases capable of producing a similar radiologic picture, especially tuberculosis and carcinomatous meningitis.

Management

Diagnosis and early treatment of neurosarcoidosis with steroids can minimize neurologic complications and decrease disease morbidity rates. With delayed diagnosis and treatment, the disease typically resolves only partially and may recur.

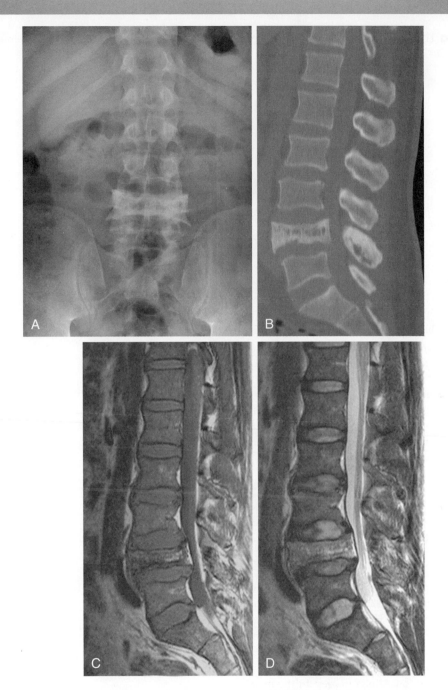

History: A 63-year-old man presents with lower back pain.

1. What should be included in the differential diagnosis? (Choose all that apply.)
   a. Paget's disease
   b. Multiple myeloma
   c. Lymphoma
   d. Fibrous dysplasia
   e. Osteoblastic metastasis

2. What is the most common spinal complication of Paget's disease?
   a. Spondylolysis
   b. Synovial cyst
   c. Pathologic fracture
   d. Sarcomatous transformation

3. Which of the following statements regarding Paget's disease is *false*?
   a. Thickening of the cortex is often seen.
   b. Associated soft tissue mass is common.
   c. The disease has three phases.
   d. 18F-FDG PET/CT has an advantage over bone scintigraphy in the imaging of Paget's disease.

4. Common radiologic findings of uncomplicated Paget's disease include all of the following *except:*
   a. Bone enlargement on CT scan
   b. Cortical thickening on CT scan
   c. Cortical destruction
   d. Disorganized trabecular thickening on CT scan

Paget's Disease in the Lumbar Spine

1. a, d, and e

2. c

3. b

4. c

References

Dell'Atti C, Cassar-Pullicino VN, Lalam RK, et al: The spine in Paget's disease, *Skeletal Radiol* 36(7):609-626, 2007.

Smith SE, Murphey MD, Motamedi K, et al: From the archives of the AFIP. Radiologic spectrum of Paget disease of bone and its complications with pathologic correlation, *Radiographics* 22(5):1191-1216, 2002.

Cross-Reference

Neuroradiology: The REQUISITES, 3rd ed, p 570.

Comment

Background

Paget's disease is one of the most common metabolically active bone diseases, second in prevalence only to osteoporosis. The overall prevalence of Paget's disease is 3% to 3.7%, and it increases with age. The spine is the second most commonly affected site (53% of cases), after the pelvis (70%). Common complications include osseous weakening (with secondary deformity and fracture); spinal stenosis from enlargement of the vertebral body, neural arch, or both; facet arthropathy; neurologic compromise; and sarcomatous transformation.

Histopathology

Paget's disease is characterized by a disturbance in bone modeling and remodeling caused by an increase in osteoblastic and osteoclastic activity. The disease is polyostotic in 66% of cases.

Imaging

Radiography is typically used for diagnostic purposes (Fig. A) and may be indicated to evaluate for fracture. Common CT findings of uncomplicated Paget's disease include bone enlargement, disorganized trabecular thickening, and cortical thickening (Fig. B). The MRI signal intensity pattern is variable. In the lytic (early, active) phase, the marrow space is heterogeneous in signal on T1-weighted and T2-weighted images. In the mixed (intermediate) phase, there is preservation of marrow fat signal (Figs. C and D). Speckled enhancement is found on images after contrast agent administration. The mixed phase is most commonly seen. In the blastic (late, inactive) phase, low signal intensity is usually found on all sequences; this corresponds to bony sclerosis. All MRI sequences must be carefully examined to exclude sarcomatous transformation.

Management

Patients presenting with neurogenic pain secondary to cord compression by expanded pagetic bone respond well to medical treatment with calcitonin and bisphosphonates. Because of the increased risk of malignancy, patients with Paget's disease should be monitored indefinitely. Chemotherapy, radiation, or both may be used to treat neoplasms that arise from pagetic bone.

Notes

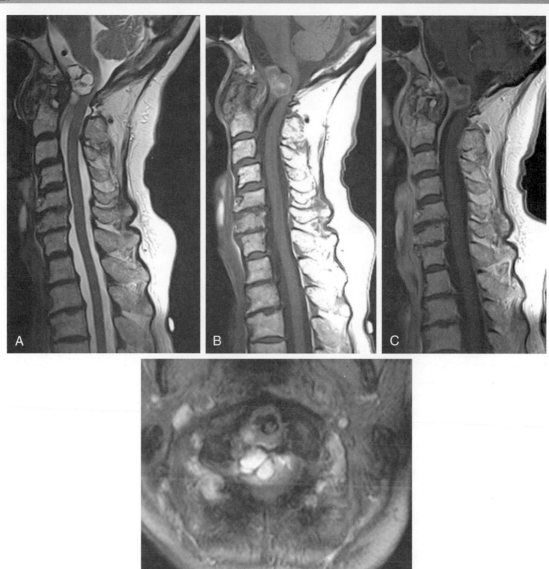

History: An 81-year-old woman with a history of lung and colon cancer presents with complaints of recurrent headaches and neck pain for the past few months.

1. What should be included in the differential diagnosis? (Choose all that apply.)
   a. Rheumatoid arthritis
   b. Metastatic disease
   c. Calcium pyrophosphate dihydrate (CPPD) deposition disease
   d. Arachnoid cyst
   e. Chordoma

2. Which of the following statements regarding CPPD deposition disease is true?
   a. The intervertebral disk is never affected.
   b. Similar to CPPD deposition disease, rheumatoid arthritis commonly has calcification of the transverse ligament.
   c. Erosion of a peripheral joint would favor CPPD deposition disease over rheumatoid arthritis.
   d. The most frequently involved location in the spine is the atlantoaxial joint.

3. Which of the following body parts is *not* commonly affected by CPPD deposition disease?
   a. Knee
   b. Spine
   c. Wrist
   d. Symphysis pubis

4. Which imaging finding favors CPPD deposition disease over rheumatoid arthritis?
   a. Erosion of the atlantoaxial joint
   b. Transverse ligament calcification
   c. Retro-odontoid mass
   d. Atlantoaxial subluxation

Calcium Pyrophosphate Dihydrate Deposition Disease

Notes

1. a, b, c, and e

2. d

3. b

4. b

References

Sethi KS, Garg A, Sharma MC, et al: Cervicomedullary compression secondary to massive calcium pyrophosphate crystal deposition in the atlantoaxial joint with intradural extension and vertebral artery encasement, *Surg Neurol* 67(2):200-203, 2007.

Steinbach LS, Resnick D: Calcium pyrophosphate dihydrate crystal deposition disease revisited, *Radiology* 200(1):1-9, 1996.

Cross-Reference

Neuroradiology: The REQUISITES, 3rd ed, p 300.

Comment

Background

CPPD deposition disease is a form of arthritis that occurs in elderly patients and affects articular and periarticular soft tissues. Involvement of the spine is rare, with the most frequent location being the atlantoaxial joint. Other locations are the ligamentum flavum and the intervertebral disk. Involvement of the disk can be severe and may mimic diskitis or osteomyelitis.

Histopathology

CPPD deposition disease is caused by the deposition of CPPD in and around the joints, especially in articular cartilage and fibrocartilage.

Imaging

Almost all reported cases of CPPD deposition disease in and around the atlantoaxial joint have calcification of the transverse ligament on CT scan. By comparison, the frequency of calcification of the transverse ligament in the general population is only about 6%. The pattern of calcification in CPPD deposition disease may be curvilinear, stippled, or, more commonly, mixed; the characteristic location in the joints around the odontoid and the lateral atlantoaxial masses may suggest the diagnosis. MRI studies (Figs. A-D) show a retro-odontoid mass that is isointense on T1-weighted images; has variable, but usually decreased, signal intensity on T2-weighted images; and shows peripheral enhancement, which may represent distended and inflamed synovial tissue surrounding the lesion. Myelopathy may result from cord compression by the mass.

Management

Treatment is surgical decompression by a transoral approach, which allows a direct approach to the site of compression and has a good clinical outcome. Posterior spinal stabilization may be needed in cases of craniovertebral instability.

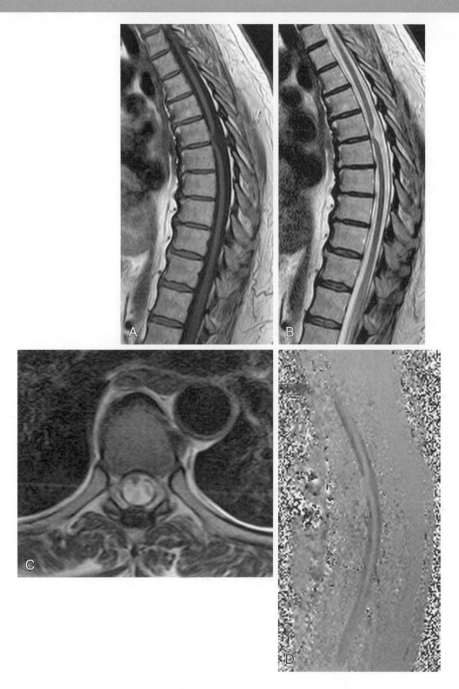

History: A 55-year-old woman presents with a history of progressive paraparesis and rapidly progressive myelopathy.

1. What should be included in the differential diagnosis? (Choose all that apply.)
   a. Spinal cord herniation
   b. Arachnoid cyst
   c. Cord tethering
   d. Diastematomyelia
   e. Dermoid cyst

2. Where does cord herniation most often occur?
   a. Cervical spine
   b. Upper thoracic spine between T1 and T4
   c. Midthoracic spine between T4 and T7
   d. Lower thoracic spine between T9 and T12

3. All of the following imaging findings may be seen in spinal cord herniation *except:*
   a. Scalloping of the vertebral body
   b. Focal cord atrophy
   c. Hyperintense T2 signal
   d. Schmorl's node

4. Which of the following imaging features has been described in patients with spinal cord herniation?
   a. "Fluid" sign
   b. "Nuclear trail" sign
   c. "Mercedes-Benz" sign
   d. "Empty-sac" sign

Idiopathic Spinal Cord Herniation

1. a, b, and c

2. c

3. d

4. b

References

Brus-Ramer M, Dillon WP: Idiopathic thoracic spinal cord herniation: Retrospective analysis supporting a mechanism of diskogenic dural injury and subsequent tamponade, *AJNR Am J Neuroradiol* 33(1):52-56, 2012.

Parmar H, Park P, Brahma B, et al: Imaging of idiopathic spinal cord herniation, *Radiographics* 28(2):511-518, 1008.

Prada F, Saladino A, Giombini S, et al: Spinal cord herniation: Management and outcome in a series of 12 consecutive patients and review of the literature, *Acta Neurochir* 154(4):723-730, 2012.

Cross-Reference

Neuroradiology: The REQUISITES, 3rd ed, p 575.

Comment

Background and Clinical Findings

Idiopathic thoracic spinal cord herniation, in contrast to spinal cord herniation with a known traumatic or postoperative origin, is an uncommon cause of thoracic myelopathy in which the anterior portion of the spinal cord herniates or prolapses through a defect in the ventral dura. Brown-Séquard syndrome is the most frequently reported clinical feature. Early manifestations include numbness and decreased temperature sensation in the legs, gait disturbances, pain, and incontinence. Symptoms often worsen over time, but timely diagnosis and treatment may allow the reversal of neurologic deficits.

Pathophysiology

The pathophysiology of this condition is unclear. Some authors suggest that it is initiated by incidental or unnoticed trauma to the anterior surface of the thoracic dura by disk protrusions or osteophytes. Subsequent herniation of spinal cord tissue through a dural defect results from the action of cerebrospinal fluid pulsation and mechanical factors, which leads to progressive myelopathy.

Imaging

Radiologic imaging is the main method of diagnosing idiopathic spinal cord herniation. On sagittal MRI, an acute anterior kink of the thoracic spinal cord is observed, with enlargement of the dorsal subarachnoid space (Figs. A and B). Cord deviation is generally limited to one or two thoracic spine segments. The dural defect occurs in the thoracic spine, most commonly between the levels of the T4 and T7 vertebrae (Fig. C). Associated cord atrophy and high T2 signal intensity may be observed within the thoracic cord. Scalloping of the vertebral body may be seen occasionally. Imaging features of spinal cord herniation generally include a dural tear through which a portion of the cord protrudes. Cerebrospinal fluid flows freely through the defect, causing increased turbulence in the fluid just dorsal to the site of herniation. The observation of this feature and the demonstration of uninterrupted flow on phase-contrast cine MRI may allow the differentiation of spinal cord herniation from an arachnoid cyst (Fig. D). The "nuclear trail" sign, a linear area of hyperintense signal on CT related to calcification of nucleus pulposus leakage from a herniated disk, has been described.

Management

The best treatment option is surgical reduction, especially in cases of progressive clinical deterioration. Patients whose symptoms are less severe may be eligible for less invasive therapy and monitoring.

Notes

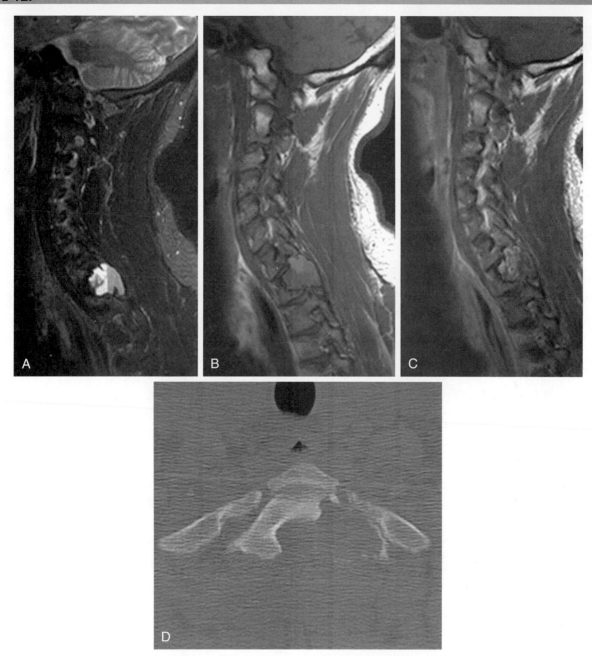

History: A 37-year-old man presents with left upper back pain and scapular pain. The patient had surgery for resection of a cystic lesion involving T1 1 year prior.

1. What should be included in the differential diagnosis? (Choose all that apply.)
   a. Aneurysmal bone cyst (ABC)
   b. Unicameral cyst
   c. Osteoblastoma
   d. Giant cell tumor
   e. Telangiectatic osteosarcoma

2. Which finding is highly suggestive of the diagnosis of ABC but is not pathognomonic?
   a. Expansile lesion
   b. Fluid-fluid levels
   c. Multiple cystic loculations
   d. Internal septations

3. Secondary ABC can be associated with all of the following tumors *except:*
   a. Nonossifying fibroma
   b. Osteoblastoma
   c. Giant cell tumor
   d. Chondroblastoma

4. Which part of the vertebra is most commonly involved with both osteoblastoma and ABC?
   a. Vertebral body
   b. Vertebral end-plate
   c. Posterior elements
   d. Pedicle

Osteoblastoma with Secondary Aneurysmal Bone Cyst

1. a, c, d, and e

2. b

3. a

4. c

Reference

Ramme AJ, Smucker JD: Balancing spinal stability and future mobility in the cervical spine: Surgical treatment of a case of osteoblastoma with secondary aneurysmal bone cyst, *Spine J* 11(5):e5-e12, 2011.

Cross-Reference

Neuroradiology: The REQUISITES, 3rd ed, pp 568-569.

Comment

Background

ABCs are benign, highly vascular osseous lesions of unknown origin. Eight percent to 30% of ABCs arise in the spine and most commonly affect the posterior elements. Distribution among the spinal segments is reportedly 75% in the thoracic and lumbar spine and 25% in the cervical spine.

Osteoblastoma accounts for 30% to 40% of all spinal tumors, with an equal distribution among the cervical, thoracic, and lumbar levels. Lesions affect mainly the posterior elements. Osteoblastoma occurs most frequently in individuals 10 to 25 years of age and has a 3:1 male predominance.

Pathophysiology

The pathophysiology of ABCs is unclear, but several mechanisms have been proposed, including a vascular degenerative process, traumatic reparative process, and nonspecific 17p13 genetic translocation. In about one third of cases, ABCs arise within a preexisting bone tumor, such as chondroblastoma, chondromyxoid fibroma, and giant cell tumor, or in a region of fibrous dysplasia. Less frequently, ABCs may arise from malignant tumors, such as osteosarcoma, chondrosarcoma, and hemangioendothelioma. Secondary changes consistent with ABC are exhibited in 10% of all osteoblastomas.

Imaging

On plain radiographs, osteoblastoma appears as an intracortical, expansile, radiolucent lesion with a "ground glass" appearance and focal density at the lesion's core. The aggressive form shows evidence of bony destruction, invasion of surrounding tissues, and disorganized calcifications. An ABC appears on plain films as a "blown-out," lytic, expansile lesion. CT scans demonstrate septated lesions surrounded by normal cortical bone (Fig. D). CT and MRI may show fluid-fluid levels within the lesion (Figs. A-C), which is not diagnostic of ABC because this finding is also associated with osteoblastoma, chondroblastoma, giant cell tumor, and telangiectatic osteosarcoma. For both osteoblastoma and ABC, CT scan is most effective in identifying the lesion location, extent of bony destruction, and involvement of surrounding complex anatomy. MRI allows visualization of the impact on surrounding soft tissues.

Management

Optimal surgical management of osteoblastoma and ABC consists of complete resection, which has the lowest rate of recurrence. Recurrence of osteoblastoma is rare after total resection, but with incomplete resection, it is 10% to 20%. Maximal recurrence of ABC occurs at 1 year after excision, with rates of 20% to 30%. A 2- to 5-year follow-up is indicated.

Notes

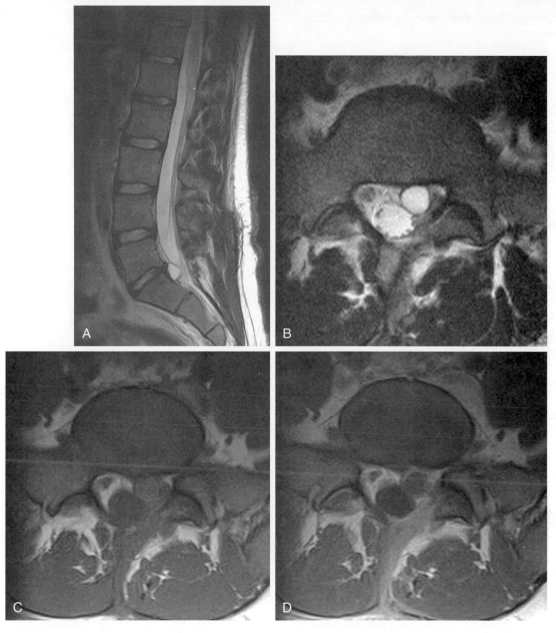

History: A 17-year-old boy presents with left leg pain 6 weeks after lumbar diskectomy at L5-S1.

1. What should be included in the differential diagnosis? (Choose all that apply.)
   a. Synovial cyst
   b. Postoperative diskal pseudocyst
   c. Epidural hematoma
   d. Migrated disk herniation
   e. Ganglion cyst of the posterior longitudinal ligament

2. Which of the following features is *not* helpful in distinguishing postoperative diskal pseudocyst from other epidural cysts such as diskal cyst?
   a. Atypical form
   b. Formation after diskectomy
   c. Spontaneous regression
   d. Paracentral ventral epidural location

3. Which technique is preferred for imaging postoperative diskal pseudocyst?
   a. Plain radiographs
   b. Ultrasound
   c. CT myelography
   d. MRI

4. Which of the following statements regarding postoperative diskal pseudocyst is true?
   a. Rim enhancement excludes the diagnosis of postoperative diskal pseudocyst.
   b. Postoperative diskal pseudocyst communicates with the herniated disk on diskography.
   c. Postoperative diskal pseudocyst is located in the posterolateral aspect of the spinal canal.
   d. Most postoperative diskal pseudocysts appear during the first week after diskectomy.

Postoperative Diskal Pseudocyst After Lumbar Diskectomy

1. b and e

2. d

3. d

4. b

Reference

Chung D, Cho DC, Sung JK, et al: Retrospective report of symptomatic postoperative discal pseudocyst after lumbar discectomy, *Acta Neurochir (Wien)* 154(4):715-722, 2012.

Cross-Reference

Neuroradiology: The REQUISITES, 3rd ed, p 531.

Comment

Background

Postoperative diskal pseudocyst develops after lumbar diskectomy and seems to have a very low incidence (1%). It has been described as a cystic lesion attached to the operated disk that is usually apparent at about 1 month after diskectomy. Postoperative diskal pseudocysts are found mostly in male patients with relatively mild disk degeneration; these patients are typically younger than those with degenerative lumbar disk herniation. The differential diagnosis includes cysts arising from the facet joint, posterior longitudinal ligament, ligamentum flavum, perineurium, arachnoid, and disk. Among these epidural cysts, diskal cysts share an origin and many other features with postoperative diskal pseudocyst.

Pathophysiology

Postoperative diskal pseudocyst is thought to be caused by an accumulation of liquid pumped from a mildly degenerated nucleus through an annular cleft, resulting in a pseudomembranous formation, during physical activity.

Imaging

Characteristic MRI findings are a well-defined round or oval lesion in the ventrolateral extradural spinal canal adjacent to a herniated disk that has cerebrospinal fluid–equivalent signal intensity on all pulse sequences (Figs. A-D) and demonstrates rim enhancement (see Fig. D). Most of the features described for diskal cysts are similar to the features of postoperative diskal pseudocysts; however, postoperative diskal pseudocyst may manifest atypically, depending on the amount of dead space that remains postoperatively. Triangular (see Fig. A), bilobed, and dumbbell-shaped postoperative diskal pseudocysts have been observed, as well as lesions spanning the midline of the intervertebral disk space. Both postoperative diskal pseudocysts and diskal cysts have been shown to communicate with the intervertebral disk on diskography.

Management

Postoperative diskal pseudocyst may regress spontaneously and can often be treated conservatively. However, recovery time is variable, and surgical treatment may be required in some cases.

Notes

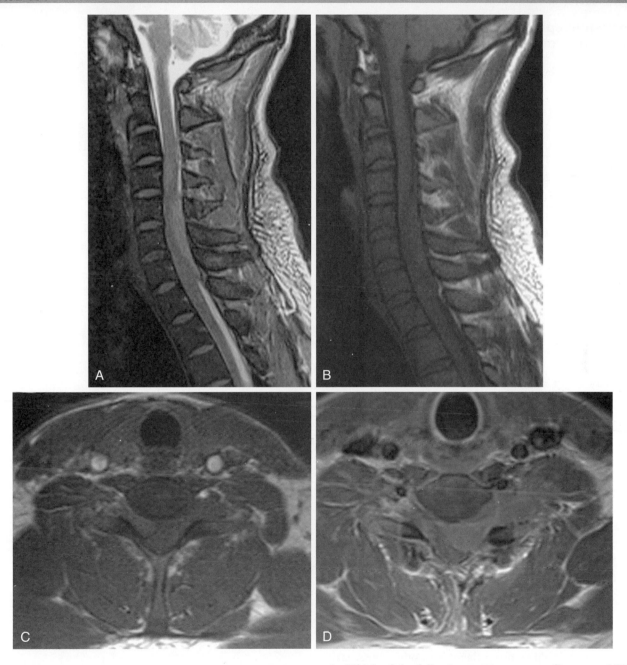

History: A 25-year-old man presents with neck pain and left arm numbness and tingling.

1. What should be included in the differential diagnosis? (Choose all that apply.)
   a. Lymphoma
   b. Ependymoma
   c. Nerve sheath tumor
   d. Astrocytoma
   e. Primitive neuroectodermal tumor (PNET)

2. Which of the following descriptions of the appearance of intraspinal PNET on CT and MRI is *false?*
   a. Isointense relative to cord on T1-weighted imaging
   b. Hyperintense relative to cord on T2-weighted imaging
   c. Calcifications on CT
   d. Heterogeneous enhancement

3. Which of the following statements regarding central PNET and intraspinal PNET is *false?*
   a. Central PNET is more aggressive than intraspinal PNET.
   b. The average age at presentation is much older for patients with intraspinal PNET than for those with intracranial PNET.
   c. Both tumors are more common in males.
   d. Peripheral PNETs are related to Ewing's sarcoma.

4. Which of the following features is *not* suggestive of primary intraspinal PNET?
   a. Cranial symptoms
   b. Local recurrence
   c. Intramedullary location
   d. Short duration of illness

Primary Intraspinal Primitive Neuroectodermal Tumor

1. a, c, and e

2. c

3. a

4. a

References

Duan XH, Ban XH, Liu B, et al: Intraspinal primitive neuroectodermal tumor: Imaging findings in six cases, *Eur J Radiol* 80(2):426-431, 2011.

Jingyu C, Jinning S, Hui M, et al: Intraspinal primitive neuroectodermal tumors: Report of four cases and review of the literature, *Neurol India* 57(5):661-668, 2009.

Cross-Reference

Neuroradiology: The REQUISITES, 3rd ed, pp 78-79.

Comment

Background

Intraspinal PNETs are rare tumors found predominantly in males. They can occur at any level of the spine, and the location can be intramedullary, intradural extramedullary, or epidural. The average age at presentation is 24 years (range, 3 months to 69 years), which is much older than the average age for intracranial PNETs. The duration of illness is often short.

Histopathology

PNETs are undifferentiated small, blue, round cell tumors divided into central and peripheral types. Both types are aggressive tumors; however, they differ in their clinical presentation, spread pattern, and immunohistochemical profile. Central PNETs are mainly intracranial, predominantly in the cerebellum.

Imaging

Intraspinal PNETs often demonstrate hyperintense signal on T2-weighted images (Fig. A) and hypointense or isointense signal on T1-weighted images (Figs. B and C), and they tend to exhibit heterogeneous enhancement. Based on signal intensity alone, it is hard to differentiate them from other intraspinal tumors. Both extradural and the intradural extramedullary lesions often extend into the paraspinal tissues through the neural foramen and form a paraspinal soft tissue mass (Figs. C and D). Extradural PNETs frequently occur in the thoracic spine and may be associated with lytic spinal bone destruction.

Management

The prognosis of intraspinal PNETs is very poor, and most patients experience a recurrence after initial treatment. The treatment of choice is total resection of the tumor and vertebral canal decompression. Radiotherapy and chemotherapy are frequently used as adjuvant therapy.

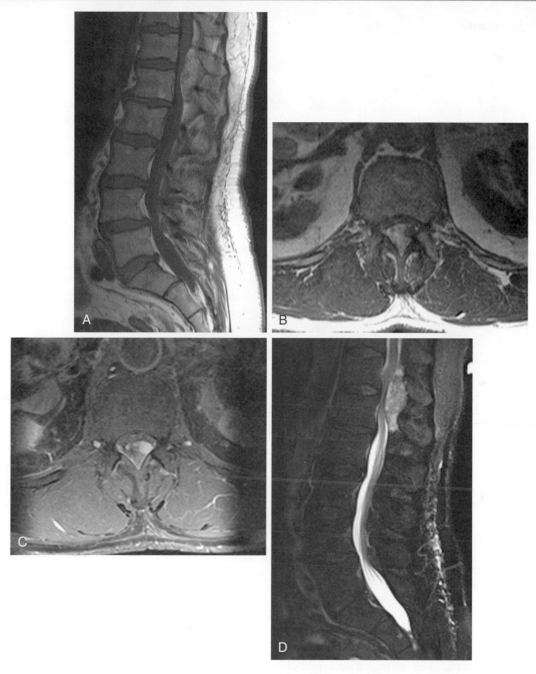

History: A 67-year-old patient presents with increasing intermittent back and leg pain over the last 2 months, which worsens when changing positions.

1. What should be included in the differential diagnosis? (Choose all that apply.)
   a. Epidural hematoma
   b. Epidural lipomatosis
   c. Epidural angiolipoma
   d. Liposarcoma
   e. Meningioma

2. What is the location of the lesion?
   a. Intramedullary
   b. Intradural extramedullary
   c. Extradural
   d. Extraspinal

3. Which of the following findings is *not* helpful in differentiating this lesion from epidural lipomatosis?
   a. Location within the posterior epidural space
   b. Inhomogeneous signal on T1-weighted images
   c. Inhomogeneous enhancement
   d. Focal mass

4. Which of the following techniques is used to suppress the fat signal on the postcontrast T1-weighted image shown?
   a. Fluid attenuated inversion recovery (FLAIR)
   b. Saturation band
   c. Frequency selective saturation
   d. Short tau inversion recovery (STIR)

Epidural Angiolipoma

1. c and d

2. c

3. a

4. c

References
Hungs M, Paré LS: Spinal angiolipoma: Case report and literature review, *J Spinal Cord Med* 31(3):315-318, 2008.

Leu NH, Chen CY, Shy CG, et al: MR imaging of an infiltrating spinal epidural angiolipoma, *AJNR Am J Neuroradiol* 24(5):1008-1011, 2003.

Nanassis K, Tsitsopoulos P, Marinopoulos D, et al: Lumbar spinal epidural angiolipoma, *J Clin Neurosci* 15(4):460-463, 2008.

Cross-Reference
Neuroradiology: The REQUISITES, 3rd ed, pp 564-565.

Comment
Background
Spinal angiolipomas are rare benign tumors that account for 0.5% of all spinal axis tumors. They are found predominantly in women, and the most common location is the epidural mid-thoracic area. Most extend over three to four vertebral levels. Pregnancy, weight gain, and hormonal factors are assumed to be aggravating factors. The onset of symptoms is in the fifth decade, and the typical clinical presentation is back pain and symptoms related to spinal cord compression. Symptoms vary in duration, with a slowly progressive course over months. A patient with a prolonged neurologic course can suddenly deteriorate as a result of vascular engorgement, enlarging or degenerated blood vessels, vascular steal phenomena, venous stasis with thrombosis, or hemorrhage into the lesion.

Histopathology
Spinal angiolipomas are composed of varying proportions of mature fat cells and abnormal capillary, sinusoidal, venous, or arterial vascular elements.

Imaging
The variability of the vascular and adipose elements of the tumor causes significant heterogeneity in imaging studies. Plain radiography is often negative but may show erosions of the pedicle and widening of the spinal canal, whereas infiltrating tumors cause trabeculation of the affected vertebral body. On CT, the tumor appears hypodense relative to the spinal cord but may contain isodense areas, likely related to the vascularized soft tissue. MRI is the imaging modality of choice. Typically, T1-weighted images (Figs. A and B) show a high-signal, inhomogeneous mass that is hypointense relative to epidural fat. The vascular soft tissue within angiolipomas likely accounts for the hypointense component on T1-weighted images and the inhomogeneous enhancement, which is best seen on post-contrast T1-weighted images obtained by using fat saturation techniques (Fig. C). Angiolipomas are least conspicuous on T2-weighted images, where signal intensity may be similar to that of the subcutaneous adipose tissue. On T2-weighted images with fat suppression (Fig. D), some parts of the lesion are hyperintense, and these enhance with gadolinium. These parts most likely represent vascularized soft tissue, favoring a diagnosis of epidural angiolipoma. A high vascular content correlates with the presence of large hypointense regions on T1-weighted images. A predominance of hypodense regions may indicate a very vascular tumor, even though these tumors do not typically contain the vascular "flow voids" that are a feature of high-flow lesions such as arteriovenous malformations.

Management
The treatment of angiolipoma is surgical removal. Most extradural noninfiltrative tumors are amenable to complete excision. The use of adjuvant chemotherapy and radiotherapy after incomplete tumor removal is controversial. Tumor recurrence is rare, and no malignant transformation has been reported.

Notes

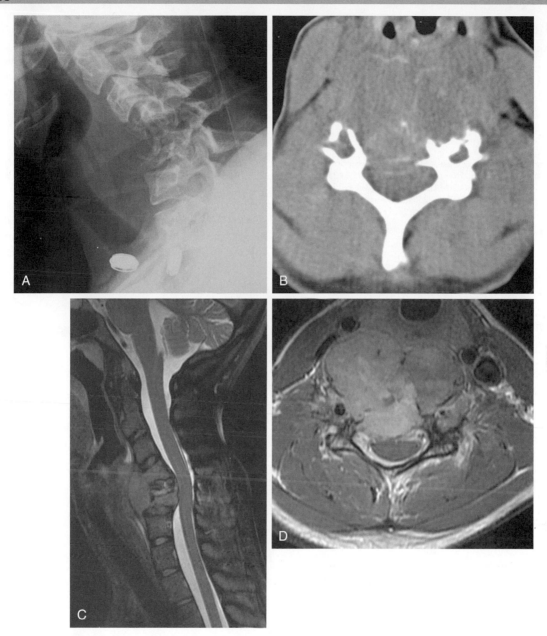

History: A 20-year-old woman presents with a history of neck pain and decreased range of motion for the past year and shooting pain in the arms for the past few months.

1. What should be included in the differential diagnosis? (Choose all that apply.)
   a. Chordoma
   b. Metastasis
   c. Aneurysmal bone cyst
   d. Osteoblastoma
   e. Diskitis osteomyelitis

2. What is the most common location of giant cell tumor involving the spine?
   a. Cervical spine
   b. Thoracic spine
   c. Lumbar spine
   d. Sacral spine

3. All of the following imaging features are helpful in differentiating giant cell tumor from other etiologies *except:*
   a. Location within the vertebral body
   b. Sparing of the intervertebral disk space
   c. Extension into the prevertebral soft tissues
   d. Hypointense signal on T2-weighted images relative to the cord

4. What is the estimated frequency of malignant giant cell tumors or malignant transformation of benign giant cell tumors?
   a. Less than 1%
   b. 10%
   c. 25%
   d. 50%

Giant Cell Tumor of the Cervical Spine

1. a, b, c, d, and e

2. d

3. c

4. b

References

Junming M, Cheng Y, Dong C, et al: Giant cell tumor of the cervical spine: A series of 22 cases and outcomes, *Spine (Phila Pa 1976)* 33(3):280-288, 2008.

Kwon JW, Chung HW, Cho EY, et al: MRI findings of giant cell tumors of the spine, *AJR Am J Roentgenol* 189(1):246-250, 2007.

Cross-Reference

Neuroradiology: The REQUISITES, 3rd ed, pp 568-569.

Comment

Background

Giant cell tumors in the vertebrae are quite rare. Most of these lesions occur in the sacrum, followed by the thoracic, cervical, and lumbar spine. Spinal lesions are more frequently found in women and affect patients in the second to fourth decades of life. The clinical symptoms are primarily neck and shoulder pain, numbness in the extremities, and weakness.

Histopathology

Pathologically, giant cell tumors consist of abundant osteoclastic giant cells intermixed throughout the spindle cell stroma. Prominent areas of fibrous tissue with a high collagen level are a frequent finding. Aneurysmal bone cyst formation may be encountered as a secondary feature in various osseous lesions, including giant cell tumors.

Imaging

Giant cell tumor commonly manifests as an osteolytic expansile lesion on radiographs. Pathologic fracture and dislocation may be observed (Fig. A). On CT scans, a thin sclerotic border surrounding the soft tissue component may be seen; however, a mineralized matrix is usually not observed (Fig. B). When a giant cell tumor occurs in the spine above the sacrum, it usually affects the vertebral body as opposed to the posterior elements, which are involved by many other neoplasms (e.g., aneurysmal bone cyst, osteoid osteoma, osteoblastoma). Extension into the posterior elements and paraspinal soft tissues and associated vertebral collapse are often apparent. The intervertebral disk space is typically not involved. Generally, the tumor is heterogeneous in signal and has low to intermediate signal intensity on T1-weighted MRI. Giant cell tumors usually have low to similar signal intensity relative to the normal spinal cord on T2-weighted images (Fig. C). This signal intensity appears to be caused by the relatively fibrous components and hemosiderin within the tumor. Although this feature is not unique to giant cell tumors of the spine, it is quite helpful in making a diagnosis because most other spinal neoplasms (e.g., metastasis, myeloma, lymphoma, chordoma) show high signal intensity on long–recovery time (TR) MRI. Evidence of hemorrhage may also be apparent, with high signal intensity on T1-weighted and T2-weighted images or fluid-fluid levels on MRI. Curvilinear low signal and cystic changes may be seen within the mass. Giant cell tumors typically enhance after contrast medium injection (Fig. D).

Management

Because giant cell tumors are locally aggressive, radical excision is the best treatment option; however, complete resection is often not feasible for tumors in the cervical spine. Giant cell tumors that cannot be excised entirely are often treated with a combination of partial curettage and radiation therapy. The estimated frequency of malignant giant cell tumors or malignant transformation of benign giant cell tumors is 10%. In most cases, malignant transformation develops after irradiation.

Notes

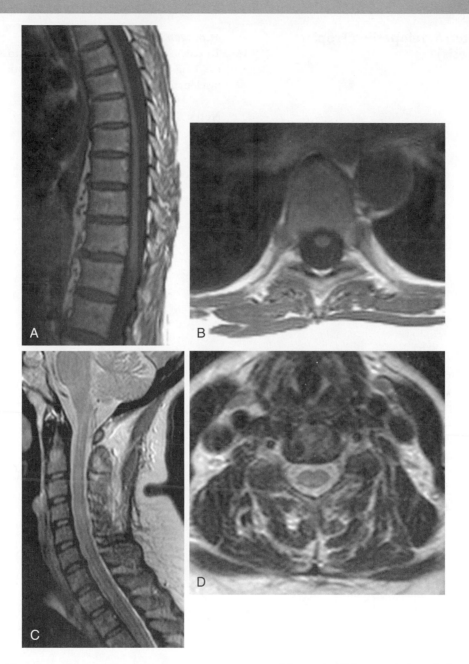

History: A 39-year-old woman from the Bahamas presents with spastic paraparesis and progressive pain in the lower extremities for the past 10 years.

1. What should be included in the differential diagnosis? (Choose all that apply).
   a. Multiple sclerosis
   b. Ependymoma
   c. Subacute combined degeneration
   d. HIV vacuolar myelopathy
   e. Human T-cell lymphotropic virus type I (HTLV-I)–associated myelopathy

2. Which of the following statements regarding HTLV-I infection is *false?*
   a. HTLV-I mainly infects CD4$^+$ T cells.
   b. An elevated HTLV-I proviral load is the best marker of symptomatic neurologic disease.

c. Maternal-child transmission via breast milk is the major mode of transmission.
d. Most infected individuals develop the disease.

3. Which of the following imaging findings in the cord is most common in patients with clinical disease?
   a. Atrophy of the cervical cord
   b. Atrophy of the thoracic cord
   c. Increased signal in the cervical cord
   d. Increased signal in the thoracic cord

4. All of the following viruses are known to infect the spinal cord *except:*
   a. Parainfluenza
   b. Herpesvirus
   c. HIV
   d. Poliovirus

HTLV-I–Associated Myelopathy (Tropical Spastic Paraparesis)

1. a, c, d, and e

2. d

3. b

4. a

References

Howard AK, Li DK, Oger J: MRI contributes to the differentiation between MS and HTLV-I associated myelopathy in British Columbian coastal natives, *Can J Neurol Sci* 30(1):41-48, 2003.

Oh U, Jacobson S: Treatment of HTLV-I-associated myelopathy/tropical spastic paraparesis: Toward rational targeted therapy, *Neurol Clin* 26(3):781-797, 2008.

Cross-Reference

Neuroradiology: The REQUISITES, 3rd ed, pp 548-550.

Comment

Background

HTLV-I is a retrovirus that preferentially infects $CD4^+$ T cells and, to a lesser extent, $CD8^+$ T cells. The virus causes an inflammatory disorder of the central nervous system termed HTLV-I–associated myelopathy or tropical spastic paraparesis. It is a chronic myelopathy characterized by a triad of motor, sensory, and bladder dysfunction; it has a progressive, unremitting course that resembles primary progressive multiple sclerosis. In endemic areas, maternal-child transmission via breast milk is the major mode of transmission of HTLV-I, followed by sexual contact. Transmission also occurs through unscreened blood transfusions and the use of contaminated intravenous needles. Most infected individuals remain lifelong asymptomatic carriers; 3.8% develop the disease. Another 2% to 3% of infected individuals develop an aggressive mature T-cell malignancy termed adult T-cell leukemia. HTLV-I immunoreactivity in the serum confirms the diagnosis.

Histopathology

Inflammatory changes are prominent histopathologic features of the disease, with demyelination, neuroaxonal degeneration, and reactive gliosis. Examination of the spinal cord reveals degeneration of the lateral columns, with variable damage to the anterior and posterior columns; the thoracic cord is typically most severely affected.

Imaging

MRI findings in the cord in patients with clinical disease are, in order of decreasing frequency, atrophy of the thoracic cord (Figs. A and B), increased signal in the cervical cord (Figs. C and D), increased signal in the thoracic cord, and atrophy of the cervical cord. Spinal cord atrophy is detected in one third of patients.

Management

To date, no therapy has been shown to significantly modify the long-term disability associated with HTLV-I–associated myelopathy.

Notes

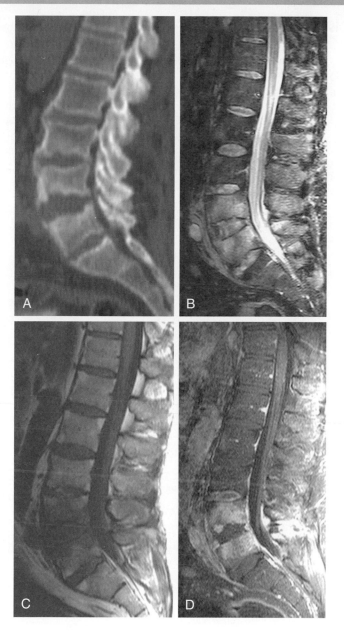

History: A 47-year-old man presents with a history of increasing back pain for the past 3 years.

1. What should be included in the differential diagnosis? (Choose all that apply.)
   a. Pyogenic diskitis osteomyelitis
   b. Ankylosing spondylitis
   c. Modic type I degenerative changes
   d. Tuberculous spondylodiskitis
   e. Metastatic disease

2. Imaging features of Andersson lesion include all of the following *except:*
   a. Disk space narrowing
   b. Destruction of vertebral end-plate
   c. Sclerosis of adjacent bone
   d. Large prevertebral fluid collection

3. Which of the following statements regarding Romanus lesions is *false?*
   a. Romanus lesions are focal destructive areas along the margin of the diskovertebral junction.
   b. Romanus lesions have been described as "shiny corners" on radiographs.
   c. MRI is less sensitive than radiographs in detecting early Romanus lesions.
   d. MRI has an important role in assessing the treatment response.

4. All of the following findings support the MRI "corner" sign secondary to ankylosing spondylitis over degenerative corner changes *except:*
   a. Small right-angled, triangular lesion
   b. No adjacent end-plate erosions
   c. Hyperintense signal on both T1-weighted and fast-spin-echo T2-weighted images
   d. Location in the thoracolumbar junction

Ankylosing Spondylitis Diskovertebral (Andersson) Lesions

1. a, b, and d

2. d

3. c

4. c

References

Bron JL, de Vries MK, Snieders MN, et al: Discovertebral (Andersson) lesions of the spine in ankylosing spondylitis revisited, *Clin Rheumatol* 28(8):883-892, 2009.

Kim NR, Choi JY, Hong SH, et al: "MR corner sign": Value for predicting presence of ankylosing spondylitis, *AJR Am J Roentgenol* 191(1):124-128, 2008.

Cross-Reference

Neuroradiology: The REQUISITES, 3rd ed, p 534.

Comment

Background

A known complication of ankylosing spondylitis is the development of diskovertebral lesions of the spine, known as Andersson lesions (also referred to as spondylodiskitis, aseptic diskitis, and pseudarthrosis). The exact etiology of these lesions is unknown; however, they are characterized by inflammation and stress fractures, resulting in the development of pseudarthrosis.

Histopathology

On pathology, nonspecific reactive changes are found in the intervertebral disk, which is replaced by hypovascular fibrous tissue, and end-plate destruction extends into the subchondral bone. Mild inflammatory changes may also be present.

Imaging

CT scan of an Andersson lesion shows irregular diskovertebral osteolysis with surrounding reactive sclerosis (Fig. A), which may mimic infection. Fractures of the posterior elements or nonfusion of the facet joints may also be seen. MRI shows increased short tau inversion recovery (STIR) signal (Fig. B) and decreased T1-weighted signal (Fig. C) of the disk space and surrounding vertebral bodies, with corresponding enhancement (Fig. D). Contrast-enhanced fat-suppression imaging allows better differentiation between fat and enhanced lesions (see Fig. D). Spinal canal stenosis may be seen, resulting from hypertrophic ligamentum flavum and facet joints and from hypertrophic callus formation in the anterior and posterior elements of the Andersson lesion. Another significant feature of ankylosing spondylitis is the MRI "corner" sign (see Fig. C), which represents enthesitis at the site where the annulus fibrosus attaches to the vertebral end-plate. These marginal erosions of the anterior vertebral corners, first described by Romanus, are related to inflammation of the anterior annulus fibrosus in patients with Andersson lesion. In the healing phase, the erosions are enclosed by a rim of sclerosis, which later results in the formation of syndesmophytes and eventually in a complete ankylosed spinal segment.

Management

Initial treatment is conservative, with nonsteroidal anti-inflammatory drugs, intensive physical therapy, or tumor necrosis factor–α inhibitors. Surgical instrumentation and fusion are considered the principal method of management in patients with symptomatic Andersson lesions that fail to resolve after conservative treatment.

Notes

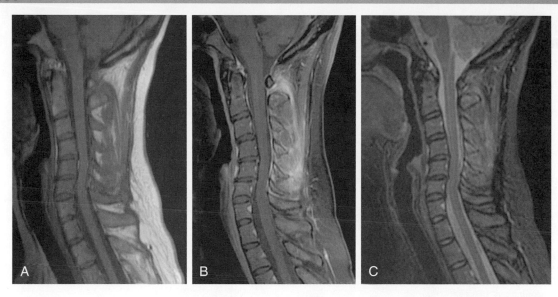

History: A 60-year-old woman reports a several-week history of severe neck and shoulder pain and morning stiffness. X-rays of the axial and peripheral skeleton are negative.

1. What should be included in the differential diagnosis? (Choose all that apply.)
   a. Psoriasis
   b. Rheumatoid arthritis
   c. Polymyalgia rheumatica (PMR)
   d. Fibromyalgia
   e. Polymyositis

2. Which imaging modality is *least* useful in the diagnosis of PMR?
   a. Plain films
   b. MRI
   c. Ultrasound
   d. Positron emission tomography (18F-FDG PET) and 18F-FDG PET/CT

3. Which of the following statements regarding patients with PMR and cervical interspinous bursitis is *false*?
   a. Areas of increased T2 signal and enhancement on MRI are usually found from C1 to C4.
   b. MRI findings of PMR in the lumbar spine are often located in the interspinous bursae of L3, L4, and L5.
   c. MRI findings of cervical and lumbar PMR interspinous bursitis are due to edema in areas of inflammation.
   d. Moderate to severe cervical or lumbar interspinous bursitis in the absence of other articular changes might support the diagnosis of PMR.

4. Which of the following statements in reference to the imaging diagnosis of PMR is *least* accurate?
   a. Imaging allows appreciation of the multifaceted nature of PMR.
   b. Imaging patterns of PMR inflammation are helpful in the diagnosis and differential diagnosis of the disease.
   c. It is unnecessary to differentiate PMR from giant cell arteritis on clinical examination and imaging.
   d. In patients with elderly-onset rheumatoid arthritis and polymyalgia-like symptoms, MRI may be helpful in differentiating these entities from PMR.

Cervical Interspinous Bursitis in Polymyalgia Rheumatica

Notes

1. c and e

2. a

3. a

4. c

References

Paroli M, Garlaschi G, Silvestri E, et al: Magnetic resonance imaging in the differential diagnosis between polymyalgia rheumatica and elderly onset rheumatoid arthritis, *Clin Rheumatol* 25(3):402-403, 2006.

Salvarani C, Barozzi L, Cantini F, et al: Cervical interspinous bursitis in active polymyalgia rheumatic, *Ann Rheum Dis* 67(6):758-761, 2008.

Salvarani C, Cantini F, Hunder GG: Polymyalgia rheumatica and giant-cell arteritis, *Lancet* 372(9634):234-245, 2008.

Cross-Reference

Neuroradiology: The REQUISITES, 3rd ed, p 136.

Comment

Background

PMR is a common condition of unknown etiology that affects elderly individuals. Whites are affected more than other ethnic groups, and PMR is twice as common in women versus men. The median age at diagnosis is 72 years. PMR is characterized clinically by proximal myalgia of the shoulders and hip girdles, with accompanying morning stiffness that lasts more than 1 hour. PMR is known to cause synovitis, bursitis, and tenosynovitis around joints such as the shoulders, hips, and knees, as well as inflammation of the interspinous bursae in the cervical and lumbar spine. Approximately 20% of patients with PMR develop giant cell arteritis, and 40% of patients with giant cell arteritis have associated PMR.

Imaging

Imaging studies and the patient's clinical presentation are helpful in distinguishing PMR from other rheumatologic conditions. Radiographs reveal either normal joints or evidence of osteoarthritis. Ultrasound may show changes characteristic of bursitis in the shoulders and hips, shoulder synovitis, and biceps tenosynovitis. MRI is excellent at revealing areas of active inflammation secondary to bursitis, tenosynovitis, and tendinitis in the shoulders (most patients have subacromial and subdeltoid bursitis and glenohumeral joint synovitis), cervical spine interspinous bursae, and trochanters (trochanteric bursitis) (Figs. A-C).

Management

Corticosteroids are considered the treatment of choice. A rapid response to low-dose corticosteroids is considered pathognomonic of PMR. The prognosis is excellent, although exacerbations may occur if corticosteroids are tapered too soon or too rapidly.

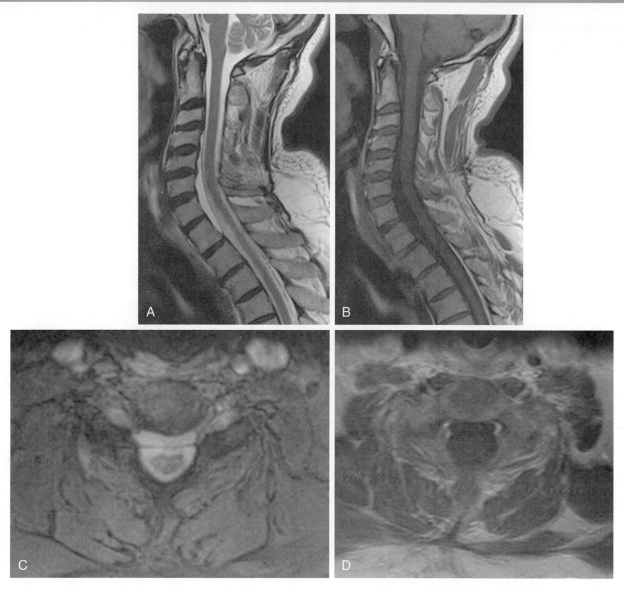

History: A 59-year-old man with a 2-year history of progressive gait dysfunction and spacticity.

1. What should be included in the differential diagnosis? (Choose all that apply.)
   a. Congenital arachnoid cyst
   b. Epidural abscess
   c. Ventral spinal meningocele
   d. Acquired arachnoid cyst
   e. Cystic schwannoma

2. Where are ventral spinal memingoceles typically located?
   a. Intramedullary
   b. Intradural extramedullary
   c. Interdural
   d. Extradural

3. Which of the following statements regarding ventral epidural meningoceles is FALSE?
   a. They communicate with the subarachnoid space.
   b. There is good correlation between the site of the dural defect and the presenting symptoms.
   c. They may be associated with concomitant spinal cord herniation.
   d. They typically extend through multiple vertebral body segments.

4. Which of the following is the imaging modality of choice for identifying the dural defect?
   a. Plain radiographs
   b. MRI
   c. CT with IV contrast
   d. CT myelography

Ventral Spinal Meningocele

1. a and c

2. c

3. b

4. d

References

Ball BG, Luetmer PH, Giannini C, et al: Ventral "spinal epidural meningeal cysts"—not epidural and not cysts? Case series and review of the literature, *Neurosurgery* 70:320-328, 2012.

Fiss I, Danne M, Hartmann C, et al: Rapidly progressive paraplegia due to an extradural lumbar meningocele mimicking a cyst. Case report, *J Neurosurg Spine* 7:75-79, 2007.

Cross-Reference

Neuroradiology: The REQUISITES, 3rd ed, p 551.

Comment

Background

Ventral spinal intradural dissecting meningoceles are rare clinical disorders. The patient typically presents with a prolonged course of symptoms including pain, myelopathy, muscle weakness, and headache.

Histopathology

The cyst wall shows collagenous tissue consistent with dura without arachnoid features. It is therefore thought that a ventral meningocele represents dissection of cerebrospinal fluid within the layers of the dura.

Imaging

The fluid collection is readily identified on routine MR imaging (Figs. A to D). Routine CT myelography shows the contrast accumulation within the meningocele. However, the exact site of communication is frequently not identified. Dynamic CT myelography, performed with the patient prone and the contrast ascent monitored, will allow the accurate localization of the dural defect.

Management

Treatment is to surgically close the dural defect intervention.

Notes

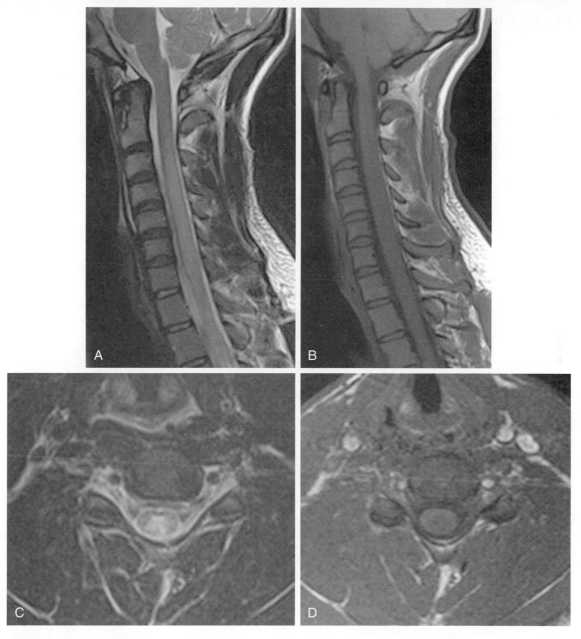

A   B   C   D

History: A 23-year-old man who panicked while scuba diving and made a quick ascent from a depth of 50 meters.

1. Which of the following should be included in the differential diagnosis for the imaging findings presented? (Choose all that apply.)
   a. Cord infarction
   b. Caisson disease (decompression sickness)
   c. Astrocytoma
   d. Multiple sclerosis
   e. Carbon monoxide poisoning

2. Which of the following clinical symptoms is classified as type I decompression sickness?
   a. Joint pain
   b. Sensory loss in the extremities
   c. Motor loss in the extremities
   d. Nystagmus

3. Which of the following MRI patterns will be unlikely in Caisson disease?
   a. Focal involvement of the grey and white matter
   b. Long segment involvement of the grey and white matter
   c. Isolated white matter involvement
   d. Isolated grey matter involvement

4. Which of the following statements regarding decompression sickness is true?
   a. Negative MRI findings exclude decompression sickness.
   b. Improvement in MRI findings correlates with clinical improvement.
   c. The diagnosis of motion sickness is clinical and the patient's transfer to a hyperbaric oxygen treatment center should not be delayed.
   d. MRI has high sensitivity in detecting spinal lesions.

281

Caisson Disease (Decompression Sickness)

1. a and b

2. a

3. d

4. c

References
Hennedige T, Chow W, Ng YY, et al: MRI in spinal cord decompression sickness, *J Med Imaging Radiat Oncol* 56:282-288, 2012.

Kei PL, Choong CT, Young T, et al: Decompression sickness: MRI of the spinal cord, *J Neuroimaging* 17:378-380, 2007.

Yoshiyama M, Asamoto S, Kobayashi N, et al: Spinal cord decompression sickness associated with scuba diving: correlation of immediate and delayed magnetic resonance imaging findings with severity of neurologic impairment—a report on 3 cases, *Surg Neurol* 67:283-287, 2007.

Cross-Reference
Neuroradiology: The REQUISITES, 3rd ed, p 571.

Comment
Background
Decompression sickness, also known as Caisson disease, is a clinical syndrome caused by rapid reduction in pressure during ascent from depth, and it can lead to spinal cord infarction. Decompression sickness is classified into two types based on clinical symptoms. Type I includes joint pain, skin rash, and localized edema. Type II has more serious complications and is further divided into four subtypes according to the organ or system affected: central nervous system, spinal cord, inner ear, and lungs. Spinal cord involvement may occur in up to 50% of patients with type II decompression sickness.

Pathophysiology
Ascending too quickly causes the dissolved nitrogen from compressed air—which accumulates in blood and tissues—to return to its gaseous form, resulting in the formation of bubbles. The pathophysiology of cord injury is not completely understood. Three possible mechanisms have been proposed: (1) venous infarction due to bubble formation in epidural veins, causing clotting and leading to obstruction; (2) autochthonous bubble formation, in which gas bubbles form space-occupying lesions within the myelin of the spinal cord, especially in the lateral and posterior columns affected secondary to high fat content; and (3) arterial gas embolization, which is considered to be a less frequent cause.

Imaging
Typical findings include patchy, increased T2-weighted signal changes that affect multiple levels (Figs. A and B) and mixed venous and arterial pattern with signal changes that involve the dorsal column white matter as well as the grey matter (Figs. C and D).

Management
Initial treatment is with 100% oxygen until hyperbaric oxygen therapy can be instituted.

Notes

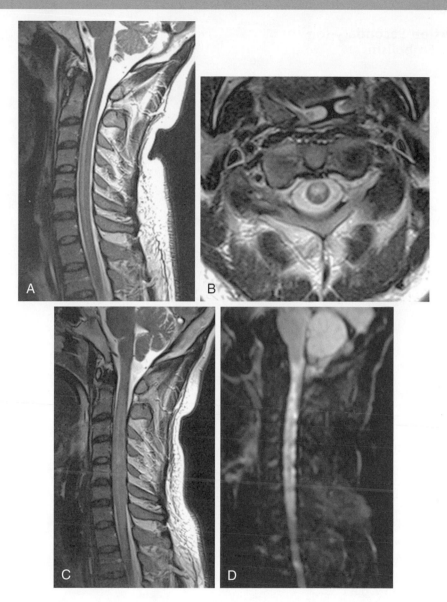

History: A 39-year-old man presents with an acute onset of neck pain, extremity weakness, and difficulty breathing requiring intubation. While in the hospital, he develops pneumonia and has a cardiac arrest, resulting in brain death. An autopsy is performed.

1. What should be included in the differential diagnosis? (Choose all that apply.)
   a. Acute longitudinal transverse myelitis
   b. Astrocytoma
   c. Cord contusion
   d. Acute disseminated encephalomyelitis
   e. Cord infarction

2. Which part of the spinal cord is most commonly involved in cases of fibrocartilaginous embolism?
   a. Cervical cord
   b. Thoracic cord
   c. Conus area
   d. Entire spinal cord

3. Which of the following statements regarding fibrocartilaginous embolism is true?
   a. A preceding severe injury to the vertebral column is usually reported.
   b. The interval between the traumatic insult and the onset of symptoms is usually days or weeks.
   c. Cerebrospinal fluid studies show increased protein in most cases.
   d. The mortality rate is higher in patients with cervical cord involvement.

4. Which of the following imaging findings favors fibrocartilaginous embolism over other causes of transverse myelitis?
   a. Diffuse hyperintense cord signal on sagittal T2-weighted images, with flow void structures on the dorsal cord surface
   b. Linear hyperintensity on sagittal T2-weighted images involving the anterior aspect of the cord
   c. Linear hyperintensity on sagittal T2-weighted images involving the dorsal columns
   d. Unilateral focal signal abnormality on axial T2-weighted images involving the lateral column

Spinal Cord Infarction Secondary to Fibrocartilaginous Embolism

1. a, d, and e

2. a

3. d

4. b

References

Han JJ, Massagli TL, Jaffe KM: Fibrocartilaginous embolism—an uncommon cause of spinal cord infarction: A case report and review of the literature, *Arch Phys Med Rehabil* 85(1):153-157, 2004.

Raghavan A, Onikul E, Ryan MM, et al: Anterior spinal cord infarction owing to possible fibrocartilaginous embolism, *Pediatr Radiol* 34(6):503-506, 2004.

Thöne J, Hohaus A, Bickel A, et al: Severe spinal cord ischemia subsequent to fibrocartilaginous embolism, *J Neurol Sci* 263(1-2):211-213, 2007.

Cross-Reference

Neuroradiology: The REQUISITES, 3rd ed, p 571.

Comment

Background

Fibrocartilaginous embolism is characterized by rapidly progressive paraplegia following an episode of back pain (usually after a minor trauma).

Pathophysiology

Several mechanisms have been proposed; the most widely accepted hypothesis is that a sudden elevation of venous and intervertebral disk pressure induces a prolapse of cartilaginous material into spinal vessels. In most cases, the anterior spinal artery is involved, with about five to six spinal segments affected by embolism. Cervical spinal cord ischemia and resulting neurologic deficits often affect the respiratory muscles. The clinical course may be dominated by respiratory insufficiency and infections of the respiratory system, which can ultimately cause lethal complications, as seen in this case.

Imaging

The earliest demonstrated signal changes can be seen a few hours after the onset of cord ischemia; typically, this appears as a linear hyperintensity involving the anterior aspect of the cord on T2-weighted sagittal images (Fig. A). Serial MRI examinations over the following days show progressive cord swelling, with increased T2 signal changes involving the anterior two thirds of the cord (Figs. B and C), diffusion restriction (Fig. D), and lack of contrast enhancement in the acute phase. Disk collapse or Schmorl's nodes at the level of injury are often present.

Management

No treatment recommendations exist. Long-term treatment includes supportive care and rehabilitative physical therapy.

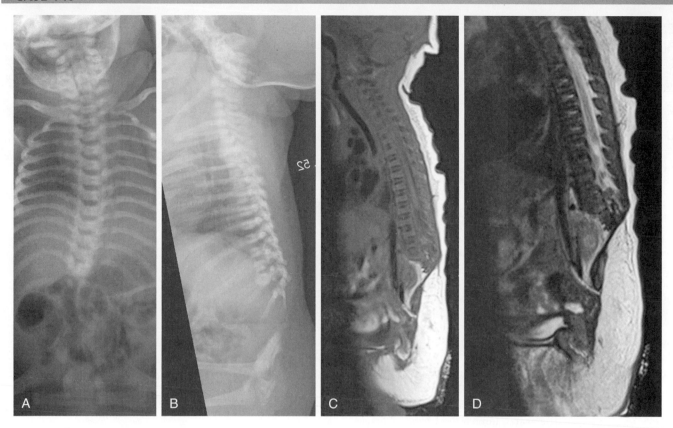

History: A 4-day-old infant has malformed lower extremities.

1. What should be included in the differential diagnosis? (Choose all that apply.)
   a. Neuroblastoma
   b. Tethered cord
   c. Myelomeningocele
   d. Sacrococcygeal teratoma
   e. Caudal regression syndrome

2. Which of the following disorders has been linked to this syndrome?
   a. Cretinism
   b. Vitamin K deficiency
   c. Rh incompatibility
   d. Maternal diabetes mellitus

3. Which of the following conditions is associated with this syndrome?
   a. Hemihypertrophy
   b. Lipomeningocele
   c. Capillary hemangioma
   d. Cystic hygroma

4. Which of the following statements regarding the two types of caudal agenesis is true?
   a. Caudal agenesis has been divided into two types, depending on the location of the conus medullaris.
   b. Vertebral dysgenesis is less severe in type II caudal agenesis than in type I.
   c. Patients with type I caudal agenesis typically present with tethered cord syndrome.
   d. Patients with type II caudal agenesis have an abrupt spinal cord terminus that is club shaped or wedge shaped.

Caudal Regression Syndrome (Caudal Agenesis)

1. e

2. d

3. b

4. a

References

Barkovich AJ, Raghavan N, Chuang S, et al: The wedge-shaped cord terminus: A radiographic sign of caudal regression, *AJNR Am J Neuroradiol* 10(6):1223-1231, 1989.

Nievelstein RAJ, Valk J, Smit LME, et al: MR of the caudal regression syndrome: Embryologic implications, *AJNR Am J Neuroradiol* 15(6):1021-1029, 1994.

Pang D: Sacral agenesis and caudal spinal cord malformations, *Neurosurgery* 32(5):755-778, 1993.

Cross-Reference

Neuroradiology: The REQUISITES, 3rd ed, p 318.

Comment

Background

Caudal agenesis or caudal regression syndrome involves total or partial agenesis of the spinal column. The congenital spectrum of vertebral abnormalities ranges from agenesis of the coccyx to absence of the sacral, lumbar, and lower thoracic vertebrae. About 16% of infants with caudal regression syndrome have diabetic mothers, and about 1% of diabetic mothers have offspring with the syndrome.

Embryology

It has been hypothesized that sacral agenesis or dysgenesis may occur as a result of hyperglycemia in a genetically predisposed fetus early in gestation. The insult may prevent canalization and retrogressive differentiation of the caudal cell mass, or it may promote excessive retrogression that results in the sacral deformity or anorectal and urogenital malformations.

Imaging

Sacral agenesis or dysgenesis has been divided into two types on the basis of conus position: type I has a high conus terminating cephalad to the L1 inferior end-plate, and type II has a low conus terminating caudal to L1. Patients with type I tend to have a large sacral defect (Figs. A-D), with the sacrum ending above S1. In about 90% of patients with type I, the conus has a blunted, wedge-shaped contour (shorter ventrally because of a deficiency of anterior horn cells) (see Figs. C and D). The spinal cord terminus is high (at the T12 level in most cases). The thecal sac tapers below the cord terminus and ends at an unusually high level (see Figs. C and D). Clinically, patients have a stable neurologic deficit. In patients with type II, the conus is often elongated as a result of tethering to a thickened filum, lipoma, or myelocystocele. Sacral dysgenesis is relatively mild; however, the clinical course is more likely to involve neurologic deterioration because of cord tethering.

Terminal myelocystoceles and lipomyelomeningoceles are associated with sacral agenesis or dysgenesis in approximately 9% and 6% of cases, respectively. Other anomalies associated with caudal regression include diastematomyelia and anterior sacral meningocele.

Management

Patients may require surgical intervention for decompression and vertebral anomalies. Some authors suggest cutting the filum in cases of cord tethering.

Notes

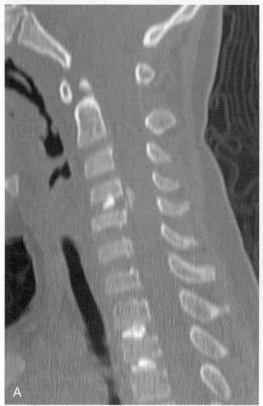

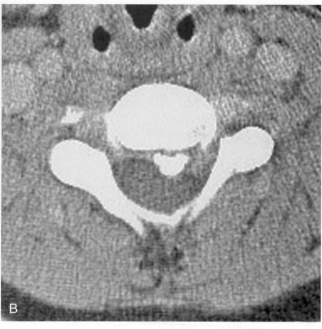

History: A 9-year-old boy presents with acute torticollis.

1. What should be included in the differential diagnosis? (Choose all that apply.)
   a. Calcified meningioma
   b. Ankylosing spondylitis
   c. Remote infection
   d. Calcified epidural hematoma
   e. Calcified intervertebral disk

2. Where are most calcified intervertebral disk herniations in children located?
   a. Cervical spine
   b. Thoracic spine
   c. Lumbar spine
   d. Equally prevalent throughout the spine

3. What is the mean age at presentation of pediatric intervertebral disk calcification?
   a. 2 years
   b. 5 years
   c. 8 years
   d. 11 years

4. What is the best management of this condition?
   a. Surgical decompression without fusion
   b. Calcitonin
   c. Steroid injections
   d. Conservative management

Cervical Disk Calcification in a Child

1. c and e

2. a

3. c

4. d

References

Dai LY, Ye H, Qian QR: The natural history of cervical disc calcification in children, *J Bone Joint Surg Am* 86-A(7):1467-1472, 2004.

Sato K, Nagata K, Park JS: Calcified intervertebral disc herniation in a child with myelopathy treated with laminoplasty, *Spinal Cord* 43(11):680-683, 2005.

Cross-Reference

Neuroradiology: The REQUISITES, 3rd ed, pp 524, 525b.

Comment

Background

Pediatric intervertebral disk calcification is more common in boys than in girls. Symptoms are usually limited to spinal irritation and include pain, stiffness, torticollis, and limitation of neck movement. There may be mild fever, leukocytosis, and elevation of the erythrocyte sedimentation rate. In rare cases, rupture of the annulus may occur, with radicular pain or deficit. The incidence of disk herniation is greater in symptomatic patients.

Pathophysiology

The etiology of disk calcification in children is unclear; however, it is likely different from the degenerative calcification seen in adults. Trauma has been implicated as a predisposing factor; however, most patients have no history of injury. Disk calcification in newborns has been reported.

Imaging

The calcified disk is usually seen on plain radiographs as a dense round or oval mass within the region of the nucleus pulposus. Calcification may be difficult to detect at the cervicothoracic junction, however, because of overlying density from the shoulders. CT or MRI may be necessary to improve visualization; these modalities can also demonstrate any associated disk herniation (Figs. A and B).

Management

Intervertebral disk calcification in children is usually a self-limited process. Symptoms persist for days to weeks. Conservative treatment is recommended, and the prognosis is excellent even when disk herniation occurs. In most cases, calcification disappears spontaneously within a few weeks to months.

Notes

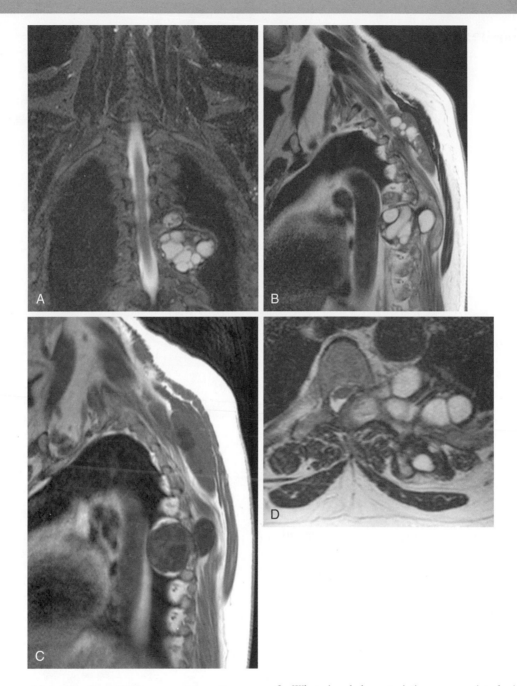

History: A 40-year-old woman from Turkey complains of increasing back pain for the past 2 years.

1. What should be included in the differential diagnosis? (Choose all that apply.)
   a. Chordoma
   b. Aneurysmal bone cyst
   c. Giant cell tumor
   d. Hydatid cyst
   e. Tuberculous abscess

2. What part of the spine is most commonly involved?
   a. Cervical
   b. Thoracic
   c. Lumbar
   d. Sacrum

3. What signal characteristics are associated with cyst viability?
   a. Hyperintense T1 signal centrally within the cyst
   b. Hypointense T1 signal of the cyst wall
   c. Hypointense T2 signal of the cyst wall
   d. Hypointense T2 signal centrally within the cyst

4. Which of the following statements regarding the histopathology of spinal hydatid disease is true?
   a. Viable cysts typically show dystrophic calcifications on radiographs.
   b. The intervertebral disks are typically involved in the early stages of the disease.
   c. The cyst is restricted to the bone and periosteum.
   d. Spinal involvement is believed to occur through vertebral–portal venous anastomosis.

Spinal Extradural Hydatid Cyst

1. d and e

2. b

3. c

4. d

References

Fahl M, Haddad FS, Huballah M, et al: Magnetic resonance imaging in intradural and extradural spinal echinococcosis, *Clin Imaging* 18(3):179-183, 1994.

Pamir MN, Ozduman K, Elmaci I: Spinal hydatid disease, *Spinal Cord* 40(4):153-160, 2002.

Prabhakar MM, Acharya AJ, Modi DR, et al: Spinal hydatid disease: A case series, *J Spinal Cord Med* 28(5):426-431, 2005.

Cross-Reference

Neuroradiology: The REQUISITES, 3rd ed, p 221.

Comment

Background

Hydatid disease in humans is caused by the cystic (larval) stage of the tapeworm *Echinococcus granulosus* in endemic countries. The infection is transmitted orally via eggs shed in the feces of infected animals. Spinal involvement in hydatid disease is rare, with an incidence of less than 1%. Neurologic complications are the result of intradural or extradural growth of the cysts, causing direct compression.

Histopathology

Spinal involvement is believed to occur through vertebral–portal venous anastomosis. Infestation of the spine progresses as a multivesicular infiltration of cancellous bone that involves the vertebral bodies, pedicles, and laminae to varying extents. The intervertebral disks are usually spared because cyst growth is confined by the periosteum.

Imaging

MRI is the best imaging modality for determining the vertebral locations of the cystic lesions, spinal levels involved, overall extent of disease along the neural axis, and completeness of resection postoperatively (Figs. A-D). Cysts are occasionally spherical, but they typically have two dome-shaped ends and look like flattened sausages (see Fig. B), with thin, regular walls and no septations (see Figs. A-D). The lumina of the cysts are usually free of debris. Intradural cysts may be single or multiple; extradural cysts are almost always multiple and involve the bone (see Fig. D). Extradural spread of hydatid cysts through a widened neural foramen into the muscle planes may be seen. The formation of daughter cysts may result in a "bunch of grapes" appearance (see Fig. D). Although most extradural hydatid cysts are multiple, the finding of a unilocular extradural cyst on MRI should suggest the possibility of hydatid disease, even if hydatid cysts are absent in the lung or liver and skin or serologic tests are negative.

Management

Surgery is considered the treatment of choice for spinal hydatid disease. The goal of surgery is intact removal of the cyst. The efficacy of albendazole for primary bone hydatid involvement is questionable, and postoperative treatment with this agent seems only to delay recurrence.

Notes

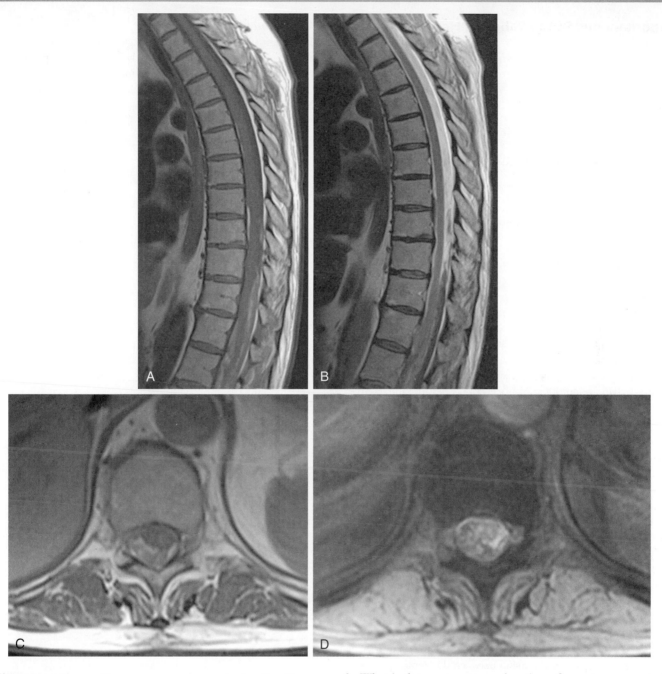

History: A 63-year-old woman reports an episode of sudden severe back pain while standing in her kitchen.

1. What should be included in the differential diagnosis? (Choose all that apply.)
   a. Lymphoma
   b. Meningioma
   c. Subdural empyema
   d. Subdural hematoma
   e. Sarcoidosis

2. What is the location of the hemorrhage?
   a. Intramedullary
   b. Subarachnoid
   c. Subdural
   d. Epidural

3. What is the most common location of spontaneous spinal subdural hematoma along the spinal axis?
   a. Cervical spine
   b. Thoracic spine
   c. Lumbar spine
   d. Sacrum

4. What stage of hemorrhage is seen in this case?
   a. Deoxyhemoglobin
   b. Intracellular methemoglobin
   c. Extracellular methemoglobin
   d. Hemosiderin

Spontaneous Spinal Subdural Hematoma

1. d

2. c

3. b

4. b

References

Dampeer RA: Spontaneous spinal subdural hematoma: Case study, *Am J Crit Care* 19(2):191-193, 2010.

Post MJ, Becerra JL, Madsen PW, et al: Acute spinal subdural hematoma: MR and CT findings with pathologic correlates, *AJNR Am J Neuroradiol* 15(10):1895-1905, 1994.

Yang NR, Kim SJ, Cho YJ, et al: Spontaneous resolution of nontraumatic acute spinal subdural hematoma, *J Korean Neurosurg Soc* 50(3):268-270, 2011.

Cross-Reference

Neuroradiology: The REQUISITES, 3rd ed, pp 173-176.

Comment

Background

Spinal subdural hematoma is rare. Causes include trauma, coagulopathy, recent lumbar puncture, and vascular malformations. Spontaneous spinal subdural hematoma (in the absence of underlying conditions) has been observed in patients after minor trauma, such as sneezing or coughing. Presenting symptoms include sudden pain radiating to the extremities, acute motor and sensory impairment, and loss of sphincter tone. It occurs most often in the thoracic spine.

Pathophysiology

The exact cause is unknown; however, spinal subdural hematoma is thought to result from an effort (often not remembered by the patient) that causes a sudden increase in pressure in the radiculomedullary veins, resulting in vein rupture in the inner surface of the dura mater. Several authors have described the presence of combined subdural and subarachnoid hemorrhage in the same patient.

Imaging

MRI is excellent in delineating the extent of spinal hemorrhage and determining the relationship between the hemorrhage and the thecal sac and cord (Figs. A-D). Distinguishing between subdural hematoma and the more common epidural hematoma is frequently difficult. Signs that favor subdural hematoma include lack of epidural fat "capping" (see Fig. A). Signal intensity of the collection is variable on both T1-weighted and T2-weighted images, although low signal is frequently seen on fast-spin-echo T2-weighted and gradient-recalled-echo T2*-weighted images (see Figs. B and D). On T1-weighted images, acute spinal hematoma is typically isointense to the cord, and subacute hematoma is hyperintense (see Figs. A and C).

Management

Treatment typically consists of surgical decompression; however, conservative treatment is advocated if the presenting symptoms are either mild or resolving.

Notes

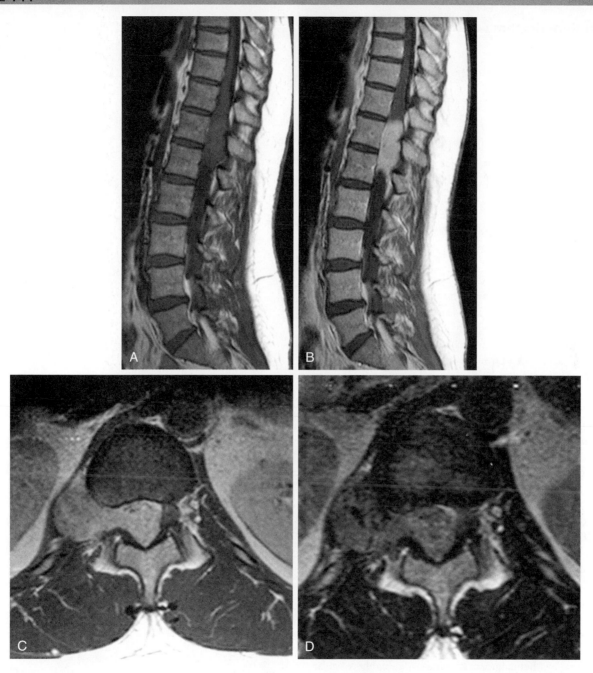

History: A 33-year-old man presents with back pain and leg numbness.

1. What should be included in the differential diagnosis? (Choose all that apply.)
   a. Meningioma
   b. Lymphoma
   c. Hemangiopericytoma
   d. Neurofibroma
   e. Metastasis

2. What is the location of the lesion?
   a. Intramedullary
   b. Intradural extramedullary
   c. Intradural
   d. Extradural

3. What is the most common location of spinal hemangioblastomas?
   a. Cervical spine
   b. Thoracic spine
   c. Lumbar spine
   d. Sacrum

4. Which MRI feature is the most helpful in diagnosing hemangioblastoma?
   a. Hypointense T1 signal relative to cord
   b. Intense enhancement
   c. Intratumoral flow voids
   d. Dumbbell shape

Hemangiopericytoma of the Lumbar Spine

1. a, b, c, and d

2. d

3. b

4. c

Reference
Santillan A, Zink W, Lavi E, et al: Endovascular embolization of cervical hemangiopericytoma with ONYX-18: Case report and review of the literature, *J Neurointerv Surg* 3(3):304-307, 2011.

Cross-Reference
Neuroradiology: The REQUISITES, 3rd ed, pp 62, 338.

Comment
Background
Hemangiopericytomas are hypervascular tumors that occur most commonly in patients between the ages of 30 and 50 years; men and women are equally affected. Hemangiopericytomas typically involve the musculoskeletal system; they are rarely found in the central nervous system, arising primarily within the epidural space. Within the spinal column, they are usually extradural in location, although intradural lesions have been described.

Histopathology
Hemangiopericytomas are thought to arise from the pericytes of Zimmerman, which are modified smooth muscle cells surrounding capillaries and postcapillary venules.

Imaging
Hemangiopericytomas are predominantly isointense to spinal cord parenchyma on T1-weighted (Fig. A) and T2-weighted (Fig. B) MRI. They may be distinguished by prominent intratumoral flow voids (see Fig. B) and intense enhancement (Figs. C and D), consistent with the known hypervascularity of these neoplasms. Preoperative identification of these tumors is important because of their aggressive nature, high rate of local recurrence, and propensity for late distant metastases. On angiography, hemangiopericytoma is a highly vascular lesion demonstrating corkscrew vessels and long-lasting, dense tumor staining.

Management
Surgical excision is the therapy of choice. Adjuvant postoperative radiotherapy has been recommended because of the high incidence of local recurrence. Preoperative embolization may prevent excessive intraoperative blood loss.

Notes

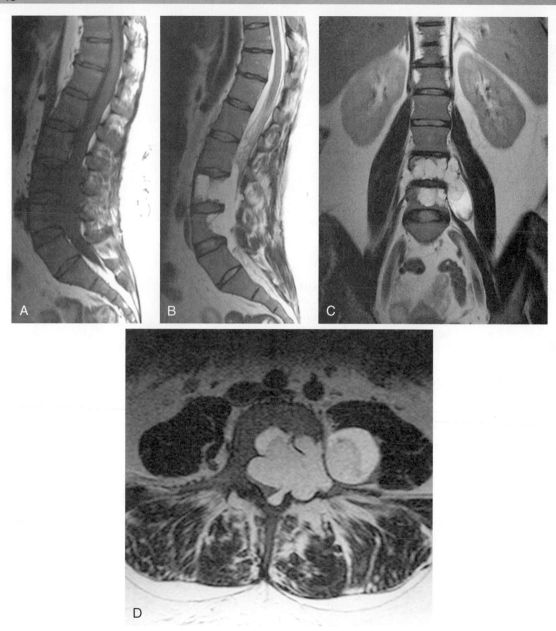

History: A 28-year-old woman presents with back pain and lower extremity pain.

1. What should be included in the differential diagnosis? (Choose all that apply.)
   a. Nerve sheath tumor
   b. Lymphoma
   c. Giant cell tumor
   d. Chordoma
   e. Diskitis osteomyelitis

2. What percentage of spinal chordomas originates in the lumbar vertebrae?
   a. 6%
   b. 15%
   c. 35%
   d. 50%

3. What finding on MRI suggests the diagnosis?
   a. Hypointense signal on T1-weighted images
   b. Hyperintense signal with multiple hypointense septa on T2-weighted images
   c. Sparing of the disk spaces
   d. Heterogeneous signal on T2-weighted images

4. Which of the following statements regarding lumbar chordomas is true?
   a. Lumbar chordomas are often diagnosed early because of symptoms arising from compression of the anterior column and roots.
   b. The most common presenting symptom of lumbar chordoma is paraplegia.
   c. The most likely cause of death in cases of lumbar chordoma is distant metastasis.
   d. Lumbar chordomas have higher metastatic rates than chordomas in any other location.

Chordoma of the Lumbar Spine

1. b, c, and d

2. a

3. b

4. d

Reference

Sivabalan P, Li J, Mobbs RJ: Extensive lumbar chordoma and unique reconstructive approach, *Eur Spine J* 20(Suppl 2):S336-S342, 2011.

Cross-Reference

Neuroradiology: The REQUISITES, 3rd ed, pp 567, 568.

Comment

Background

Chordomas are rare, slow-growing, locally invasive malignant tumors. The mean age at diagnosis is 56 years (range, 27 to 80 years). Symptoms most commonly arise from compression of the anterior column and roots. The most frequent complaint in patients with lumbar chordomas is pain and paresthesia. Symptoms often appear to be caused by a diskogenic or nonspecific pathology, resulting in delayed diagnosis.

Histopathology

Chordomas are thought to arise from notochord remnants (mesodermal precursor of the vertebral column). They appear as lobules of cells arranged in long strands or "cords," with a mucinous background separated by fibrous bands.

Imaging

Chordomas appear hypointense or isointense on T1-weighted images (Fig. A). Lesions demonstrating high signal intensity on T1-weighted images have also been reported. Signal intensity is usually inhomogeneous because there is often a combination of cystic and solid components. On T2-weighted images (Figs. B-D), inhomogeneous signal intensity is also observed, with some regions of the tumor equaling or exceeding the intensity of cerebrospinal fluid. Septa of low signal intensity radiating throughout the predominantly high-signal-intensity mass on T2-weighted images (see Fig. D) may help in differentiating chordomas from more common paraspinal or spinal masses.

Management

Chordomas are well known for their high local recurrence rates, and distant metastases following treatment are reported in more than 40% of patients. Complete surgical en bloc resection with wide, histologically proven tumor-free margins is the treatment of choice.

Notes

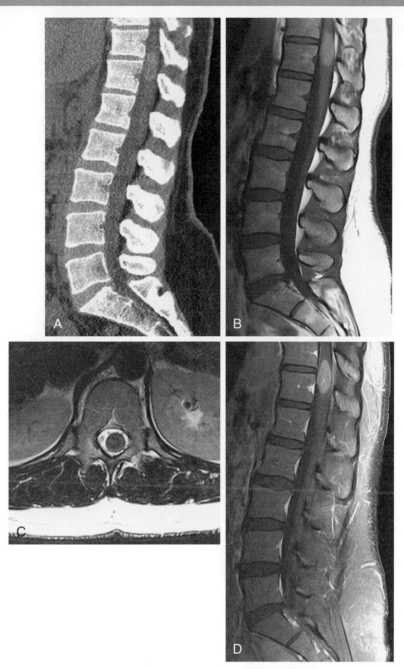

History: A 42-year-old woman presents with back pain for 2 years and burning sensation in her left leg for the past 2 weeks.

1. What should be included in the differential diagnosis? (Choose all that apply.)
   a. Meningioma
   b. Lipoma
   c. Meningeal melanocytoma
   d. Subacute hemorrhage
   e. Schwannoma

2. What is the most common location of this tumor along the spinal axis?
   a. Cervical spine
   b. Thoracic spine
   c. Lumbar spine
   d. Sacral spine

3. Which of the following is *not* expected to appear hyperintense on T1-weighted images?
   a. Fat
   b. Hemosiderin
   c. Methemoglobin
   d. Melanin

4. Which of the following pigmented neoplasms is *least* likely to occur with a primary localized mass?
   a. Melanotic schwannoma
   b. Pigmented meningioma
   c. Meningeal melanocytoma
   d. Primary leptomeningeal melanomatosis

Meningeal Melanocytoma

1. a, c, d, and e

2. a

3. b

4. d

References

Painter TJ, Chaljub G, Sethi R, et al: Intracranial and intraspinal meningeal melanocytosis, *AJNR Am J Neuroradiol* 21(7):1349-1353, 2000.

Turhan T, Oner K, Yurtseven T, et al: Spinal meningeal melanocytoma: Report of two cases and review of the literature, *J Neurosurg* 100(3 Suppl Spine):287-290, 2004.

Cross-Reference

Neuroradiology: The REQUISITES, 3rd ed, pp 62, 567.

Comment

Background

Meningeal melanocytoma is an uncommon pigmented lesion of the spinal leptomeninges. This lesion can manifest at any age. It is included in the group of primary leptomeningeal melanocytic proliferations, which can be diffuse or focal. The diffuse proliferations are usually a manifestation of neurocutaneous melanosis syndrome, a congenital neuroectodermal dysplasia involving the neural crest. The focal proliferations are meningeal melanocytoma and primary leptomeningeal melanoma.

Histopathology

Melanocytes originate in the neural crest and are found throughout the leptomeninges. Primary melanocytic neoplasms arise from the transformation of normally occurring leptomeningeal melanocytes.

Imaging

On CT, the lesion may be isodense or hyperdense (Fig. A), with variable contrast enhancement. The MRI features of meningeal melanocytoma depend on the amount of melanin and the presence or absence of hemorrhage. Paramagnetic effects secondary to melanin pigment are considered to be responsible for the decreased T1 and T2 relaxation times of melanocytoma. The lesion is typically isointense to hyperintense relative to cord on T1-weighted images (Fig. B), is isointense to slightly hypointense on T2-weighted images (Fig. C), and tends to enhance strongly and homogeneously after contrast agent administration (Fig. D).

Management

Total excision of the lesion is the treatment of choice.

Notes

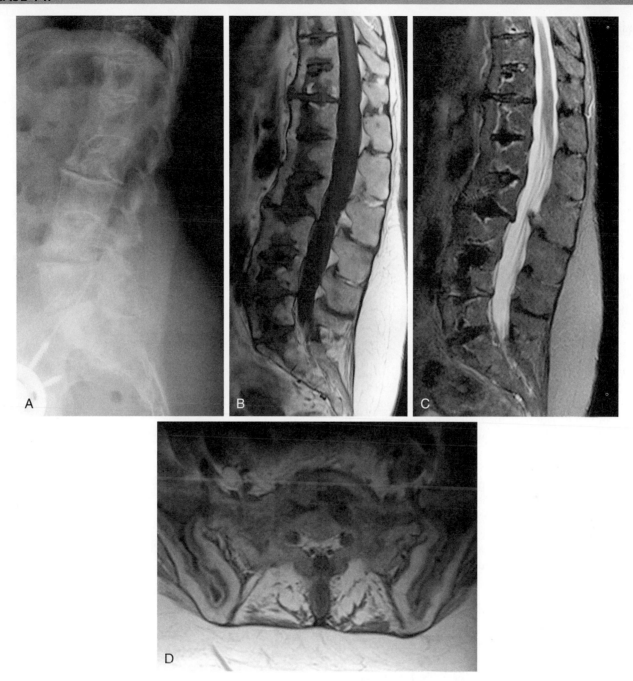

History: A 56-year-old man presents with back pain.

1. What should be included in the differential diagnosis? (Choose all that apply.)
   a. Metastasis
   b. Multiple myeloma
   d. Lymphoma
   d. Sickle cell disease
   e. Gaucher disease

2. H-shaped vertebrae are classically seen in which condition?
   a. Hurler's syndrome
   b. Scheuermann's disease
   c. Renal osteodystrophy
   d. Sickle cell disease

3. All of the following are skeletal manifestations of Gaucher disease *except:*
   a. Osteopoikilosis
   b. Osteonecrosis
   c. Osteosclerosis
   d. Osteopenia

4. Which of the following MRI marrow signal changes are seen in Gaucher disease?
   a. Hyperintense T1 and T2 signals
   b. Hypointense T1 and T2 signals
   c. Hyperintense T1 signal and hypointense T2 signal
   d. Hypointense T1 signal and hyperintense T2 signal

Gaucher Disease

1. d and e

2. d

3. a

4. b

References

Ozcan HN, Kara M, Kara O, et al: Severe skeletal involvement in a patient with Gaucher's disease, *J Orthop Sci* 14(4):465-468, 2009.

Wenstrup RJ, Roca-Espiau M, Weinreb NJ, et al: Skeletal aspects of Gaucher disease: A review, *Br J Radiol* 75(Suppl 1):A2-A12, 2002.

Cross-Reference

Neuroradiology: The REQUISITES, 3rd ed, p 272.

Comment

Background

Gaucher disease is the most prevalent inherited lysosomal storage disease and occurs most commonly in Ashkenazic Jews.

Pathophysiology

Gaucher disease is a rare autosomal recessive lysosomal storage disorder caused by β-glucocerebrosidase deficiency, which leads to an accumulation of the lipid glucocerebroside in the reticuloendothelial system. The symptoms and pathology of Gaucher disease result from the accumulation of Gaucher cells in various organ systems. Musculoskeletal complications include osteopenia, abnormal bone remodeling, delayed bone healing, pathologic fracture, increased propensity for infection, and bleeding from involvement of the bone marrow.

Imaging

Radiologic findings include Erlenmeyer flask deformity, osteopenia, osteosclerosis, osteonecrosis, pathologic fractures, and bone marrow infiltration (Fig. A). H-shaped vertebrae may be seen in Gaucher disease and are secondary to infarction of the end vessels supplying the vertebral body, causing growth retardation of the central aspect of the vertebral body (Fig. B). MRI shows reduced T1 and T2 signals secondary to bone marrow infiltration and features of osteonecrosis (Figs. C and D).

Management

Depending on the status of the patient, the mainstay of treatment is enzyme replacement and substrate reduction.

Notes

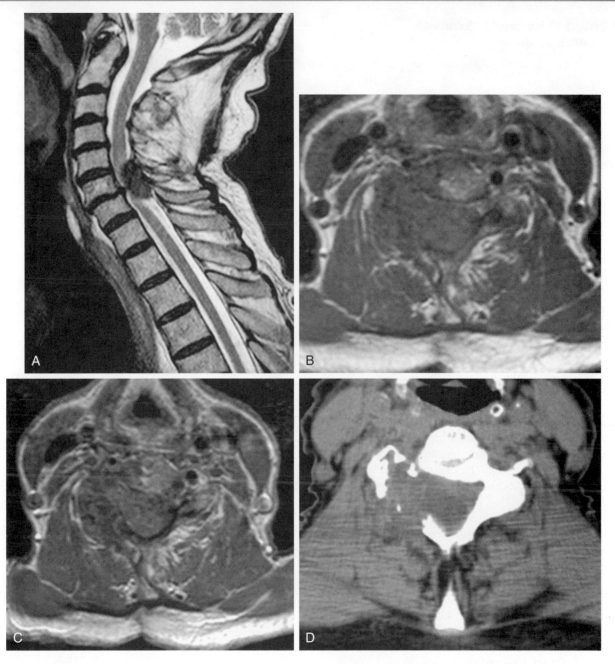

History: A 70-year-old woman presents with a history of back pain and left leg numbness.

1. What should be included in the differential diagnosis? (Choose all that apply.)
   a. Chondrosarcoma
   b. Lymphoma
   c. Schwannoma
   d. Pigmented villonodular synovitis (PVNS)
   e. Metastatic disease

2. What is the most common site of involvement of PVNS in the spinal axis?
   a. Cervical spine
   b. Thoracic spine
   c. Lumbar spine
   d. Sacrum

3. Which part of the vertebra is most commonly involved in PVNS?
   a. Vertebral body
   b. Facet joint
   c. Lamina
   d. Spinous process

4. Which of the following statements regarding imaging findings in PVNS is true?
   a. Postcontrast MRI images rarely demonstrate enhancement.
   b. Most PVNS lesions affecting the spine show hyperintense T2 signal.
   c. Most PVNS lesions are hypodense on CT scan.
   d. Calcifications are not a feature of PVNS affecting the lumbar spine.

Pigmented Villonodular Synovitis of the Cervical Spine

Notes

1. d and e

2. a

3. b

4. d

References

Hsieh YC, Chen WY, Hsieh TY, et al: Pigmented villonodular synovitis of the lumbar spine, *J Clin Rheumatol* 18(5):274-275, 2012.

Motamedi K, Murphey MD, Fetsch JF, et al: Villonodular synovitis (PVNS) of the spine, *Skeletal Radiol* 34(4):185-195, 2005.

Parmar HA, Sitoh YY, Tan KK, et al: MR imaging features of pigmented villonodular synovitis of the cervical spine, *AJNR Am J Neuroradiol* 25(1):146-149, 2004.

Cross-Reference

Neuroradiology: The REQUISITES, 3rd ed, p 531.

Comment

Background

PVNS, also known as giant cell tumor of the synovium, is a slow-growing mass lesion of the synovium characterized by villous and nodular overgrowth of the synovial membranes of tendon sheaths, bursae, and joints. PVNS affects a wide age range of patients, with no definite sex predilection. It most frequently involves the hip and knee joints but may occur in any joint of the appendicular skeleton. In the spine, it usually arises from the facet joints. The exact cause of PVNS is unclear. Trauma has been considered as a possible etiology.

Histopathology

The lesion is characterized by the proliferation of synovial cells, macrophage infiltration, the presence of multinucleated giant cells, and hemosiderin deposition.

Imaging

The best imaging modalities to evaluate and characterize PVNS are CT and MRI. PVNS typically appears as a space-occupying lesion or mass in close relationship with the facet joints (Figs. A-C). CT scan typically shows a hyperdense lesion (Fig. D). Erosive changes of the facet joints adjacent to the lesion are typically found (see Fig. D). On MRI, low signal on T2-weighted images is seen (see Fig. A) because of the chronic presence of blood products. Enhancement is variable.

Management

The treatment of choice for PVNS is surgical, with gross total resection of the lesion and as much of the affected adjacent structures as possible. Management may also include radiation therapy, although its role is limited. Local recurrence is common (up to 20%), and close follow-up imaging is needed.

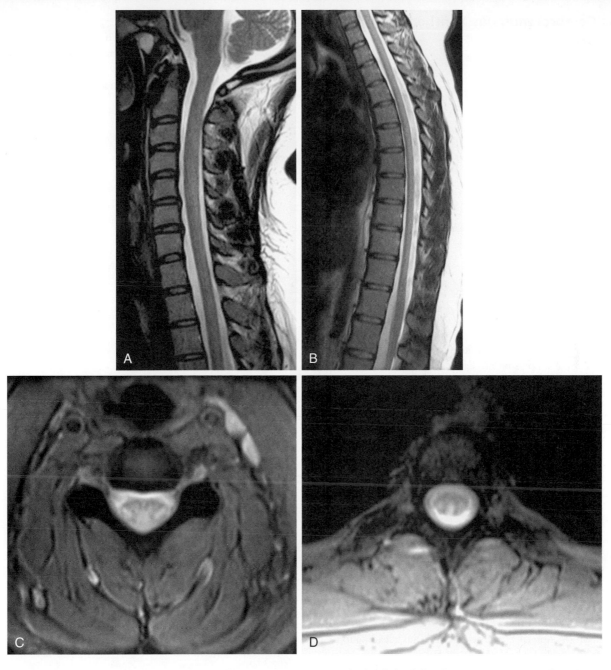

History: A 27-year-old woman with a history of cataracts as a child developed lower extremity weakness 7 years ago and recently developed bumps over her Achilles tendons.

1. What should be included in the differential diagnosis? (Choose all that apply.)
   a. Subacute combined degeneration
   b. Cerebrotendinous xanthomatosis (CTX)
   c. Multiple sclerosis
   d. HIV myelitis
   e. Cord infarct

2. Which of the following is not a feature of CTX?
   a. Juvenile cataracts
   b. Dislocation of the lens
   c. Achilles tendon xanthoma
   d. Peripheral neuropathy

3. Which of the following statements regarding CTX is true?
   a. The inheritance pattern is autosomal dominant.
   b. Low plasma cholestanol levels are diagnostic.
   c. The spinal form of CTX is more common than the classic form.
   d. Teenagers with the disease typically develop tendon xanthomas.

4. Which of the following is *not* a typical imaging feature of CTX?
   a. Cord enlargement
   b. High T2 signal in the dorsal columns
   c. High T2 signal in the lateral tracts
   d. Increased T2 signal in the dentate nuclei

Spinal Cerebrotendinous Xanthomatosis

1. a, b, c, and d

2. b

3. d

4. a

References

Barkhof F, Verrips A, Wesseling P, et al: Cerebrotendinous xanthomatosis: The spectrum of imaging findings and the correlation with neuropathologic findings, *Radiology* 217(3):869-876, 2000.

Bartholdi D, Zumsteg D, Verrips A, et al: Spinal phenotype of cerebrotendinous xanthomatosis—a pitfall in the diagnosis of multiple sclerosis, *J Neurol* 251(1):105-107, 2004.

Verrips A, Nijeholt GJ, Barkhof F, et al: Spinal xanthomatosis: A variant of cerebrotendinous xanthomatosis, *Brain* 122(Pt 8):1589-1595, 1999.

Cross-Reference

Neuroradiology: The REQUISITES, 3rd ed, pp 546-550.

Comment

Background

CTX is an autosomal recessive lipid storage disorder. High bile alcohols in urine or plasma cholestanol levels are diagnostic. Disease onset is usually in childhood, and manifestations often include bilateral cataracts and diarrhea. Later, during the teenage years, neurologic abnormalities and tendon xanthomas manifest. The neurologic symptoms and signs include cerebellar and pyramidal dysfunction, dementia, epilepsy, and polyneuropathy. There are two forms of CTX: classic and spinal. The classic phenotype includes juvenile cataracts; cerebellar involvement; dementia; tendon xanthoma formation, particularly of the ankle tendons; and peripheral neuropathy early in the disease process. The spinal form is characterized by extensive white matter lesions in the lateral corticospinal tracts and in the gracile tracts. This form typically has a milder course.

Pathophysiology

CTX is characterized by abnormal bile acid synthesis caused by deficiency of the enzyme sterol-27-hydroxylase. There is decreased production of chenodeoxycholic acid, leading to the accumulation of cholesterol and cholestanol in various tissues, particularly in the central and peripheral nervous systems, eye lenses, and tendons.

Imaging

Imaging features of the classic form include symmetric high-T2-signal lesions in the cerebellar white matter, cerebral atrophy, diffuse nonspecific periventricular white matter abnormalities, and bilateral lesions in basal ganglia. Imaging features of the spinal form have been sparsely described in the literature. Findings include spinal cord atrophy and T2-weighted signal abnormalities in the lateral tracts and dorsal columns (Figs. A-D).

Management

Antispastic agents such as baclofen aid in treating the symptoms of CTX. In addition, maximum therapy with lipid-lowering agents such as simvastatin has shown success. Alternatively, the administration of chenodeoxycholic acid has demonstrated success in low-powered trials.

Notes

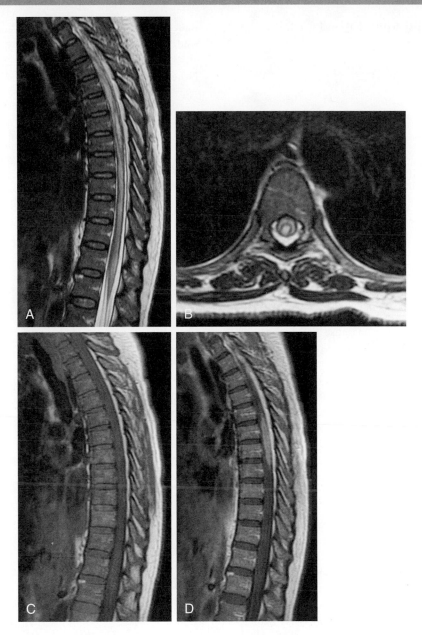

History: A 53-year-old woman with AIDS presents with severe upper back pain between the shoulders and progressive weakness of the lower extremities.

1. What should be included in the differential diagnosis for the imaging findings presented? (Choose all that apply.)
   a. HIV vacuolar myelopathy
   b. *Toxoplasma* myelitis
   c. Intramedullary abscess
   d. Tuberculoma
   e. Lymphoma

2. Which of the following infectious causes of intramedullary and meningeal lesions does not occur with increased frequency in patients with AIDS?
   a. Cytomegalovirus
   b. Herpesvirus
   c. Syphilis
   d. Human T-cell lymphotrophic virus

3. What imaging modality would you recommend next?
   a. MRI of the brain
   b. Single photon emission computed tomography (SPECT) with thallium-201
   c. Ultrasound of the abdomen
   d. CT myelography

4. Which of the following statements regarding immune restoration inflammatory syndrome (IRIS) is *false?*
   a. Patients with IRIS experience clinical deterioration despite improvement of their immune system function.
   b. IRIS typically occurs 6 months after initiation of highly active antiretroviral therapy (HAART).
   c. Most cases of IRIS in patients with AIDS are attributed to bacterial, viral, or fungal infections.
   d. In most patients with IRIS, the condition is self-limited.

Toxoplasmosis of the Spinal Cord

1. b, c, d, and e

2. d

3. a

4. b

References

Garcia-Gubern C, Fuentes CR, Colon-Rolon L, et al: Spinal cord toxoplasmosis as an unusual presentation of AIDS: Case report and review of the literature, *Int J Emerg Med* 3(4):439-442, 2010.

Kung DH, Hubenthal EA, Kwan JY, et al: Toxoplasmosis myelopathy and myopathy in an AIDS patient: A case of immune reconstitution inflammatory syndrome? *Neurologist* 17(1):49-51, 2011.

Cross-Reference

Neuroradiology: The REQUISITES, 3rd ed, p 209.

Comment

Background

Toxoplasmosis is the most common cause of cerebral mass lesions in patients with AIDS. *Toxoplasma* affecting the spinal cord has been reported infrequently and is usually associated with multiple lesions in the brain. Reports of isolated spinal cord toxoplasmosis are rare. *Toxoplasma* myelitis manifests with symptoms of myelopathy, including a sensory level, paraparesis, incontinence, and changes in deep tendon reflexes. Cerebrospinal fluid and serum *Toxoplasma* IgG and IgM levels can be helpful diagnostically if they are elevated, but they may not be positive.

Pathophysiology

Initial infection with *Toxoplasma gondii* is usually the result of ingesting oocysts from contaminated food or ingesting raw pork containing tissue bradyzoites. The ingested oocysts become tachyzoites, which invade systemically. The initial infection is usually asymptomatic or causes mild lymphadenopathy. Reactivation of toxoplasmosis in patients with AIDS typically occurs with $CD4^+$ lymphocyte counts less than 100 cells/mL. Initiation of antiretroviral therapy in patients with HIV leads to the recovery of $CD4^+$ counts and the restoration of a protective immune response; however, in a subset of patients, a dysregulated immune response after the initiation of therapy leads to IRIS. The hallmark of this syndrome is paradoxic worsening of an existing infection soon after initiation of therapy. The most common forms of IRIS are associated with mycobacterial infections, fungi, and herpesviruses.

Imaging

MRI typically shows localized enhancing intramedullary lesions in the cervical or thoracic cord associated with edema and cord enlargement (Figs. A-D).

Management

Definitive diagnosis must be made by biopsy. If unrecognized, toxoplasmosis of the spinal cord can be devastating in a short time. Treatment is with anti-*Toxoplasma* medications and steroids to decrease cord edema.

Notes

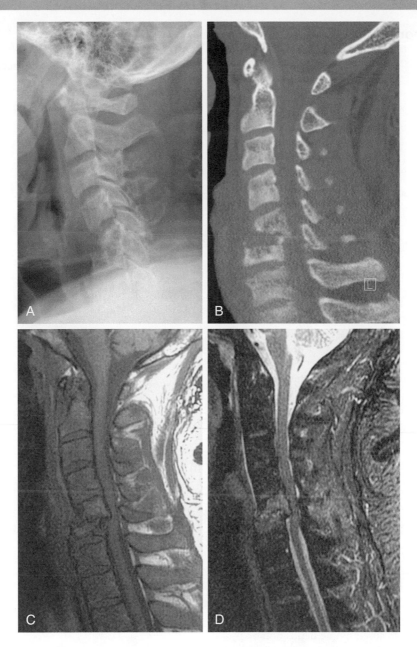

History: A 55-year-old man with end-stage renal disease who is on long-term hemodialysis presents with recent severe neck pain, upper extremity numbness, and weakness.

1. What should be included in the differential diagnosis? (Choose all that apply.)
   a. Diskitis osteomyelitis
   b. Neuropathic spondyloarthropathy (Charcot spine)
   c. Dialysis-induced spondyloarthropathy
   d. Degenerative spondyloarthritis
   e. Metastatic disease

2. All of the following are underlying mechanisms of dialysis-induced spondyloarthropathy *except:*
   a. β_2-Microglobulin amyloidosis
   b. Crystal-induced arthropathy
   c. Aluminum-induced spondyloarthropathy
   d. Calcium toxicity

3. Which MRI finding is characteristic in dialysis-induced spondyloarthropathy?
   a. Erosive end-plate changes
   b. High T2 end-plate signal
   c. High T2 signal in the disk
   d. High T1 end-plate signal

4. What is the most reliable way to differentiate between an infectious and a noninfectious cause in patients with chronic renal disease and rapidly progressive spondyloarthropathy?
   a. CT
   b. MRI
   c. Laboratory data (sedimentation rate and white blood cell count)
   d. Biopsy

Dialysis-Induced Spondyloarthropathy

1. a and c

2. d

3. a

4. d

References
Danish FR, Klinkmann J, Yokoo H, et al: Fatal cervical spondyloarthropathy in a hemodialysis patient with systemic deposition of beta2-microglobulin amyloid, *Am J Kidney Dis* 33(3):563-566, 1999.

Kaplan P, Resnick D, Murphey M, et al: Destructive noninfectious spondyloarthropathy in hemodialysis patients: A report of four cases, *Radiology* 162 (1 Pt 1):241-244, 1987.

Kiss E, Keusch G, Zenetti M, et al: Dialysis-related amyloidosis revisited, *AJR Am J Roentgenol* 185(6):1460-1467, 2005.

Cross-Reference
Neuroradiology: The REQUISITES, 3rd ed, p 543.

Comment
Background
In patients undergoing long-term dialysis for chronic renal disease, a destructive spondyloarthropathy that resembles infection may develop. The process tends to affect primarily the cervical spine, followed by the thoracic spine and thoracolumbar junction. Clinically, patients present with pain, radiculopathy, and signs of compressive myelopathy in the absence of symptoms of obvious infection.

Histopathology
Dialysis-induced spondyloarthropathy may be related to the deposition of crystals in the intervertebral disks and adjacent end-plates, as demonstrated by transmission electron microscopy. It is now known that aluminum toxicity and accumulation in the disk space and diskovertebral junction can produce similar destructive changes and secondary hyperparathyroidism in patients with renal osteodystrophy, leading to subperiosteal and subchondral reabsorption of bone and erosive arthropathy. Dialysis-related amyloidosis is caused by the deposition of β_2-microglobulin as amyloid fibrils, which are known to accumulate in synovial membranes and osteoarticular sites, particularly in the spine, evoking an inflammatory reaction that leads to destructive osteoarthropathy.

Imaging
Characteristic imaging features include marked disk space narrowing, vertebral body erosions, and sclerosis on CT or plain films; Schmorl's node formation in the absence of significant osteophyte formation; and epidural spinal masses (Figs. A and B). On MRI, the disk typically displays a low or minimally bright signal on T2-weighted images. There is also evidence of abnormal low T1 signal and low T2 signal of the eroded subchondral end-plates, although occasionally, owing to the presence of inflammatory cells, the subchondral end-plates may show bright T2 signal, making differentiation from infection very difficult (Figs. C and D).

Management
Treatment includes medical care and, in more severe cases, decompression and surgical stabilization.

Notes

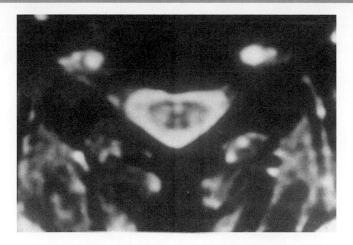

History: A 35-year-old man presents with loss of strength in the fingers.

1. What should be included in the differential diagnosis? (Choose all that apply.)
   a. Spinal cord arterial infarction
   b. Wallerian degeneration
   c. Amyotrophic lateral sclerosis (ALS)
   d. Multiple sclerosis
   e. Subacute combined degeneration

2. Which associated intracranial finding may be seen?
   a. Hyperintense T2 signal in the callososeptal interface
   b. Hyperintense signal in the splenium of the corpus callosum
   c. Optic nerve enhancement
   d. Precentral gyrus hypointense signal and corticospinal tract hyperintense signal on T2-weighted images

3. In this disorder, which region of the cord is most likely to demonstrate marked atrophy?
   a. Anterior horn cell region
   b. Posterior horn cell region
   c. Lateral funiculus
   d. Posterior funiculus

4. What percentage of ALS cases is familial?
   a. 1%
   b. 5% to 10%
   c. 20% to 25%
   d. 50%

Amyotrophic Lateral Sclerosis

1. b, c, and d

2. d

3. a

4. b

References

Sperfeld AD, Bretschneider V, Flaith L, et al: MR-pathologic comparison of the upper spinal cord in different motor neuron diseases, *Eur Neurol* 53(2):74-77, 2005.

Waragai M, Shinotoh H, Hayashi M, et al: High signal intensity on T1-weighted MRI of the anterolateral column of the spinal cord in amyotrophic lateral sclerosis, *J Neurol Neurosurg Psychiatry* 62(1):88-91, 1997.

Cross-Reference

Neuroradiology: The REQUISITES, 3rd ed, pp 263, 550.

Comment

Background

ALS is the most common degenerative motor neuron disease. It gained recognition and is best known as Lou Gehrig's disease, named after the famous baseball player. It is a syndrome of upper and lower motor neuron dysfunction of the arms, legs, and bulbar or respiratory motor system in adults that slowly progresses over months to years; there is no primary involvement of any other part of the nervous system and no specific cause.

Histopathology

The cause of ALS is unknown. Histopathologic examination shows selective degeneration of the somatic motor neurons of the brainstem nuclei and spinal cord (anterior horn cells), as well as the large pyramidal neurons of the motor cortex. Associated degeneration of the corticospinal tracts has been tracked in postmortem specimens from the cerebral cortex to the conus medullaris.

Imaging

High signal intensity of the corticospinal tracts on T2-weighted images has been tracked from the centrum semiovale to the lower cervical spine in patients with ALS (see the figure); however, this is likely an infrequent feature of ALS (and other motor neuron diseases). The symmetry of the hyperintensity distinguishes these findings from multiple sclerosis and other demyelinating diseases, as well as from wallerian degeneration resulting from infarction or trauma. High signal intensity on T1-weighted images in the anterolateral columns of the spinal cord has also been reported in patients with ALS.

Management

ALS is a fatal disease and is incurable. A glutamate pathway antagonist is the only medication that has shown efficacy in extending life in patients with ALS.

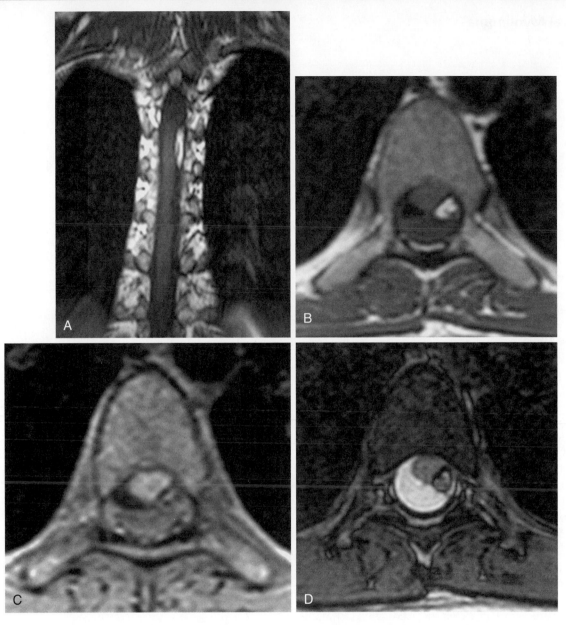

History: A 25-year-old, previously healthy woman presents with a 4-year history of progressive pain and disturbance of temperature sensation in her right leg and recent heaviness in her left leg.

1. What should be included in the differential diagnosis? (Choose all that apply.)
   a. Schwannoma
   b. Myolipoma
   c. Cavernoma
   d. Meningioma
   e. Dermoid

2. Where are intradural lipomas most likely to be located relative to the cord parenchyma?
   a. Anterior
   b. Posterior
   c. Lateral and to the right
   d. Lateral and to the left

3. Which of the following is responsible for the dark rim surrounding the lesion?
   a. Pseudocapsule
   b. Rim calcification
   c. Hemosiderin deposition
   d. Chemical shift

4. What imaging finding may explain the 4-year history of progressive pain and loss of temperature sensation and bilateral lower extremity weakness?
   a. Cord hemorrhage
   b. Cord compression
   c. Cord tethering
   d. Demyelination

Intradural Myolipoma

1. b and e

2. b

3. d

4. c

Reference
Brown PG, Shaver EG: Myolipoma in a tethered cord: Case report and review of the literature, *J Neurosurg* 92(2 Suppl):214-216, 2000.

Cross-Reference
Neuroradiology: The REQUISITES, 3rd ed, pp 564-565.

Comment
Background
Intradural myolipoma is a rare congenital tumor that usually manifests in children 8 years old or younger. In most reported cases, the tumor is located in the lumbosacral region.

Histopathology
Myolipoma is a benign tumor consisting of fully differentiated striated muscle fibers mingled with fat.

Imaging
On T1-weighted images, myolipomas are hyperintense (Figs. A and B); they suppress on T1-weighted images with fat saturation (Fig. C). They typically contain hypointense areas, which correspond to bundles of smooth muscle intermixed with adipose tissue (see Fig. B). The signal intensity of cerebrospinal fluid on T1-weighted images is not uniformly low at the level of the tumor and inferior to it, presumably because of fluid flow artifacts resulting from the presence of tumor and cord tethering. On gradient-echo images (Fig. D), a dark rim may be seen owing to the chemical shift difference between fat and water (approximately 3.5 parts per million); this is caused by cancellation of the signals from fat and water at their interface because they are out of phase (at the echo time [TE] of the pulse sequence).

Management
In symptomatic patients, treatment involves surgical removal and cord untethering.

Notes

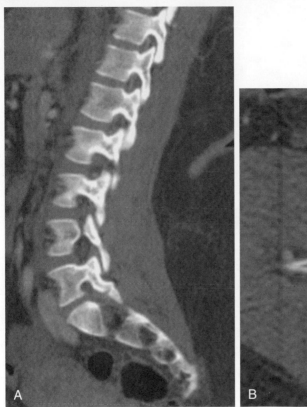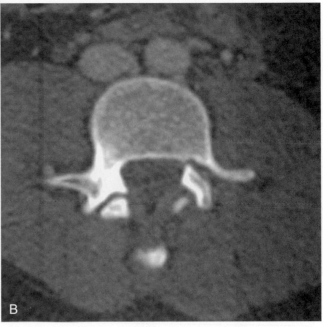

History: A 25-year-old woman was involved in a motor vehicle collision.

1. What should be included in the differential diagnosis? (Choose all that apply.)
   a. Osteoid osteoma
   b. Fracture of the pedicle
   c. Retrosomatic cleft
   d. Pars interarticularis defect
   e. Congenital absence of the pedicle

2. Where along the spinal axis is congenital absence of the pedicle most common?
   a. Cervical spine
   b. Thoracic spine
   c. Lumbar spine
   d. Sacrum

3. Osseous abnormalities frequently reported in association with a congenitally absent pedicle include all of the following *except:*
   a. Spina bifida occulta
   b. Vertebral body fusion
   c. Additional hypoplastic pedicles
   d. Limbus vertebra

4. All of the following findings on plain radiographs are useful in differentiating congenital absence of the pedicle from a lytic lesion *except:*
   a. Hypertrophy of the contralateral pedicle
   b. Compression deformity of the vertebral body
   c. Displacement of the spinous process
   d. Anomalies of the articular process

Congenital Absence of the Pedicle

1. e

2. c

3. d

4. b

Reference

Kaito T, Kato Y, Sakaura H, et al: Congenital absence of a lumbar pedicle presenting with contralateral lumbar radiculopathy, *J Spinal Disord Tech* 18(2):203-205, 2005.

Cross-Reference

Neuroradiology: The REQUISITES, 3rd ed, pp 516-517.

Comment

Background

Congenital absence of the pedicle or hypoplasia of a lumbar pedicle is an uncommon anomaly. Most cases are asymptomatic and are discovered incidentally or are found when patients present with low back pain. The anomaly occurs most frequently in the lumbar spine, followed by the cervical spine. It has been observed in association with genitourinary and other congenital abnormalities and in patients with neurofibromatosis.

Pathophysiology

In a patient with congenital absence of the pedicle, the biomechanical dysfunction from the concomitant deformity or abnormal function of the facet joint causes lumbar spine instability in axial rotation and flexion. In addition, because the facet shares the axial load at a specific level, the contralateral joint in patients with congenital absence of the pedicle must bear a greater load, resulting in the development of severe degenerative changes.

Imaging

CT scan is performed to detect bony anomalies (Figs. A and B). Three-dimensional CT is effective in determining the relationships between the deformed bones. MRI helps distinguish this condition from pedicle destruction by tumor or infection by the presence of fat, nerves, and vessels rather than a soft tissue mass in the intervertebral foramen and by the dorsally positioned abnormal articular processes.

Management

Most patients are asymptomatic or complain of low back pain that can be managed with conservative therapy. In rare cases with neurologic impairment, surgical intervention may be required.

Notes

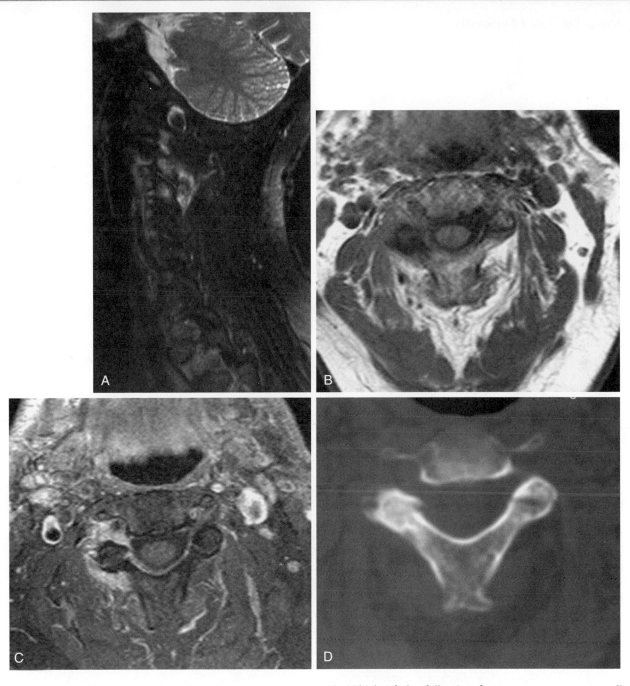

A

B

C

D

History: A 60-year-old man presents with neck pain.

1. What should be included in the differential diagnosis? (Choose all that apply.)
   a. Metastatic disease
   b. Degenerative facet disease
   c. Facet joint septic arthritis
   d. Osteoid osteoma
   e. Malignant fibrous histiocytoma

2. What is the most likely cause of the increased signal in the posterior epidural space on the postcontrast axial image?
   a. Epidural fat
   b. Epidural veins
   c. Enhancing soft tissue
   d. Epidural blood

3. Which of the following features suggests a nonmalignant etiology in this case?
   a. Enhancement of paraspinal soft tissues
   b. Age of the patient
   c. Sclerosis of the superior and inferior articular facet
   d. Unilateral findings

4. All of the following soft tissue tumors are included in the differential diagnosis for the findings presented *except:*
   a. Malignant fibrous histiocytoma
   b. Liposarcoma
   c. Fibromatosis
   d. Hemangiopericytoma

Degenerative Facet Synovitis

1. a, b, c, d, and e

2. c

3. c

4. d

Reference
Czervionke LF, Haughton VM: Degenerative disease of the spine. In Atlas SW, editor: *Magnetic resonance imaging of the brain and spine*, ed 3, Philadelphia, 2002, Lippincott Williams & Wilkins, pp 1633-1713.

Cross-Reference
Neuroradiology: The REQUISITES, 3rd ed, pp 516-517.

Comment

Pathophysiology

Degeneration of the facet joint, which has a thin synovial lining, is characterized by loss of cartilage from the articular surface. Subsequent degenerative changes include subarticular erosions, sclerosis of bone, and hypertrophy.

Imaging

Osseous and cartilaginous changes in the degenerated joint are well shown by CT scan, but acute and chronic inflammation induced in the capsule and adjacent soft tissues (myositis) is better demonstrated by MRI, especially when fat-suppression techniques (frequency selective fat saturation or short tau inversion recovery [STIR] sequences) are used (Figs. A-D). Exuberant inflammatory facet osteoarthropathy has been referred to as facet synovitis, and differentiation between sterile and infectious etiologies may be difficult in some cases. In this case, the patient underwent a biopsy because of the uncertainty of the findings.

Management

Spine interventionalists have found that in patients with symptoms related to degenerative facets in the cervical or lumbar spine, the pain often correlates with the site of hyperintensity on fat-suppressed T2-weighted images and enhancement on fat-suppressed postcontrast T1-weighted images, as shown here (see Fig. C). Patients are more likely to experience relief of symptoms when therapeutic injections are directed to the facet joints with this MRI appearance.

Notes

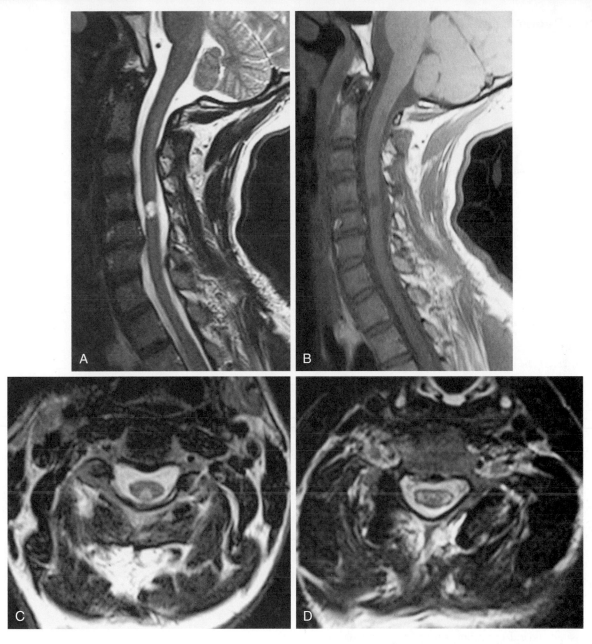

History: A 61-year-old man presents with a history of a boat accident 6 months earlier, resulting in cord injury and paralysis.

1. What should be included in the differential diagnosis? (Choose all that apply.)
   a. Subacute combined degeneration
   b. Vacuolar myelopathy
   c. Multiple sclerosis
   d. Wallerian degeneration
   e. Astrocytoma

2. Which of the following statements regarding wallerian degeneration is true?
   a. MRI signal abnormalities are in the lateral columns above the injury site.
   b. MRI signal abnormalities are in the posterior columns above the injury site.

c. MRI signal abnormalities are in the lateral columns and dorsal columns below the injury site.
d. MRI signal abnormalities are in the lateral columns and dorsal columns above the injury site.

3. How long after cord injury does wallerian degeneration become visible on MRI?
   a. 7 days
   b. 2 weeks
   c. 5 weeks
   d. 7 weeks

4. What is the most common cause of wallerian degeneration in the spinal cord?
   a. Trauma
   b. Infarct
   c. Hemorrhage
   d. Neoplasm

Wallerian Degeneration

1. a, b, c, and d

2. b

3. d

4. a

References

Becerra JL, Puckett WR, Hiester ED, et al: MR-pathologic comparisons of wallerian degeneration in spinal cord injury, *AJNR Am J Neuroradiol* 16(1):125-133, 1995.

Valencia MP, Castillo M: MRI findings in posttraumatic spinal cord wallerian degeneration, *Clin Imaging* 30(6):431-433, 2006.

Cross-Reference

Neuroradiology: The REQUISITES, 3rd ed, p 243.

Comment

Background

Wallerian degeneration involves the disintegration of axons and myelin sheaths and results from injury to the proximal portion of the axon or its cell body. It is most commonly seen in the brain, where the main cause is infarct. In the spinal cord, it occurs mainly after trauma.

Pathophysiology

Myelin breakdown in the posterior columns above the injury level and in the lateral corticospinal tracts below the injury level occurs 8 to 12 days after injury. Wallerian degeneration becomes visible on routine MRI 7 weeks after injury.

Imaging

The patient in this case has had posterior fusion from C3 to C6. The focal area of abnormal cord signal at C4-5 is isointense to cerebrospinal fluid on T1-weighted and T2-weighted images (Figs. A and B), and there is associated mild cord atrophy at this level. These findings are consistent with posttraumatic cystic myelomalacia. In patients with wallerian degeneration, there is a region of abnormal signal contiguous with the focal area of cord tissue loss and extending superiorly in the territory of the posterior columns; this region is isointense (to uninvolved cord) on T1-weighted axial images and hyperintense on T2-weighted axial images extending cephalad. In the present case (Fig. C), this region extends to the cervicomedullary junction and is consistent with wallerian degeneration in the posterior columns. Below the level of cord tissue loss, hyperintense T2 signal is noted in the lateral posterior aspect of the cord, corresponding with the lateral corticospinal tracts (Fig. D).

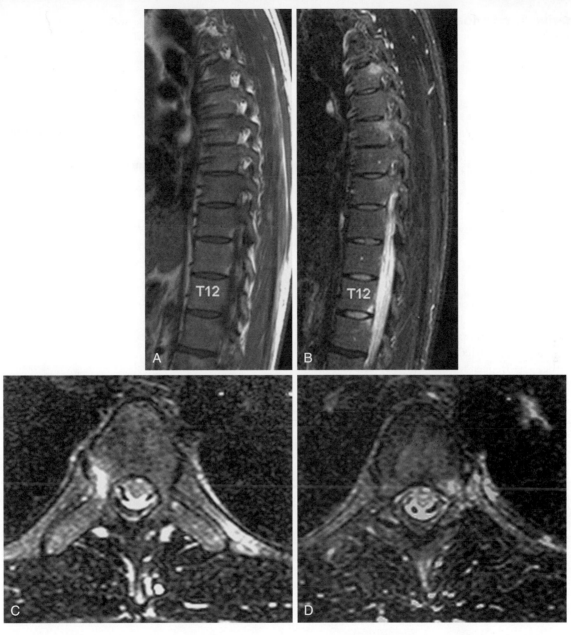

History: A 35-year-old man presents with a 2-month history of back pain, initially radiating to the right midback and then, 1 month later, radiating to the left midback.

1. What should be included in the differential diagnosis? (Choose all that apply.)
   a. Diffuse idiopathic skeletal hyperostosis
   b. Diskitis osteomyelitis
   c. Ankylosing spondylitis
   d. Rheumatoid arthritis
   e. Inflammatory bowel disease

2. In patients with Crohn's disease, sacroiliitis is most likely to be which of the following?
   a. Unilateral
   b. Bilateral and symmetric
   c. Bilateral and asymmetric
   d. Not present

3. Which of the following findings is typically seen in patients with Crohn's disease spondyloarthropathy?
   a. Romanus lesion
   b. Andersson lesion
   c. Schmorl's node
   d. Annular fissure

4. What is the frequency of spondyloarthropathy in patients with Crohn's disease 30 years after diagnosis?
   a. More than 90%
   b. 50%
   c. 20%
   d. Less than 10%

Seronegative Spondyloarthritis (Crohn's Disease)

1. c and e

2. b

3. a

4. c

Reference

Hermann KG, Althoff CE, Schneider U, et al: Spinal changes in patients with spondyloarthritis: Comparison of MR imaging and radiographic appearances, *Radiographics* 25(3):559-569, 2005.

Cross-Reference

Neuroradiology: The REQUISITES, 3rd ed, p 534.

Comment

Background

Arthritis is one of the most common extraintestinal manifestations of inflammatory bowel disease, with a 10% to 35% prevalence reported in patients diagnosed with Crohn's disease. Axial involvement includes spondylitis, which is usually asymmetric. The frequency with which spondyloarthritis occurs in patients with Crohn's disease is not well studied. In a population-based report from Norway, the prevalence of ankylosing spondylitis was 3.7% in patients seen 6 years after diagnosis of inflammatory bowel disease.

Histopathology

Five subgroups of seronegative spondyloarthritis are distinguished: ankylosing spondylitis, reactive arthritis (Reiter's syndrome), psoriatic arthritis, arthritis associated with inflammatory bowel disease, and undifferentiated spondyloarthritis. The spinal changes associated with spondyloarthritis are florid anterior or posterior spondylitis (Romanus lesion), diskitis (Andersson lesion), ankylosis, insufficiency fractures of the ankylosed spine, syndesmophytes, arthritis of the apophyseal and costovertebral joints, and enthesitis of the interspinal ligaments.

Imaging

Of the spinal changes, only syndesmophytes may be better seen by radiography than MRI. Active Romanus lesions involving the posterior vertebral edges (called posterior spondylitis) typically show hypointensity on T1-weighted sagittal images (Fig. A) and hyperintensity on short tau inversion recovery (STIR) sagittal images (Fig. B). Involvement of the anterior vertebral edges is called anterior spondylitis, whereas involvement of the anterior and posterior edges is called marginal spondylitis. Inactive Romanus lesions typically show hyperintensity on T1-weighted images (see Fig. A) and suppression of signal on STIR images (see Fig. B). These represent circumscribed regions of postinflammatory fatty bone marrow degeneration (note the similarity in MRI signal intensity between these lesions and type 2 degenerative end-plate changes). Arthritis affecting the facet joints as well as the costovertebral and costotransverse joints (Figs. B-D) is characterized by joint effusion, synovitis, erosions, and bone marrow edema (osteitis).

Management

Treatment includes physical therapy to promote spinal extension and mobility. Drug treatment options are nonsteroidal anti-inflammatory drugs, steroid injections, and antirheumatic drugs. Biologic blockade with tumor necrosis factor–α antagonist is very effective in treating the spinal symptoms of spondyloarthritis.

Notes

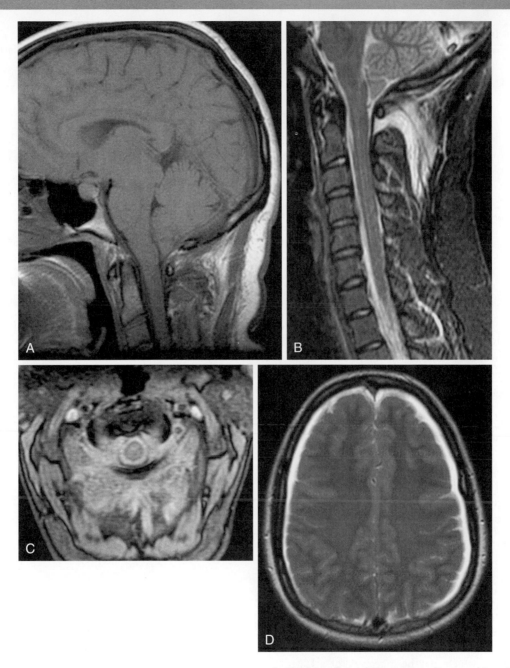

History: A 25-year-old woman presents with a 4-month history of severe postural headaches.

1. What should be included in the differential diagnosis? (Choose all that apply.)
   a. Chiari I malformation
   b. Meningitis
   c. Dandy-Walker variant
   d. Intracranial hypotension
   e. Idiopathic intracranial hypertension

2. What is the mechanism of pachymeningeal enhancement in patients with intracranial hypotension?
   a. Enlargement of the epidural space
   b. Dural thickening
   c. Dural inflammatory changes
   d. Subdural hemorrhage

3. Which of the following studies would assist in identifying the cause of the problem?
   a. Contrast-enhanced CT scan of the brain
   b. Myelography and postmyelography CT scan
   c. Cine cerebrospinal fluid (CSF) flow study
   d. MRI of the lumbar spine

4. What is a treatment option for this condition?
   a. Ventriculoperitoneal shunt placement
   b. Epidural blood patch
   c. Posterior fossa decompression
   d. Lumbar drain

Spontaneous Intracranial Hypotension

1. a and d

2. a

3. b

4. b

References

Chiapparini L, Farina L, D'Incerti L, et al: Spinal radiological findings in nine patients with spontaneous intracranial hypotension, *Neuroradiology* 44(2):143-150, 2002.

Medina JH, Abrams K, Falcone S, et al: Spinal imaging findings in spontaneous intracranial hypotension, *AJR Am J Roentgenol* 195(2):459-464, 2010.

Cross-Reference
Neuroradiology: The REQUISITES, 3rd ed, p 178.

Comment

Background

The syndrome of intracranial hypotension is a single pathophysiologic entity of diverse origin. Usually, it is characterized by an orthostatic headache—a headache that occurs or worsens with an upright posture—although patients with chronic headaches or even no headache have been described.

Pathophysiology

Most cases of intracranial hypotension result from a persistent CSF leak. This CSF leak most commonly occurs after dural puncture for a diagnostic lumbar puncture, myelography, or spinal anesthesia. In some cases, the syndrome occurs spontaneously. Evidence indicates that several of the abnormalities seen on imaging studies are the result of vascular dilatation to compensate for reduced CSF volume.

Imaging

The MRI findings are characteristic of this syndrome. Intracranial findings are diffuse thickening and enhancement of the pachymeninges, engorgement of the venous sinuses, subdural fluid collections, enlargement of the pituitary gland, and downward displacement of the brain with a low position of the cerebellar tonsils, which may be mistaken for a Chiari I malformation (Figs. A-D). Intraspinal findings include collapse of the dural sac around the cord, resulting in a paucity of CSF signal; a "festooned" appearance (see Fig. C) of the tethered dura mater; and dilatation of the epidural venous plexus, with marked enhancement after contrast agent administration. An epidural fluid collection, which appears isointense to CSF (or slightly hyperintense on T2-weighted images), demonstrates no postcontrast enhancement and is usually found in the cervical or thoracic region (or both). Another important finding is the C1-C2 sign, seen on MRI of the cervical spine as an area of fluid signal intensity between the spinous processes of C1 and C2 (see Fig. B). Visualization of this finding can lead to the diagnosis; however, this area is not indicative of the leakage site. Resolution of these abnormalities on MRI parallels an improvement in clinical symptoms.

Management

Treatment includes bed rest, intravenous caffeine, theophylline, and autologous epidural blood patch.

Notes

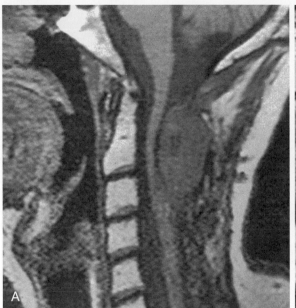 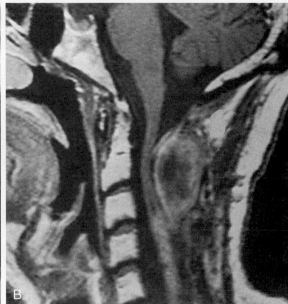

History: A 63-year-old woman with a history of an ependymoma resected 10 years earlier presents with cervical myelopathy.

1. What should be included in the differential diagnosis? (Choose all that apply.)
   a. Malignant fibrous histiocytoma
   b. Meningioma
   c. Metastatic lesion
   d. Abscess
   e. Lymphoma

2. All of the following are sequelae of spinal irradiation that may be seen on MRI *except:*
   a. Hyperintense vertebra on T1-weighted images
   b. H-shaped vertebrae
   c. Abnormal cord signal intensity
   d. Secondary malignancies

3. The most common types of latent, postradiation, secondary malignancies include all of the following *except:*
   a. Osteosarcoma
   b. Fibrosarcoma
   c. Liposarcoma
   d. Spindle cell sarcoma

4. What is the latency period between initial radiation therapy and diagnosis of radiation-induced sarcoma of the head and neck?
   a. 6 months
   b. 1 year
   c. 5 years
   d. Longer than 9 years

Radiation-Induced Malignant Fibrous Histiocytoma

1. a, c, and e

2. b

3. c

4. d

References
Nadeem SQ, Feun LG, Bruce-Gregorios JH, et al: Post radiation sarcoma (malignant fibrous histiocytoma) of the cervical spine following ependymoma (a case report), *J Neurooncol* 11(3):263-268, 1991.
Satomi T, Watanabe M, Kaneko T: Radiation-induced malignant fibrous histiocytoma of the maxilla, *Odontology* 99(2):203-208, 2011.

Cross-Reference
Neuroradiology: The REQUISITES, 3rd ed, p 551.

Comment
Background
Malignant fibrous histiocytoma is one of the most common soft tissue sarcomas in adults and has been reported in various organs; however, postradiation malignant fibrous histiocytoma is very rare. Most postradiation malignancies are sarcomas. Central nervous system tumors that may develop after radiation therapy (in some cases combined with chemotherapy) include meningiomas and astrocytomas. Radiation-induced sarcomas are characterized by aggressive behavior, with a high incidence of local recurrence and distant metastasis.

Histopathology
Malignant fibrous histiocytoma is composed of an admixture of spindle-shaped fibroblastic tumor cells and bizarre mononuclear histiocytic tumor cells arranged in a storiform pattern, with some multinucleated giant cells.

Imaging
The precontrast and postcontrast T1-weighted images shown here (Figs. A and B) reveal diffuse hyperintensity involving the cervical vertebrae. This finding represents the conversion of normal bone marrow to fatty marrow as a result of spinal irradiation, and it is key to formulating a differential diagnosis in this case. In addition to radiation therapy, an extensive laminectomy (C1-C7) has been performed. The cord demonstrates abnormal enhancement, without enlargement, at C4 and C5 (see Fig. B). The most plausible explanation for these findings is that the patient has been treated for an intramedullary neoplasm, either an ependymoma or an astrocytoma. The cord enhancement could result from radiation myelitis, recurrent intramedullary tumor, or possibly cord invasion from the posterior, peripherally enhancing mass. Although the differential diagnosis includes lymphoma, metastatic disease, and invasive primary bone malignancy, the radiation changes should prompt a diagnosis of radiation-induced malignancy.

Management
Treatment is surgical resection with wide margins and adjuvant chemotherapy.

Notes

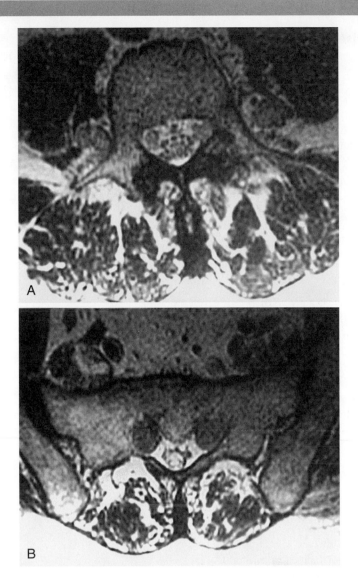

History: A 36-year-old woman presents with diminished lower extremity touch sensation and atrophy of the peroneal musculature.

1. Which of the following should be included in the differential diagnosis? (Choose all that apply.)
   a. Neurofibromatosis type 1
   b. Dejerine-Sottas disease
   c. Amyotrophic lateral sclerosis
   d. Arachnoiditis
   e. Charcot-Marie-Tooth (CMT) disease

2. Which imaging technique can be used evaluate the lumbo-sacral plexus and other peripheral nerves?
   a. Diffusion-weighted imaging
   b. Susceptibility-weighted imaging
   c. Perfusion-weighted imaging
   d. Magnetic resonance (MR) neurography

3. The abnormality in this patient is caused by a dysfunction in which cells?
   a. Schwann cells
   b. Upper motor neurons
   c. Lower motor neurons
   d. Muscle spindle cells

4. Which of the following therapies holds promise for the treatment of this condition?
   a. Folate
   b. Vitamin B$_{12}$
   c. Ascorbic acid
   d. Vitamin E

Charcot-Marie-Tooth Disease

1. a, b, and e
2. d
3. a
4. c

References

Cellerini M, Salti S, Desideri V, et al: MR imaging of the cauda equina in hereditary motor sensory neuropathies: correlations with sural nerve biopsy, *AJNR Am J Neuroradiol* 21:1793-1798, 2000.

Patzko A, Shy ME: Charcot-Marie-Tooth disease and related genetic neuropathies, *Continuum* 18:39-59, 2012.

Cross-Reference

Neuroradiology: The REQUISITES, 3rd ed, pp 563-564.

Comment

Background

Charcot-Marie-Tooth (CMT) disease is a group of progressive hereditary disorders that affect the peripheral nerves. CMT disease is characterized by chronic degeneration of peripheral nerves and roots with subsequent muscle atrophy and sensory impairment in a distal distribution. Onset is in late childhood or adolescence, but may occur anytime from early childhood through late adulthood. Symptoms vary in severity and include imbalance, clumsiness, and muscle weakness.

Histopathology

CMT disease is caused by mutation in many different genes involved in the function of peripheral nerves. The inheritance pattern varies, but it is usually inherited as an autosomal dominant trait. Some forms are autosomal recessive and some have an X-linked pattern of inheritance.

There are several types of CMT disease. CMT disease type I (CMT I) is characterized by abnormalities in myelin. CMT disease type II (CMT II) is characterized by abnormalities in the axon. CMT type III is a severe, early childhood form also known as Dejerine-Sottas disease. CMT type IV affects either the axon or myelin and is distinguished from the other types by its pattern of inheritance.

Imaging

MR findings differ from patient to patient, with variable combinations of nerve enlargement, hyperintensity on T2-weighted images, and postcontrast enhancement in most patients, and negative findings in others (Figs. A and B). In a study of seven CMT patients, Cellerini and colleagues found that hypertrophic nerves in CMT I tended to enhance, and correlations with biopsy results indicate that the enhancement is not related to inflammatory infiltrates, but rather to disruption of the blood-nerve barrier from congenital and/or demyelinating processes. In patients with CMT II, peripheral nerves had normal size, electrical conduction, and appearance on MR imaging.

Management

Treatments aim to improve motor impairment and sensory disturbances.

Notes

Page numbers followed by *f* refer to figures.